PHOSPHOLIPIDS AND ATHEROSCLEROSIS

Phospholipids and Atherosclerosis

Editors

Pietro Avogaro, M.D.
Primario Divisione Medica
Ospedale Generale Regionale
Venice, Italy

Mario Mancini, M.D.
Istituto Semeiotica Medica
IIᵃ Facoltà di Medicina
Naples, Italy

Giorgio Ricci, M.D.
Istituto di Terapia Medica
Sistematica
della Università
Rome, Italy

Rodolfo Paoletti, M.D.
Istituto di Farmacologia e
Farmacognosia
della Università
Milan, Italy

Scientific Coordinator

Alberico L. Catapano, Ph.D.
Istituto di Farmacologia e
Farmacognosia
della Università
Milan, Italy

Raven Press ■ New York

Raven Press, 1140 Avenue of the Americas, New York, New York 10036

Made in the United States of America

Library of Congress Cataloging in Publication Data
Main entry under title:

Phospholipids and atherosclerosis.

Includes index.
1. Atherosclerosis. 2. Phospholipids—Physiological effect. I. Avogaro, Pietro. II. Catapano, Alberico L. [DNLM: 1. Arteriosclerosis—Physiopathology. 2. Phospholipids—Physiology. 3. Phospholipids—Metabolism. QU 93 P5756]
RC692.P48   1983   615'.71   83-9678
ISBN 0-89004-842-8

Preface

The present volume includes a series of reviews, written by experts from different countries and scientific backgrounds, on the biochemistry and pharmacology of phospholipids, in particular on the role of phospholipids in modulating membrane properties and their pharmacological actions with respect to the development of atherosclerotic phenomena.

In our opinion, this book is timely because of the recent discoveries on the effect of phospholipids in cell regulation and the relation between phospholipids and hormonal actions as well as between phospholipids and plasma lipoproteins. The volume therefore should be of interest not only to laboratory investigators devoted to basic research on phospholipids and their relation to atherosclerotic phenomena, but also to clinicians interested in dietary and drug interactions with membrane phospholipids, and how these naturally occurring compounds can modulate membrane properties and enzyme action.

The Editors

Acknowledgment

The editors wish to thank Dr. A. L. Catapano for acting as scientific secretary in this project.

Contents

PHOSPHOLIPIDS AND ATHEROSCLEROSIS

Contributors

Olaf Adam
Forschergruppe Ernährung
Medizinische Poliklinik der Universität
München, West Germany

G. Assmann
Zentrallaboratorium der Medizinischen
 Einrichtungen der Westfälischen
 Wilhelms-Universität
Domagkstr. 3
D-4400 Münster/Westfälischen,
 West Germany

Pietro Avogaro
Primario Divisione Medica
Ospedale Regionale
Venice, Italy

A. Baritussio
Department of Internal Medicine
Policlinico
Via Giustiniani 2
35100 Padova, Italy

L. Bellina
Department of Internal Medicine
Policlinico
Via Giustiniani 2
35100 Padova, Italy

Sebastiano Calandra
Istituto Patologia Generale
Università degli Studi di Modena
Via Campi 287
41100 Modena, Italy

Martin C. Carey
Department of Medicine
Harvard Medical School
Brigham and Women's Hospital
Boston, Massachusetts 02115

R. Carraro
Department of Internal Medicine
Policlinico
Via Giustiniani 2
35100 Padova, Italy

G. Enzi
Department of Internal Medicine
Policlinico
Via Giustiniani 2
35100 Padova, Italy

L. Favaretto
Department of Internal Medicine
Policlinico
Via Giustiniani 2
35100 Padova, Italy

J. M. Fox
Faculty of Medicine
University of Saarland
D-6650 Homburg, West Germany

C. Galli
Institute of Pharmacology
 and Pharmacognosy
University of Milan
Via A. Del Sarto 21
20129 Milano, Italy

Ermanno Gherardi
Istituto Patologia Generale
Università degli Studi di Modena
Via Campi 287
41100 Modena, Italy

Gianfrancesco Goracci
Department of Biochemistry
Medical School
University of Perugia
Via del Giochetto
06100 Perugia, Italy

Antonio M. Gotto, Jr.
Department of Medicine
Baylor College of Medicine
Houston, Texas 77030

L. McGregor
Inserm, Unit 63
22 Ave. Doyen Lépine
69500 Bron, France

E. Monico
Department of Internal Medicine
Policlinico
Via Giustiniani 2
35100 Padova, Italy

R. Morazain
Inserm, Unit 63
22 Ave. Doyen Lépine
69500 Bron, France

A. Petroni
Institute of Pharmacology
and Pharmacognosy
University of Milan
Via A. Del Sarto 21
20129 Milano, Italy

Giuseppe Porcellati
Department of Biochemistry
Medical School
University of Perugia
Via del Giochetto
06100 Perugia, Italy

Henry J. Pownall
Department of Medicine
Baylor College of Medicine
Houston, Texas 77030

S. Renaud
Inserm, Unit 63
22 Ave. Doyen Lépine
69500 Bron, France

M. Rosseneu
Department of Clinical Biochemistry
Ar. St. Jan
Ruddershovelaan 10
B-8000 Brugge, Belgium

Gianfranco Salvioli
Ospedale Estense
Viale Vittorio Veneto 9
41100 Modena, Italy

Angelo M. Scanu
Departments of Medicine and
Biochemistry
The University of Chicago Pritzker
School of Medicine
Chicago, Illinois 60637

Jürgen Schneider
Department of Internal Medicine
Phillipps-University
355 Marburg, West Germany

H. Schriewer
Zentrallaboratorium der Medizinischen
Einrichtungen der Westfälischen
Wilhelms-Universität
Domagkstr. 3
D-4400 Münster/Westfällischen,
West Germany

Noris Siliprandi
Institute of Biological Chemistry
University of Padova
Via Marzolo 3
35100 Padova, Italy

C. R. Sirtori
Center E. Grossi Paoletti and
Chemotherapy Chair
University of Milan
Via A. Del Sarto 21
20129 Milano, Italy

Wilhelm Stoffel
Institut für Physiologische Chemie der
Universität zu Köln
West Germany

Patrizia Tarugi
Istituto Patologia Generale
Università degli Studi di Modena
Via Campi 287
41100 Modena, Italy

Gilbert R. Thompson
Medical Research Council
Lipid Metabolism Unit
Hammersmith Hospital
Ducane Road
London W12 OHS, England

Günther Wolfram
Forschergruppe Ernährung Medizinische
Poliklinik der Universität
München, West Germany

Ottfried Zierenberg
A. Nattermann & Cie. GmbH
Abt. Biochemie
Köln, West Germany

Nepomuk Zollner
Forschergruppe Ernährung Medizinische
Poliklinik der Universität
München, West Germany

Phospholipids and Atherosclerosis, edited by
P. Avogaro, M. Mancini, G. Ricci, and
R. Paoletti. Raven Press, New York © 1983.

Dynamic Aspects of Phosphatidylcholine in Biological Membranes

Giuseppe Porcellati and Gianfrancesco Goracci

*Department of Biochemistry, The Medical School, University of Perugia,
06100 Perugia, Italy*

Most membrane functions require a certain physical state of the membrane. For instance, membrane fluidity has been found to influence processes occurring at the membrane level (enzymic reactions and transport). Membrane fluidity depends on several factors, including the fatty acid composition of phospholipid. It increases when higher proportions of polyunsaturated molecular species are present.

The analyses of the phospholipid composition of membranes from different tissues and of the relative proportion of their subclasses and molecular species show evidence that their composition is maintained at a steady state typical for the tissue or subcellular component considered. On the other hand, membrane components, particularly phospholipids, are continuously renewed. Their renewal is due to catabolic and biosynthetic reactions, which underlie, as a final task, the compositional maintenance of the membrane and, consequently, its functional integrity.

The study of the metabolic processes connected with the turnover and rearrangement of membrane phospholipids is rather puzzling since, concurrently with the synthesis *ex novo* of phospholipid molecules, several reactions take place, leading to the interconversion of one molecule into another. This metabolic event appears quite evident since, in most cases, different portions of a phospholipid molecule turn over at different rates.

This chapter provides a brief outline of the problem connected with the renewal of membrane phospholipids. Particular attention will be given to phosphatidylcholine, which is the most abundant phospholipid in animal tissues, and to brain tissue, because the metabolism of phospholipids in the brain has been extensively studied in this laboratory.

DE NOVO SYNTHESIS OF CHOLINE PHOSPHOGLYCERIDES

As mentioned above, choline phosphoglycerides represent the major class of phospholipids in the membranes of most animal tissues (1). This class is rather heterogeneous in regard to the type of linkage between the hydrocarbon chain and

1

the C_1 of glycerol. On this basis, three subclasses can be distinguished: 1,2-diacyl-*sn*-glycero-3-phosphorylcholine (diacyl-GPC); 1-*O*-alkyl-2-acyl-*sn*-glycero-3-phosphorylcholine (alkylacyl-GPC); and 1-alk-1'-enyl-2-acyl-*sn*-glycero-3-phosphorylcholine (alkenylacyl-GPC or choline plasmalogen). Their structures are indicated in Fig. 1. The relative concentration ratios of these subclasses vary noticeably in different tissues, but generally diacyl-GPC is present at much higher concentrations (44). Within each subclass, several molecular species have been found, depending on the different length and degree of unsaturation of the hydrocarbon chains bound to glycerol.

Diacyl-GPC is synthesized *ex novo* from choline and glycerol or dioxyacetone phosphate (Fig. 2) by the cytidine pathway (28,49). Choline is first converted into cytidine diphosphate (CDP)-choline by two consecutive reactions. The former is catalyzed by choline kinase (EC 2.7.13.2) and the latter by phosphorylcholine cytidylytransferase (EC 2.7.7.15). The second reaction is rate-limiting (37). Phosphorylcholine is then transferred from CDP-choline to diacylglycerol by cholinephosphotransferase (EC 2.7.8.2) producing diacyl-GPC and cytidine monophosphate (CMP). This reaction is reversible in several tissues (5,20,26,41,49). Diacylglycerol can be formed from glycerol phosphate or dioxyacetone phosphate, and phosphatidic acid is its direct precursor. This last reaction is catalyzed by phosphatidate phosphohydrolase (EC 3.1.3.4). The synthesis *ex novo* of one molecule of phosphatidylcholine requires a relatively high amount of energy since the cleavage of high-energy bonds is necessary if choline, glycerol, and two acyl-CoA are considered as precursors.

Since phosphatidylcholine is formed from diacylglycerol and phosphatidic acid, one would expect that the molecular species of these two lipids would be very similar. Actually this is not the case. Table 1 gives the composition of the molecular species of phosphatidylcholine, diacylglycerol, and phosphatidic acid of brain tissue. Phosphatidylcholine comprises monoenoic, tetraenoic, and saturated molecular species, and the diglycerides are mostly tetraenoics (39). The compositions of phosphatidic acid and diglyceride are also rather different, despite one being the metabolic precursor of the other.

In order to explain these apparent contradictions, other factors should be taken into consideration: the specificity of biosynthetic enzymes for different molecular species; the parallel occurrence of other reactions that produce or utilize phosphatidic acid, diglyceride, and phosphatidylcholine; the cell compartmentation of biosynthetic enzymes; and, in the case of membrane-bound enzymes, their relative localization. These last two factors are of particular interest since they could be connected with the availability of substrates to these enzymes and to the existence of metabolic pools of precursors and intermediates. All of these factors, in addition to the steady state composition of membrane lipids, contribute to the explanation of different molecular compositions.

Regarding the specificity of the biosynthetic enzymes, phosphatidate phosphohydrolase and cholinephosphotransferase, several studies have been carried out using different precursors and different tissues (3,14,27). The distribution of labeled

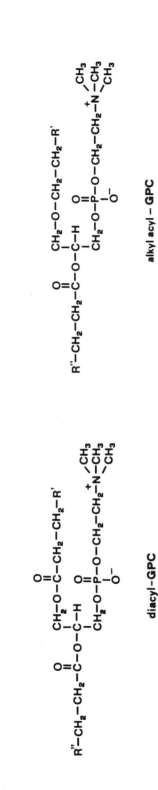

FIG. 1. Structures of cholinephosphoglycerides. Diacyl-GPC, 1,2-diacyl-*sn*-glycero-3-phosphorylcholine; alkylacyl-GPC, 1-*O*-alkyl-2-acyl-*sn*-glycero-3-phosphorylcholine; alkenylacyl-GPC, 1-alk-1′-enyl-2-acyl-*sn*-glycero-3-phosphorylcholine.

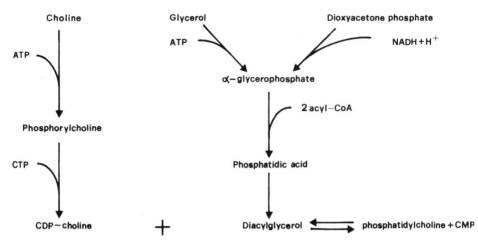

FIG. 2. Synthesis *ex novo* of phosphatidylcholine. ATP, adenosine triphosphate; CMP, cytidine monophosphate; CoA, coenzyme A; NAD, nicotinamide adenine dinucleotide (NADH, reduced form).

TABLE 1. *Composition of brain lipid molecular species[a]*

Fraction	Phosphatidylcholine	Phosphatidic acid	Diglyceride
Saturated	20.2	9.5	2.7
Monoenoic	33.7	14.2	5.1
Dienoic	0.5	13.7	5.0
Trienoic	1.2	4.5	0.9
Tetraenoic	32.5	13.2	71.2
Pentaenoic	3.5	10.1	
Hexaenoic	8.4	34.8	14.2

[a]Data expressed as percentage of the class.
From Porcellati and Binaglia (39), with permission.

choline among molecular species of brain phosphatidylcholine has been studied *in vivo* by Arienti et al. (2). Labeling was determined after very short time intervals from the injection of the radioactive precursor (10–300 sec). The results are shown in Table 2. After 10 sec from injection, monoenoic phosphatidylcholine possesses the highest specific radioactivity followed, in the order, by the tetraenoic and hexaenoic species. Rather low labeling was detected in the saturated molecular species. The time course of the incorporation of labeled choline indicated that monoenoic and tetraenoic phosphatidylcholine are preferentially synthesized, thus resembling the steady state composition (Table 1). If monoenoic diglyceride represents only 5% of the total, then it must have a certain specificity for these molecular species or be more readily available to synthesize enzymes. Another consideration is that choline can be incorporated into phosphatidylcholine by base exchange. This aspect will be discussed later.

TABLE 2. *Specific radioactivities of different phosphatidylcholines after the intracerebral injection of radioactive choline into rats[a]*

Fraction	Time after injection (sec)			
	10	30	60	300
Saturated	0.029	0.162	0.226	
Monoenoic[b]	0.831	6.370	6.560	84.960
Tetraenoic[c]	0.653	4.180	5.450	46.46
Hexaenoic	0.540	1.070	6.05	21.70

[a]The data are expressed as percent of the total recovered radioactivity incorporated in each fraction /μmole $\times$ 10^3 (mean values from 10 individual rats).
[b]Plus dienoic.
[c]Plus pentaenoic.
From Arienti et al. (2), with permission.

Other data on the synthesis of choline phosphoglycerides by cholinephosphotransferase have been reported by Roberti et al. (40). They labeled microsomal diglyceride from [^{14}C]glycerophosphate *in vitro* and incubated the labeled microsomes with CDP-choline for different time intervals. In this case, labeled diglycerides were formed from phosphatidic acid only, and the initial distribution of the label into phosphatidylcholine molecular species was very similar to that of diglycerides before incubation. However, a certain specificity for monoenoic diglycerides was also found (40).

All these data are consistent with the hypothesis that the composition of available diglycerides is as important as the specificity of biosynthetic enzymes, at least for the last metabolic step of phosphatidylcholine synthesis. In other words, cholinephosphotransferase can utilize only a certain pool of diglycerides which probably differ in molecular species composition from the total pool present in a particular membrane.

Binaglia et al. (4) have approached this problem by using different experimental models and have concluded that brain microsomal membranes have two pools of diglycerides. The first can be utilized very fast by cholinephosphotransferase since it is probably formed in the membrane area close to the enzyme. The second pool is utilized at a slower rate because it may need a diffusion process which is rate-limiting or may "flip-flop" from one side of the membrane to the other.

Roberti et al. (40) have also reported data on the incorporation of labeled diglycerides, produced *in vitro* from phosphatidic acid, into ethanolamine phosphoglycerides and particularly into their molecular species. In this case, a rather high specificity for polyenoic molecular species of diglycerides could be observed.

It is not known, however, whether the different behavior of choline- and ethanolaminephosphotransferases, concerning the specificity for molecular species of diglycerides, is due to the enzyme or to a differential availability of diglycerides connected to their relative localization in the membrane. Furthermore, the pool size and composition of diglycerides depend also on the relative concentration of CDP-choline, CDP-ethanolamine, and CMP. Cholinephosphotransferase is competitively inhibited by CDP-ethanolamine; ethanolaminephosphotransferase, by CDP-choline. CMP, which is the product of the phosphotransferase reactions, inhibits the incorporation of CDP-choline and CDP-ethanolamine into the corresponding phosphoglycerides (8,15,16). The inhibition is probably connected with the reversibility of both phosphotransferases (5,20,26,41,49). Furthermore, microsomal membranes possess diglyceride lipase activity, which breaks down diglycerides; very little is known about their specificity and regulation (9,10,22). Diglyceride can be also converted to phosphatidic acid by diglyceride kinase.

From this brief discussion several factors, often interrelated, most likely influence the synthesis *ex novo* of phosphatidylcholine.

SYNTHESIS OF PHOSPHATIDYLCHOLINE BY INTERCONVERSION REACTIONS AT THE POLAR HEAD LEVEL

Several reactions that convert one phospholipid molecule into another take place in the cell. These reactions are extremely important since new phospholipid molecules are formed with low expenditures of energy. Furthermore, at least in some cases, this conversion occurs at the site where a new molecule is required.

One phospholipid can be converted into another by reactions that produce changes at the polar head level. These reactions are responsible for the interconversion of phospholipid classes. Conversion is performed either directly by a single reaction or indirectly by a certain number of reactions. Phosphatidylcholine can be formed from other phospholipids in this way. The most important reactions are summarized in Fig. 3.

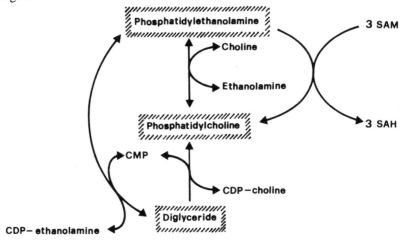

FIG. 3. Synthesis of phosphatidylcholine by interconversion reactions at the polar head level. SAM, *S*-adenosylmethionine; SAH, *S*-adenosylhomocysteine; CMP, cytidine monophosphate.

As shown, phosphatidylcholine is produced from choline and another phospholipid molecule, mainly phosphatidylethanolamine by base-exchange or by *N*-methylation, with *S*-adenosylmethionine (SAM) being the methyl donor. Both mechanisms represent an example of direct conversion of a phospholipid molecule into another since a single reaction is required for the conversion. In the case of the *N*-methylation of phosphatidylethanolamine, three consecutive reactions are necessary; nevertheless, the mono- and dimethylated intermediates are also phospholipids.

Phosphatidylethanolamine can be converted into phosphatidylcholine by another mechanism, which can be considered an indirect conversion since the intermediate is not a phosphoglyceride but a diglyceride. More precisely, diglyceride can be produced from phosphatidylethanolamine by the reversal of the ethanolaminephosphotransferase reaction; then diglyceride can be utilized by cholinephosphotransferase for the synthesis of phosphatidylcholine. Diglyceride could be also formed by phospholipase C, but in this case its origin would be phosphatidylinositol for in animal tissue the enzymes involved show a specificity for this phospholipid class (30).

Base-Exchange Reactions

Base-exchange reactions, shown in Fig. 4, allow the rapid conversion of one phospholipid molecule into another at the membrane level without an apparent requirement of energy. Serine, ethanolamine, and choline can be used as exchanging bases even if the reaction rates are different, with ethanolamine and serine being better substrates than choline. Although other divalent cations are uneffective or strongly inhibitory, Ca^{2+} is required for enzyme activity. Regarding subcellular localization of the base-exchange enzymes, they are mainly localized in the microsomal fraction (38), but a relatively high activity has been found also in the neuronal plasma membrane (19).

A small pool of phospholipids is available for base-exchange. An estimation of the size of this pool has been provided by prelabeling brain microsomal phosphoglycerides with ethanolamine, serine, or choline by base-exchange and then measuring the extent of the displacement of the labeled bases after a short incubation with unlabeled or differently labeled bases (18). The results indicate that microsomal phosphatidylethanolamine can be a substrate for the incorporation of choline by base-exchange, but only 5 to 6% of the total ethanolamine phosphoglyceride is available for the exchange reaction. On the other hand, if microsomal phosphati-

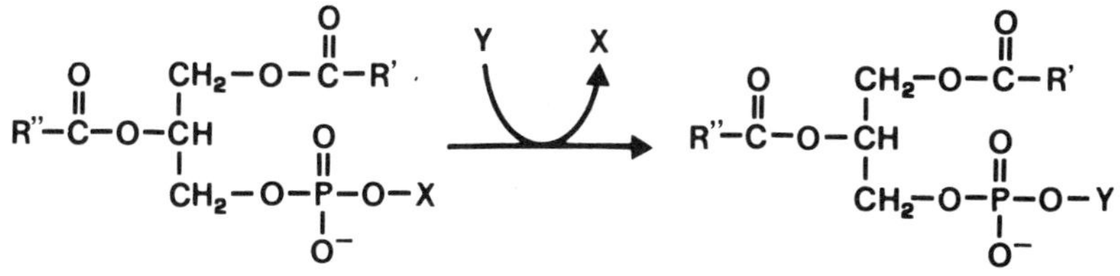

FIG. 4. Base-exchange reactions.

dylethanolamine is prelabeled *in vitro* by the cytidine pathway, choline cannot displace the labeled ethanolamine. Other studies have shown that choline is better incorporated into tetraenoic molecular species (12). There are several indications that base-exchange reactions can take place also *in vivo* (2,36,45), thus supporting the hypothesis that they might have a physiological role unknown at present.

Methylation Pathway

The *N*-methylation pathway for the synthesis of phosphatidylcholine was demonstrated in liver by Bremer and Greenberg in 1961 (6). Later, methyltransferase activities were found in other tissues (11,23,24,31,42,51). Particularly, Hirata and Axelrod (23) have shown that the conversion of phosphatidylethanolamine to phosphatidylcholine in erythrocyte membranes is carried out by two methyltransferases and that the methyl donor is *S*-adenosylmethionine. The reactions are shown in Fig. 5. Methyltransferase I requires Mg^{2+} and is localized on the cytoplasmic site of the membrane. Methyltransferase II, which catalyzes the other two methylations (Fig. 5), is present in the external surface.

According to these authors, this peculiar localization of the two enzymes could facilitate the transfer of phosphatidylcholine to the outer side of the membrane, thus contributing to the maintenance of the asymmetrical distribution of phospholipid in the erythrocyte membrane.

The existence of the *N*-methylation pathway in nervous tissue has been ruled out for several years, but recently it has been demonstrated in different laboratories (11,31,32,51). Mozzi and Porcellati (31,32) have reported that the methyl groups of *S*-adenosylmethionine can be incorporated into phosphatidylcholine of a rat brain

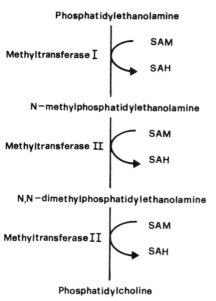

FIG. 5. Biosynthesis of phosphatidylcholine by *N*-methylation pathway. SAM, *S*-adenosylmethionine; SAH, *S*-adenosylhomocysteine.

homogenate. The addition of *N,N*-dimethylphosphatidylethanolamine greatly enhanced the formation of phosphatidylcholine by this pathway. Using rat brain microsomes the incorporation of methyl groups showed two pH optima at 7 and 8.2 (33), thus indicating the existence of two methyltransferases in brain also. Interestingly, choline plasmalogens can be synthesized by the *N*-methylation of ethanolamine plasmalogens (33,35); the metabolic pathway leading to the biosynthesis of this phospholipid is still largely unknown.

Brain methyltransferase activities seem to be age-dependent and concentrated in particular brain areas (33,34) indicating the possible involvement of this mechanism in physiological processes. Crews et al. (11) have reported that phosphatidylcholine in brain synaptosomes can be synthesized by the methylation pathway.

Stepwise methylation seems to contribute little quantitatively to the formation of phosphatidylcholine. Nevertheless, this pathway may provide a mechanism for the formation of choline from ethanolamine. In nervous tissue this mechanism might be connected with the synthesis of acetylcholine (51). Furthermore, the conversion of phosphatidylethanolamine to phosphatidylcholine produces molecular species rich in polyunsaturated fatty acids, perhaps affecting the change in membrane fluidity (43). This variation might affect ion movement and enzyme activities in restricted areas of specialized membranes.

Back-Reaction of Phosphotransferases

As mentioned above, the reactions catalyzed by ethanolaminephosphotransferase and cholinephosphotransferase are both reversible. The reverse reactions, also called back-reactions, utilize membrane-bound phospholipids, which react with CMP and produce CDP-ethanolamine or CDP-choline and diglycerides. These nucleotides or diglycerides can be reutilized for the synthesis of new phospholipids. The interconversion reactions of phosphatidylcholine into phosphatidylethanolamine and vice versa are shown in Fig. 6.

Sundler et al. (46) have found in liver that 26% of 1,2-diacylglycerol available for the synthesis of phosphatidylethanolamine originates from lecithin by a back-reaction. In brain, the reversibility of cholinephosphotransferase has been recently demonstrated and some evidence has been reported for the reversibility of ethanolaminephosphotransferase (20–22). In this tissue, diglycerides produced by back-reactions are rapidly hydrolyzed to fatty acids and glycerol by the combined action

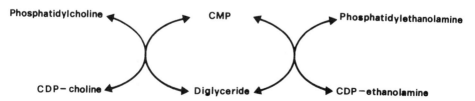

FIG. 6. Interconversion of choline- and ethanolaminephosphoglycerides by back-reaction of phosphotransferases.

of di- and monoglyceride lipase, both present in the microsomal membrane (22). However, by blocking lipase activities, diglycerides accumulate and are available for the synthesis of new phospholipid molecules (27).

These interconversion reactions lead to rearrangements of phospholipid molecules at the membrane level. Moreover, the direction of the reactions probably depends on the relative concentrations of cytidine nucleotides and on the energy state of the cell.

SYNTHESIS OF PHOSPHATIDYLCHOLINE BY INTERCONVERSION REACTIONS AT THE HYDROCARBON CHAIN LEVEL

Other reactions that produce changes at the hydrocarbon chain level are involved in the interconversion of molecular species of the same phospholipid class. Phospholipase A_1 and A_2 produce monoacylglycerophospholipids which can be reacylated by specific acyltransferases (29,47). As shown in Fig. 7, the deacylation-reacylation mechanism can lead to the interconversion of molecular species if the lysoderivative is reacylated by a different fatty acid. This mechanism has been mostly studied in liver, and the results have indicated that arachidonate is mainly introduced into lecithin by the acylation of 1-acyl-glycero-3-phosphorylcholine (25,50). Two molecules of lysolecithin can be utilized for the synthesis of phosphatidylcholine by a transesterification reaction (13,48). This mechanism seems to contribute to the synthesis of dipalmitoyl-*sn*-glycero-3-phosphocholine in lung. Recent studies have indicated that lysophosphatidylcholine transacylase activity is not present in brain tissue (17).

CONCLUSIONS

Several reactions can lead to the synthesis of phosphatidylcholine. The bulk of this phospholipid class is formed by the net synthesis, but this pathway alone does not account for the steady state composition of lecithin in various membranes. A very important role is played, therefore, by interconversion reactions through base-exchange, stepwise methylation, phosphotransferase reversal, and deacylation-reacylation cycle.

The discovery of these pathways in most tissues has provided the following concept: once a certain phospholipid molecule has been synthesized by net synthesis, it can then be modified in the polar head or hydrophobic tail of the molecule. These changes are probably connected with the functional properties of the membrane, thus affecting the transport of ions or other substances, modulating membrane-bound enzymic activities, and influencing the affinity of receptors for transmitters or hormones. Unfortunately, the regulation of the enzymic activities involved in these pathways, their relative localization in the cells and membranes, and their connections with specific functions are still largely unknown.

Attaining complete knowledge of the dynamic aspects of phospholipids in cells is a very difficult task. Too many changes can occur potentially in a certain molecule; furthermore, phospholipids migrate from one cellular compartment to another, along

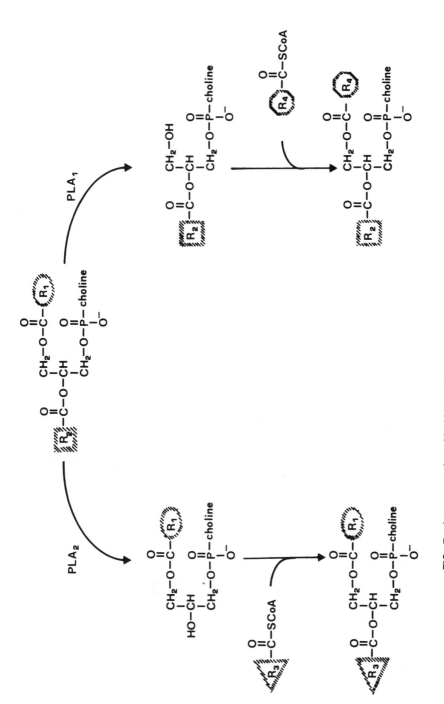

FIG. 7. Interconversion of lecithin molecular species by deacylation-reacylation.

membranes, from one side of the membrane to the other, and from one cell to another. These migrations can take place without changes; however, transport of a phospholipid molecule from one place to another may require a rearrangement in structure. For instance, nerve cells synthesize phospholipids in the endoplasmic reticulum of the cell body. They migrate successively along the axons to the nerve endings. Studies carried out by Brunetti et al. (7) on the transport of phospholipids in the oculomotor nerve of the chicken have shown that choline phosphoglycerides are axonally transported. A small portion of these phospholipids translocates from the axon to the myelin sheet, probably as intact molecules. Furthermore, Schwann cells seem to reutilize the breakdown products of the transported choline phosphoglycerides, with choline much better reincorporated into myelin than glycerol. This model aptly illustrates the complex mechanisms involved in the dynamics of phosphatidylcholine in tissues.

ACKNOWLEDGMENT

This work has been carried out by research Grant 81.0031804/115 from the Consiglio Nazionale delle Ricerche, Rome.

REFERENCES

1. Ansell, G. B., Hawthorne, J. N., and Dawson, R. M. C., eds. (1973): *Form and Function of Phospholipids.* Elsevier, Amsterdam.
2. Arienti, G., Corazzi, L., Woelk, H., and Porcellati, G. (1976): Biosynthesis of rat brain phosphatidylcholines from intracerebrally injected choline. *J. Neurochem.*, 27:203–210.
3. Binaglia, L., Roberti, R., and Porcellati, G. (1978): A study on the turnover of rat brain phosphatidic acid through the glycerol-phosphate pathway. In: *Enzymes of Lipid Metabolism*, edited by S. Gatt, L. Freysz, and P. Mandel, pp. 353–366. Plenum Press, New York.
4. Binaglia, L., Roberti, R., Vecchini, A., and Porcellati, G. (1980): Studies on rat brain microsomal choline-phosphotransferase. *Ital. J. Biochem.*, 29:360–361.
5. Bjørnstad, P., and Bremer, J. (1966): In vivo studies on pathways for the biosynthesis of lecithin in the rat. *J. Lipid Res.*, 7:38–45.
6. Bremer, J., and Greenberg, D. (1961): Methyltransferring enzyme of microsomes in the biosynthesis of lecithin. *Biochim. Biophys. Acta*, 46:205–216.
7. Brunetti, M., Di Giamberardino, L., Porcellati, G., and Droz, B. (1981): Contribution of axonal transport to the renewal of myelin phospholipids. *Brain Res.*, 219:73–84.
8. Call, F. L., and Rubert, M. (1975): Synthesis of ethanolamine phosphoglycerides by human platelets. *J. Lipid Res.*, 16:352–359.
9. Cabot, M. C., and Gatt, S. (1976): Hydrolysis of neutral glycerides by lipases of rat brain microsomes. *Biochim. Biophys. Acta*, 431:105–115.
10. Cabot, M. C., and Gatt, S. (1977): Hydrolysis of endogenous diacylglycerol and monoacylglycerol by lipases in rat brain microsomes. *Biochemistry*, 16:2330–2334.
11. Crews, F. T., Hirata, F., and Axelrod, J. (1980): Identification and properties of methyltransferases that synthesize phosphatidylcholine in rat brain synaptosomes. *J. Neurochem.*, 34:1491–1498.
12. De Medio, G. E., Woelk, H., Gaiti, A., Porcellati, G., and Fratini, F. (1975): The Ca^{2+}-dependent incorporation of nitrogenous bases into brain microsomal phospholipid sub-species *in vitro*. *Ital. J. Biochem.*, 24:335–350.
13. Erbland, J. F., and Marinetti, G. V. (1965): The enzymatic acylation and hydrolysis of lysolecithin. *Biochim. Biophys. Acta*, 106:128–138.
14. Fallon, H. J., Barwick, J., and Lamb, R. G. (1976): Studies on the specificity of the reactions of glycerol lipid biosynthesis in rat liver using membrane-bound substrates. In: *Lipids*, edited by R. Paoletti, G. Porcellati, and G. Jacini, Vol. 1, pp. 67–74. Raven Press, New York.

15. Freysz, L., and Mandel, P. (1974): Etude comparative de la biosynthèse des phosphatidylcholines dans les neurones et les cellules gliales du cerveau de poulet. *FEBS Lett.*, 40:110–113.
16. Freysz, L., Horrocks, L. A., and Mandel, P. (1978): Ethanolamine and choline phosphotransferases of chicken brain. In: *Enzymes of Lipid Metabolism*, edited by S. Gatt, L. Freysz, and P. Mandel, pp. 253–268. Plenum Press, New York.
17. Freysz, L., and Van den Bosch, H. (1980): Biosynthesis and subcellular distribution of disaturated phosphatidylcholine in rat brain. *Seventh Meeting of the International Society for Neurochemistry*, Jerusalem (Abstr. 334).
18. Gaiti, A., Brunetti, M., and Porcellati, G. (1975): The relationship between the phospholipid pool and the base-exchange reaction in the Ca^{2+}-stimulated incorporation of ethanolamine into brain microsomal phospholipids. *FEBS Lett.*, 49:361–364.
19. Goracci, G., Blomstrand, C., Arienti, G., Hamberger, A., and Porcellati, G. (1973): Base-exchange enzymic system for the synthesis of phospholipids in neuronal and glial cells and their subfractions: a possible marker for neuronal membranes. *J. Neurochem.*, 20:1167–1180.
20. Goracci, G., Horrocks, L. A., and Porcellati, G. (1977): Reversibility of ethanolamine and choline phosphotransferases (EC 2.7.8.1 and EC 2.7.8.2) in rat brain microsomes with labeled alkylglycerols. *FEBS Lett.*, 80:41–44.
21. Goracci, G., Francescangeli, E., Horrocks, L. A., and Porcellati, G. (1978): CMP-dependent degradation of membrane-bound brain choline phosphoglycerides. *Ital. J. Biochem.*, 27:284–286.
22. Goracci, G., Francescangeli, E., Horrocks, L. A., and Porcellati, G. (1981): The reverse reaction of cholinephosphotransferase in rat brain microsomes. A new pathway for degradation of phosphatidylcholine. *Biochim. Biophys. Acta*, 664:373–379.
23. Hirata, F., and Axelrod, J. (1978): Enzymatic synthesis and rapid translocation of phosphatidylcholine by two methyltransferases in erythrocyte membrane. *Proc. Natl. Acad. Sci. USA*, 75:2348–2352.
24. Hirata, F., Viveros, O. H., Diliberto, E. J., and Axelrod, J. (1978): Identification and properties of two methyltransferases in conversion of phosphatidylethanolamine to phosphatidylcholine. *Proc. Natl. Acad. Sci. USA*, 75:1718–1721.
25. Kanoh, H. (1969): Biosynthesis of molecular species of phosphatidylcholine and phosphatidylethanolamine from radioactive precursors in rat liver slices. *Biochim. Biophys. Acta*, 176:756–763.
26. Kanoh, H., and Ohno, K. (1973): Utilization of endogenous phospholipids by backreaction of CDP-choline (-ethanolamine): 1,2-diglyceride choline (ethanolamine) phosphotransferase in rat liver microsomes. *Biochim. Biophys. Acta*, 306:203–217.
27. Kanoh, H., and Ohno, K. (1975): Substrate selectivity of rat liver microsomal 1,2-diacylglycerol: CDP-choline (-ethanolamine) choline (ethanolamine) phosphotransferase in utilizing endogenous substrates. *Biochim. Biophys. Acta*, 380:199–207.
28. Kennedy, E. P., and Weiss, S. B. (1956): The function of cytidine coenzymes in the biosynthesis of phospholipids. *J. Biol. Chem.*, 222:193–214.
29. Lands, W. E. M. (1960): Metabolism of phospholipids. II. The enzymatic acylation of lysolecithin. *J. Biol. Chem.*, 235:2233–2237.
30. Lapetina, E. G., and Michell, R. M. (1973): A membrane bound activity catalysing phosphatidylinositol breakdown to 1,2-diacylglycerol, D-myoinositol 1:2 cyclic phosphate and D-myoinositol-1-phosphate. *Biochem. J.*, 131:433–442.
31. Mozzi, R., and Porcellati, G. (1979): Conversion of phosphatidylethanolamine to phosphatidylcholine in rat brain by the methylation pathway. *FEBS Lett.*, 100:363–366.
32. Mozzi, R., and Porcellati, G. (1979): *N*-methylation of phosphatidylethanolamine in rat brain. *IRCS Med. Sci. Libr. Compend.*, 7:98.
33. Mozzi, R., Andreoli, V., and Porcellati, G. (1980): Involvement of *S*-adenosylmethionine in brain phospholipid metabolism. In: *Natural Sulphur Compounds*, edited by D. Cavallini, G. E. Gaull, and V. Zappia, pp. 41–54. Plenum Press, New York.
34. Mozzi, R., Siepi, D., Andreoli, V., Piccinin, G. L., and Porcellati, G. (1981): *N*-methylation of phosphatidylethanolamine in different brain areas of the rat. *Bull. Mol. Biol. Med.*, 6:6–15.
35. Mozzi, R., Siepi, D., Andreoli, V., and Porcellati, G. (1981): Synthesis of diacyl- and alkenylacyl-glycerophosphorylcholines by the methylation pathway in brain microsomes. *Ital. J. Biochem.*, 30:311–312.
36. Orlando, P., Arienti, G., Cerrito, F., Massari, P., and Porcellati, G. (1977): Quantitative evaluation of two pathways for phosphatidylcholine biosynthesis in rat brain *in vivo*. *Neurochem. Res.*, 2:191–201.

37. Porcellati, G. (1972): Aspects of regulatory mechanisms in phospholipid biosynthesis of nervous tissue. In: *Advances of Enzyme Regulation*, Vol. 10, edited by G. Weber, pp. 83–100. Academic Press, New York.
38. Porcellati, G., Arienti, G., Pirotta, M., and Giorgini, D. (1971): Base-exchange reactions for the synthesis of phospholipids in nervous tissue: The incorporation of serine and ethanolamine into the phospholipids of isolated brain microsomes. *J. Neurochem.*, 18:1395–1417.
39. Porcellati, G., and Binaglia, L. (1976): Metabolism of phosphoglycerides and their molecular species. In: *Lipids*, Vol. 1, edited by R. Paoletti, G. Porcellati, and G. Jacini, pp, 75–88. Raven Press, New York.
40. Roberti, R., Binaglia, L., and Porcellati, G. (1980): Synthesis of glycerophospholipids from diglyceride-labeled brain microsomes. *J. Lipid Res.*, 21:449–454.
41. Sarzala, G., and Van Golde, L. M. G. (1976): Selective utilization of endogenous unsaturated phosphatidylcholines and diacylglycerols by cholinephosphotransferase of mouse lung microsomes. *Biochim. Biophys. Acta*, 441:423–432.
42. Schneider, W. J., and Vance, D. E. (1979): Conversion of phosphatidylethanolamine to phosphatidylcholine in rat liver. Partial purification and characterization of the enzymatic activities. *J. Biol. Chem.*, 254:3886–3891.
43. Skurdal, D. N., and Cornatzer, W. E. (1975): Cholinephosphotransferase and phosphatidylethanolamine methyltransferase activities. *Int. J. Biochem.*, 6:579–583.
44. Snyder, F., ed. (1972): *Ether Lipids, Chemistry and Biology*. Academic Press, New York.
45. Sundler, R., Arvidson, G., and Åkesson, B. (1972): Pathways for the incorporation of choline into rat liver phosphatidylcholines *in vivo*. *Biochim. Biophys. Acta*, 280:559–568.
46. Sundler, R., Åkesson, B., and Nilsson, Å. (1974): Sources of diacylglycerols for phospholipid synthesis in rat liver. *Biochim. Biophys. Acta*, 337:248–254.
47. Van den Bosh, H. (1974): Phosphoglyceride metabolism. *Ann. Rev. Biochem.*, 43:243–277.
48. Van den Bosh, H., Bonte, H. A., and Van Deenen, L. L. M. (1965): On the anabolism of lysolecithin. *Biochim. Biophys. Acta*, 98:648–661.
49. Weiss, S. B., Smith, S. W., and Kennedy, E. P. (1958): The enzymatic formation of lecithin from cytidine diphosphate choline and D-1,2-diglyceride. *J. Biol. Chem.*, 231:53–64.
50. Yamashita, S., Nakaya, N., Miki, Y., and Numa, S. (1975): Separation of 1-acylglycerophosphate acyltransferase and 1-acylglycerolphosphorylcholine acyltransferase of rat liver microsomes. *Proc. Natl. Acad. Sci. USA*, 72:600–603.
51. Zeisel, S. H., Blusztajn, J. K., and Wurtman, R. J. (1979): Brain lecithin biosynthesis: Evidence that bovine brain can make choline molecules. In: *Nutrition and the Brain*, Vol. 5, edited by A. Barbeau, J. M. Grawdon, and R. J. Wurtman, pp. 47–55. Raven Press, New York.

Phospholipids and Atherosclerosis, edited by
P. Avogaro, M. Mancini, G. Ricci, and
R. Paoletti. Raven Press, New York © 1983.

Overview of the Molecular Mechanisms for the Biological Role and Pharmacological Actions of Phosphatidylcholine

A. Petroni and C. Galli

Institute of Pharmacology and Pharmacognosy, University of Milan, 20129 Milan, Italy

Phosphatidylcholine (PC) is present in many biological systems, mainly as a surface component in lipoprotein complexes, which are part of membrane structures or part of circulating lipid-carrying particles. The largely uncharacterized molecular mechanisms through which PC possibly helps to regulate important biochemical processes in various biological systems, such as the cardiovascular or the nervous system, may be relevant in promoting some of the actions which are produced by the pharmacological use of lecithin in large doses. This chapter will briefly summarize the main accepted pathways involving endogenous PC in different biological processes and will consider some of the pharmacological actions of exogenous PC on the cardiovascular system and on the CNS.

The major biological roles of PC at the molecular level are summarized below:

Structural (lipoprotein complexes)
    Biological membranes
    Circulating particles
Metabolic
    Choline metabolism
    Long-chain polyunsaturated fatty acids → prostaglandins
    Methylation processes

PC AS ENDOGENOUS COMPONENT

Phosphatidylcholine in Biological Membranes

The presence of PC in most cellular and subcellular membranes is widely recognized. Together with other polar lipid components (glyco- and phospholipids) and cholesterol, PC contributes to the organization of the lipid bilayer in biological membranes, in which biochemically active proteins are embedded. Phospholipids are asymmetrically distributed in most biological membranes and PC is mainly oriented toward the outside (12,47). The lipid bilayer provides a fluid matrix for protein organization and movement (50).

Phosphatidylcholine in Circulating Lipoprotein Particles

Phosphatidylcholine is the major phospholipid present in plasma, where it is transported through lipoproteins (LP) of higher density. Phospholipids in association with unesterified cholesterol and proteins (apoproteins) are localized on the surface of LP particles, whereas triglycerides and esterified cholesterol (nonpolar lipids) constitute the core compartment of the LP ("lipid core" model).

Circulating lipoproteins are a lipid-transport system where the major lipid class being transported is a triglyceride of exogenous (dietary) and endogenous origin. During the lipid transport process, LP undergo complex metabolic transformations involving both the lipid and the protein moieties of the molecules. Interactions among LP and between LP and enzymes or cells should be regarded as participations by the whole particle. Transformation of the LP particles during lipid transport consists mainly of a delipidation process with progressive loss of the "lipid core" from very low-density lipoprotein (VLDL) particles, with subsequent formation of smaller particles (intermediate density lipoproteins and LDL) containing less nonpolar lipids (triglycerides and cholesterol esters) and more surface constituents (phospholipids, cholesterol, apoproteins) (41,48,49). Lipid transport in LP involves the activity of several enzyme systems and the interaction of particles with tissue cells.

Lipoprotein lipase (LPL) (hepatic and extrahepatic) modulates the removal of triglycerides and contains activities against monoglycerides and glycerophosphatides (3). A second enzyme system found in plasma and active on lipoprotein lipids is the lecithin-cholesterol acyltransferase (LCAT). This enzyme transfers an acyl group from lecithin molecules to unesterified cholesterol to form lysolecithin and cholesterol ester molecules (23). The combined activity of the two enzyme systems, the LPL and LCAT, affects all lipid classes in LP and promotes the progressive conversion of VLDL to LDL and finally to high-density lipoprotein (HDL). The delipidation path associated with removal of surplus surface constituents from LP is the key event of the process. Several aspects, especially those involved in the contribution of "surface remnants" to the formation of HDL are still obscure. However, an important mechanism which may transform the discoidal HDL precursors, presumably a primary fragment of the VLDL outer shell, to spherical particles is the LCAT reaction (25).

Phosphatidylcholine, during the various transformation steps from VLDL to LDL to HDL, also undergoes exchanges and metabolic transformations. Owing to the presence of a plasma protein fraction, probably analogous to the phospholipid exchange proteins found in liver cell cytosol (36), PC exchanges between VLDL and LDL in plasma (16). Also, lipolysis of VLDL through LPL results in removal of PC, partly through hydrolysis to lyso-PC and partly in an unhydrolyzed form transferred to HDL.

Phospholipid in HDL is not a substrate for LPL (17). PC plays instead a key role for the activity of LCAT, an enzyme which is synthesized in liver and circulates in plasma [and acts on HDL, mainly the HDL_2 subfraction (22)]. LCAT transfers fatty acids (mainly unsaturates) from the 2-positions of PC to unesterified cholesterol, forming lyso-PC and cholesterol esters that largely contain unsaturated fatty acids. The LCAT reaction has been suggested to be part of a mechanism for transporting cholesterol from peripheral cells to the liver (22). However, recent work in several laboratories has indicated that interactions between LP and peripheral cells are much more complex. A modified hypothesis on the effects of the LCAT reaction on peripheral cell membranes considers LCAT as one factor controlling the content of lipids on cell surface membranes to the extent that these lipids can equilibrate with HDL.

EFFECTS OF EXOGENOUS PC ON SERUM LIPOPROTEINS AND CHOLESTEROL METABOLISM

Phosphatidylcholine, especially in a form containing a high percentage of linoleic acid not only in the 2-position but also in the 1-position of glycerol (polyenoyl-PC or PPC), has been shown to exert antiatherosclerotic activity in several animal species with experimental hypercholesterolemia. A detailed report on the observations of this activity of PPC, not only at the experimental but also at the clinical level, is presented in Sirtori's chapter of this volume.

The extent of the protective action of PC in respect to the atherosclerotic process and the mechanism(s) involved have not been clarified. However, (a) the increased removal of cholesterol from arterial cells (52) and the increased activity of cholesterol ester hydrolase in arterial walls (35,55) and of serum enzymes, such as TG lipase (10,21) or LCAT (2), on one side and (b) the increased turnover of cholesterol and increased HDL/LDL ratio (46) on the other are responsible for this effect. Some of the effects and mechanisms may differ depending on the animal species and route of administration of PC.

In lymph-cannulated rats, after oral administration of twice-labeled PC (fatty acid and choline moiety), 50% of the choline label and 90% of the fatty acid label were recovered in the lymph chylomicra. The choline label occurred completely in plasma PC, but only 24% of the fatty acid label was recovered in this fraction (20). About 50% of the ingested PC was absorbed with the 1-position intact; whereas, the 2-position underwent hydrolysis for absorption and reacylation in the mucosa to form intact PC again (20). After oral or i.v. administration of labeled PC to rats, about one-third of the radioactivity was in the HDL fraction at 6 hr; whereas, in dogs a higher percentage (over 60%) of incorporation in HDL was found at shorter time intervals after oral administration (57). In dogs, i.v. injections of PC resulted in an incorporation of over 80% in HDL. In humans, intraduodenal infusions of PPC resulted in an elevation mainly of VLDL, in contrast with the predominant elevation of chylomicrons after administration of equivalent amounts of safflower oil (5). In the same study oral administration of PC reduced the absorption of choline in the intestinal tract.

Theoretically, administration of PC, rich in polyunsaturated fatty acids, results in an elevation of cholesterol esterified with polyunsaturated fatty acids, largely through the activity of LCAT. Cholesteryl esters are more soluble in plasma than nonesterified cholesterol (39), and the "sclerogenic" properties of cholesteryl esters are lower for the most unsaturated compounds (40). This may explain the protective activity of polyenoic fatty acids and of unsaturated PC against experimental atherosclerosis. The major question, which has been partly answered by the study of Beil and Grundy (5), is whether or not PC is sufficiently well absorbed across the digestive tract to exert biological effects. Obviously, this problem does not arise when PC is administered by i.v. infusion.

Phosphatidylcholine and Central Cholinergic Mechanisms

Another aspect concerning the biological role of PC is that plasma levels of choline and of the major choline-containing compound, lecithin, affect cholinergic functions. Small increases of the amino acid tryptophan in plasma cause rapid increases in brain levels of the neurotransmitter serotonin (19). This was the first surprising observation that neurotransmitter synthesis is affected by plasma composition. In addition, increases in plasma choline levels, within the range of choline concentrations observed post-prandially in humans eating PC-rich foods (33), enhance central cholinergic transmission (53). The evidence accumulated in the last decade for a possible link between the metabolism of choline lipids (notably, choline glycerophospholipids) and the cholinergic system in brain provides some basis for the interpretation of the central effects of dietary lecithin.

Studies on the pool of free choline, which is the only immediate source for acetylcholine synthesis, in brain revealed that this pool is very small but very active (26). Intracerebrally injected labeled choline is very rapidly acetylated (11) and phosphorylated (1). A relatively large amount of choline passes through the brain in the blood as PC and lyso-PC (51), and these phospholipids may release choline or may indirectly contribute to the brain phospholipid pool releasing choline. Choline is continuously released from the PC pool (43), and lyso-PC yields free choline which is then phosphorylated and acetylated (36). Choline appears, however, to be produced from an endogenous source also (7).

Several reports have shown that large doses of choline raise levels of free choline and acetylcholine in the brain. Administration by needle (13,26), stomach tube (34), or dietary supplement (14) produces sequential elevation in serum choline, brain choline, and brain acetylcholine levels. Choline appears to enhance the rate of acetylcholine formation in neurons (34) and also to promote an increased release of neurotransmitter (44,54).

These observations may provide a biochemical basis for the interpretation of the reported beneficial effects of large doses of choline and, especially, of phosphatidylcholine in the treatment of various neurological disorders. Administrations of choline and lecithin have been shown to ameliorate tardive dyskinesia (18,24,38,56), Friedreich's ataxia (45), and, more generally, memory and mood disorders (4).

Phosphatidylcholine as Donor of Prostaglandin-Precursor Fatty Acids

Formation of oxygenated derivatives of 20 carbon polyunsaturated fatty acids, such as arachidonic acid (AA), through the activity of the cyclo- and lipoxygenase pathways (prostaglandins and related compounds on one side and leukotrienes and other oxygenated products on the other) appears to require the release of the fatty acid substrate mainly from phospholipids through phospholipases. Studies carried out by measuring the incorporation of labeled AA in various lipid classes in isolated cells (platelets, leukocytes, neutrophils, and so on) and of the subsequent release of the label after appropriate stimulation revealed that most of the radioactivity was initially associated with and subsequently lost from phosphatidylcholine (8,9). This observation may indicate a role of PC as the donor phospholipid in the modulation of prostaglandin (PG) synthesis through the activation of a phospholipase A_2 acting on the 2-position of the glyceride moiety. However, the high incorporation of exogenously labeled fatty acid substrates in cellular PC may reflect the location of this phospholipid on cell surfaces, which should facilitate unspecific exchanges of the label with the medium. In order to assess whether AA released from PC is the major precursor of PG, the specific activities of the products of the cyclooxygenase and lipoxygenase should be compared with that of the labeled phospholipid precursor pool. Also, evidence obtained from platelets, as well as from other systems, suggests that phosphatidylinositol, a phospholipid with a high stimulus-dependent turnover rate (42), is the precursor of AA for PG synthesis. The initial step is the activation of a phospholipase-C type of reaction (phosphoinositide hydrolase) followed by the activation of a lipase acting on the diglyceride moiety thus formed (6). It appears hence that further research is needed to elucidate the actual role of endogenous PC as a store of PG-precursor fatty acids and its participation in the precursor-release processes after appropriate stimulation in various biological systems.

Phosphatidylcholine in Methylation Processes

A recently recognized, important biological role of endogenous PC is in the transmission of biochemical signals through membranes. The recognition and binding of specific receptor macromolecules on the outer surface of cell membranes with biochemical messages (neurotransmitters, hormones, ligands, and so on) are followed by chemical and physical changes in membranes. This is essential for the cells to carry out their specific functions. Hirata and Axelrod have shown that stepwise enzymatic methylation of phospholipids plays a role in the transduction of receptor-mediated signals through the membranes of a variety of cells (28,32). Phosphatidylethanolamine is converted by successive methylation to phosphatidylcholine through the activities of two methyltransferase systems—first detected in the adrenal medulla (27) and subsequently in several other tissues [brain (15), erythrocytes (27), lymphocytes (31), mast cells (29), and basophils and neutrophils (30)]. These two enzymes are asymmetrically distributed in the membrane and their stepwise activity results in the translocation of the polar phospholipid phosphatidylethanolamine from the inside of the membrane to the outside surface after its conversion into the less polar PC. The methylation process is stimulated by a variety of biochemical messages. This results in a reduction of membrane viscosity. Several receptor-mediated, specific biochemical changes in several biological systems appear to be associated with the methylation process, suggesting that this process is a factor in the transmission of many signals through membranes. Thus, Ca^{2+} influx, release of prostaglandins, generation of cyclic adenosine monophosphate (cAMP) in many cell types, and various events participating in inflammatory processes (such as histamine release in mast cells and basophils, mutagenesis in lymphocytes, and chemotaxis in neutrophils) are the major cellular responses associated with PC formation in cells through methylation processes (28). Also, the translocation of phospholipids from the inside to the outside of cellular membranes by sequential methylation provides an understanding of the molecular mechanisms responsible for the transport of PC in plasma membranes, from the site of synthesis to the final location, and also of the asymmetric distribution of phospholipids in the membrane.

CONCLUSIONS

Phosphatidylcholine plays several, not yet fully clarified key roles at the cellular level, not only as a structural phospholipid but also in the modulation of (a) basic responses of several cell types to receptor stimulation, through modification of membrane properties at selective sites, and (b) precursor pools in the formation of the neurotransmitter acetylcholine and, possibly, of prostaglandins. Studies on the correlation between PC metabolism in cells and major, basic molecular processes taking place during cellular responses to specific stimuli may indicate future lines of research for possible pharmacological uses of phosphatidylcholine, in addition to its accepted application in the treatment of mild lipoprotein abnormalities and neurological disorders.

REFERENCES

1. Ansell, G. B., and Spanner, S. (1968): The metabolism of Me-^{14}C choline in the brain of the rat in vivo. *Biochem. J.*, 110:201–206.
2. Assmann, G., Schmitz, G., Doneth, N., and LeKim, D. (1978): Phosphatidyl choline substrate specificity of LCAT. *Scand. J. Clin. Lab. Invest.*, 38(Suppl. 150):16–20.
3. Augustin, J., and Greten, H. (1979): Hepatic triglyceride lipase in tissue and plasma. In: *Progress in Biochemical Pharmacology—Lipoprotein Metabolism, Vol. 15*, edited by R. Paoletti. Karger, Basel, pp. 5–40.
4. Barbeau, A., Growdon, J. H., and Wurtman, R. J., eds. (1979): *Nutrition and the Brain, Vol. 5*. Raven Press, New York.
5. Beil, F. U., and Grundy, S. M. (1980): Studies on plasma lipoproteins during absorption of exogenous lecithin in man. *J. Lipid Res.*, 21:525–536.
6. Bell, R. L., Stanford, N., Kennerly, D. A., and Majerus, P. W. (1980): Diglyceride lipase: A pathway for arachidonate release from human platelets. In: *Advances in Prostaglandin and Thromboxane Research, Vol. 6*, edited by B. Samuelsson, P. W. Ramwell, and R. Paoletti. Raven Press, New York, pp. 219–224.

7. Bhatnagar, S. P., and McIntosh, F. C. (1967): Effects of quaternary bases and inorganic cations on acetylcholine synthesis in nervous tissue. *Can. J. Physiol. Pharmacol.*, 45:249–268.

8. Bills, T. K., Smith, J. B., and Silver, M. J. (1976): Metabolism of (^{14}C) arachidonic acid by human platelets. *Biochim. Biophys. Acta*, 424:303–314.

9. Blackwell, G. J., Duncombe, W. G., Flower, R. J., Parsons, M. F., and Vane, J. R. (1977): The distribution and metabolism of arachidonic acid in rabbit platelets during aggregation and its modification by drugs. *Br. J. Pharmacol.*, 59:353–366.

10. Blaton, V., Vandamme, D., and Peeters, H. (1974): Activation of lipoprotein lipase in vitro by unsaturated phospholipids. *FEBS Lett.*, 44:185–188.

11. Chakrin, L. W., and Whittaker, V. P. (1969): The subcellular distribution of N-Me-^{3}H acetylcholine synthesis by brain in vivo. *Biochem. J.*, 113:97–107.

12. Chap, H. J., Zwaal, R. F. A., and Van Deenen, L. L. M. (1977): Action of highly purified phospholipase on blood platelets. Evidence for an asymmetric distribution of phospholipids in the surface membranes. *Biochim. Biophys. Acta*, 467:146–164.

13. Cohen, E. L., and Wurtman, R. J. (1975): Brain acetylcholine: Increase after systemic choline administration. *Life Sci.*, 16:1095–1102.

14. Cohen, E. L., and Wurtman, R. J. (1976): Brain acetylcholine: Control by dietary choline. *Science*, 191:561–562.

15. Crews, F. T., Hirata, F., and Axelrod, J. (1980): Identification and properties of methyltransferases that synthesize phosphatidylcholine in rat brain synaptosomes. *J. Neurochem.*, 39:1491–1498.

16. Eisenberg, S. (1978): Effect of temperature and plasma on the exchange of apolipoproteins and phospholipids between rat plasma very low and high density lipoproteins. *J. Lipid Res.*, 19:229–236.

17. Eisenberg, S., Shurr, D., Goldmann, H., and Olivecrona, T. (1978): Comparison of the phospholipase activity of bovine milk lipoprotein lipase against rat plasma very low density and high lipoprotein. *Biochim. Biophys. Acta*, 531:344–361.

18. Fann, W. E., Lake, C. R., Gerber, C. T., and Miller, R. D. (1974): Cholinergic suppression of tardive dyskinesia. *Psychopharmacologia*, 37:101–107.

19. Fernstrom, J. D., and Wurtman, R. J. (1971): Brain serotonin content: physiological dependence on plasma tryptophan levels. *Science*, 174:149–152.

20. Fox, J. M., Betzing, H., and LeKim, D. (1979): Pharmacokinetics of orally ingested phosphatidylcholine. In: *Nutrition and the Brain, Vol. 5*, edited by A. Barbeau, J. H. Growdon, and R. J. Wurtman. Raven Press, New York, pp. 95–108.

21. Fruchart, J. C., Desreumax, C. F., Nouvelot, A., Sezille, G., and Jaillard, J. (1978): Studies on the assay of lipoprotein lipase from different sources. Effect of nature of phospholipids used in substrate preparations. European Atherosclerosis Group Meeting, Paris.

22. Glomset, J. A. (1968): The plasma lecithin: Cholesterol acyltransferase reaction. *J. Lipid Res.*, 9:155–167.

23. Glomset, J. A. (1979): Lecithin: Cholesterol acyltransferase. In: *Progress in Biochemical Pharmacology—Lipoprotein Metabolism, Vol. 15*, edited by R. Paoletti. Karger, Basel, pp. 41–66.

24. Growdon, J. H., Gelenberg, A. J., Doller, J., Hirsch, M. J., and Wurtman, R. J. (1978): Lecithin can suppress tardive dyskinesia. *N. Engl. J. Med.*, 297:524–527.

25. Hamilton, R. L., Havel, R. J., Kane, J. P., Blaurock, A. E., and Sata, T. (1971): Cholestasis: lamellar structure of the abnormal human serum lipoprotein. *Science*, 172:475–478.

26. Hambrich, D. R., and Chippendale, T. J. (1977): Regulation of acetylcholine synthesis in nervous tissue. *Life Sci.*, 20:1465–1478.

27. Hirata, F., and Axelrod, J. (1978): Enzymatic synthesis and rapid translocation of phosphatidylcholine by two methyltransferases in erythrocyte membranes. *Proc. Natl. Acad. Sci. USA*, 75:2348–2352.

28. Hirata, F., and Axelrod, J. (1980): Phospholipid methylation and biological signal transmission. *Science*, 209:1082–1090.

29. Hirata, F., Axelrod, J., and Crews, F. R. (1979): Concanavalin A stimulates phospholipid methylation and phosphatidylserine decarboxylation in rat mast cells. *Proc. Natl. Acad. Sci. USA*, 76:4813–4816.

30. Hirata, F., Corcoran, B. A., Venkatasubramanian, K., Schiffmann, E., and Axelrod, J. (1979): Chemoattractans stimulate degradation of methylated phospholipid and release of arachidonic acid in rabbit leukocytes. *Proc. Natl. Acad. Sci. USA*, 76:2640–2643.

31. Hirata, F., Toyoshima, S., Axelrod, J., and Waxdal, M. J. (1980): Phospholipid methylation: A biochemical signal modulating lymphocyte mitogenesis. *Proc. Natl. Acad. Sci. USA*, 77:862–865.

32. Hirata, F., Viveros, O. H., Diliberto, E. J., Jr., and Axelrod, J. (1978): Identification and properties of two methyltransferases in conversion of phosphatidyl ethanolamine to phosphatidyl choline. *Proc. Natl. Acad. Sci. USA*, 75:1718–1721.

33. Hirsch, M. J., Growdon, J. H., and Wurtman, R. J. (1978): Relations between dietary choline or lecithin intake, serum choline levels and various metabolic indices. *Metabolism*, 27:953–960.

34. Hirsch, M. J., Ulus, I. H., Wurtman, R. J. (1976): Elevation of brain and adrenal acetylcholine levels and of adrenal tyrosine hydroxylase activity following administration of choline via stomach tube. *Neurosci. Abstr.*, II(2):765.

35. Howard, A. N., Patelski, J., Bowyer, D. E., and Gresham, G. A. (1974): Mechanisms of antiatherosclerotic action of intravenous polyunsaturated PC. *Scand. J. Clin. Lab. Invest.*, 114:64.

36. Illingworth, D. R., and Portman, O. W. (1972): The uptake and metabolism of plasma lysophosphatidylcholine in vivo by the brain of squirrel monkeys. *Biochem. J.*, 130:557–567.

37. Illingworth, D. R., and Portman, O. W. (1972): Independence of phospholipid and protein exchange between plasma lipoproteins in vivo and in vitro. *Biochim. Biophys. Acta*, 280:281–289.

38. Jackson, I. V., Davis, L. G., Cohen, R. K., and Nuttal, E. A. (1981): Lecithin administration in tardive dyskinesia: Clinical and biomedical correlates. *Biol. Psychiatry*, 16:85–89.

39. Kritchevsky, D. (1976): Lipid and arterial metabolism. In: *Nutrition and Cardiovascular Disease*, edited by E. B. Feldman. Appleton-Century-Crofts, New York, pp. 19–29.

40. Krumdieck, C., and Butterworth, C. E., Jr. (1974): Ascorbate-cholesterol-lecithin interactions: factors of potential importance in the pathogenesis of atherosclerosis. *Am. J. Clin. Nutr.*, 27:866–876.

41. Lossow, J. J., Lindgren, F. T., Murchio, J. C., Stevens, G. R., and Jensen, J. C. (1969): Particle size and protein content of six fractions of the S_f 20 plasma lipoproteins isolated by density gradient centrifugation. *J. Lipid Res.*, 10:68–79.

42. Michell, R. H. (1975): Inositol phospholipids and cell surface receptor function. *Biochim. Biophys. Acta*, 415:81.

43. Miller, S. L., Benjamins, J. A., and Morrell, P. (1977): Metabolism of glycerophospholipids of myelin and microsomes in rat brain. *J. Biol. Chem.*, 252:4025–4037.

44. Morley, B. J., Robinson, G. R., Brown, G. B., Kemp, G. E., and Bradley, R. J. (1977): Effect of dietary choline on nicotinic acetylcholine receptors in brain. *Nature*, 266:848–859.

45. Pentland, B., Martyn, C. N., Steer, C. R., and Christie, J. E. (1981): Lecithin treatment in Friedreich's ataxia. *Br. Med. J.*, 282:1197–1198.

46. Rosseneu, M., Declercq, B., Vandamme, D., Vercaemst, R., Soetewey, F., Peeters, H., and Blaton, V. (1979): Influence of oral polyunsaturated and saturated phospholipid treatment on the lipid composition and fatty acid profile of chimpanzee lipoproteins. *Atherosclerosis*, 32:141–153.

47. Rothman, R. E., and Lenard, J. (1977): The nature of membrane asymmetry provides clues to the puzzle of how membranes are assembled. *Science*, 195:743–753.

48. Sata, T., Havel, R. J., and Jones, A. L. (1972): Characterization of subfractions of triglyceride-rich lipoproteins separated by gel chromatography from blood plasma of normolipemic humans. *J. Lipid Res.*, 13:757–768.

49. Shen, B. W., Scanu, A. M., and Kezdy, F. J. (1977): Structure of human serum lipoproteins inferred from compositional analysis. *Proc. Natl. Acad. Sci. USA*, 74:837–841.

50. Singer, S. J., and Nicolson, G. L. (1972): The fluid mosaic model of the structure of cell membranes. *Science*, 175:720–731.

51. Spanner, S., Hall, R. C., and Ansell, G. B. (1976): Arterio-venous differences of choline and choline lipids across the brain of rat and rabbit. *Biochem. J.*, 154:133–140.

52. Stein, O., Vanderhock, J., and Stein, Y. (1976): Cholesterol content and sterol synthesis in human skin fibroblasts and rat aortic smooth muscle cells exposed to lipoprotein depleted serum and high-density-apolipoprotein/phospholipid mixtures. *Biochim. Biophys. Acta*, 431:347–358.

53. Ulus, I. H., Hirsch, M. J., and Wurtman, R. J. (1976): Trans-synaptic induction of adrenomedullary tyrosine hydroxylase activity by choline: evidence that choline administration increases cholinergic transmission. *Proc. Natl. Acad. Sci. USA*, 74:798–800.

54. Ulus, I. H., and Wurtman, R. J. (1976): Choline administration: Activation of tyrosine hydroxylase in dopaminergic neurons of rat brain. *Science*, 194:1060–1061.

55. Waligora, Z., Patelski, J., Brown, B. D., and Howard, A. N. (1975): Effect of a hypercholesterolaemic diet and a single injection of polyunsaturated PC solution on the activities of lipolytic enzymes, acyl-CoA-cholesterol acyltransferase in rabbit tissue. *Biochem. Pharmacol.*, 24:2263–2267.

56. Zeisel, S. H., Gelenberg, A. J., Growdon, J. H., and Wurtman, R. J. (1980): Use of choline and lecithin in the treatment of tardive dyskinesia. In: *Advances in Biochemical Psychopharmacology, Vol. 24: Long-Term Effects of Neuroleptics*, edited by F. Cattabeni, G. Racagni, P. F. Spano, and E. Costa, pp. 463–470. Raven Press, New York.
57. Zierenberg, O., Odenthal, J., and Betzing, H. (1979): Incorporation of polyenephosphatidylcholine into serum lipoproteins after oral or intravenous administration. *Atherosclerosis*, 34:259–276.

Phospholipids and Atherosclerosis, edited by
P. Avogaro, M. Mancini, G. Ricci, and
R. Paoletti. Raven Press, New York © 1983.

Current Concepts on the Role of Endogenous and Exogenous Phospholipids

Noris Siliprandi

*Institute of Biological Chemistry, University of Padova and C.N.R. Unit
for the Study of Mitochondrial Physiology, 35100 Padova, Italy*

PHOSPHOLIPIDS IN BIOMEMBRANES

The rapidly increasing interest in phospholipids is largely due to an improved knowledge of biological membranes and of membrane-bound enzymes, and to the progress in the methodology dealing with water-insoluble compounds. As the most common and typical amphipathic lipids, phospholipids represent the main molecular components of living organisms. Phospholipids provide the structure (membranes) that allows compartmentation, endowing them with dynamic and vectorial properties (16).

The physical state of phospholipids is directly relevant to several important properties of biomembranes (26). At body temperature, lipids in biomembranes are found in a quasi-liquid-crystalline state. A decrease in temperature induces a transition to a rigid crystalline state. Transition temperature depends largely on the nature of the component fatty acids: at decreasing chain length and at increasing unsaturation, lipids "melt" at lower temperatures (9). For mixed lipids (as with lipids in most biomembranes) the transition is gradual, and at physiological temperature fluid and solid states coexist in the same membrane (31).

However, when biomembranes are exposed to temperatures around 0°C and are simultaneously submitted to considerable gravitational forces, as during the isolation of subcellular organelles, profound changes in their organization ensue. These membrane alterations and the consequent perturbations of their native permeability properties are currently underevaluated in experiments on isolated organelles (mitochondria, synaptosomes, sarcoplasmic reticulum, and so on). For instance, it is generally assumed that sucrose does not enter synaptosomes and that the integrity of synaptosomes is preserved in the presence of various physiological media. By monitoring the physical integrity of synaptosomes using the technique of "enzyme osmometry," wherein the release of an occluded enzyme is determined as a function of the hypotonicity of the medium, Janardana Sarma (21) found a near quantitative

25

equilibration of external sucrose with internal space. The entry of sucrose because of changes in the permeability characteristics of membranes during centrifugation at low temperature indicates a potential general fallacy in studies on uptake mechanisms in synaptosomes. A critical reappraisal is needed. The problem is one of general validity since analogous observations have been made by Sambasiva Rao (30) on mitochondria and other subcellular organelles.

To explain these effects of combined gravitational field and low temperature, Sitaramam (34) proposed a "pulsatile model" of membrane, wherein the energized membrane is in a quasi-micellar state in the presence of a vectorial field. This model accounts for the heterogeneity of lipid domain. The consequent alterations in a number of membrane-associated parameters and the wider generality of the model explains and predicts a variety of phenomena hitherto unaccounted for by the Singer–Nicholson model (33).

The general validity of the "fluid mosaic" model of Singer and Nicholson has been recently questioned also by Cullis and De Kruijff (11). So far, within the terms of this classic membrane model, active and facilitated transport and other functions vital to cell or organelles viability are assumed to be mediated by proteins extending into or through the lipid bilayer. However, according to Cullis et al. (12) the resulting view of phospholipids as building blocks of biomembranes is incomplete in the sense that phospholipids may participate directly in functional processes, particularly in the facilitated transport of polar molecules (14) and in transport involving membrane fusion, such as exo- and endocytosis.

The possibility of the formation of micellar Ca^{2+}-phospholipid complexes, associated with increased permeability of inner mitochondrial membrane to this cation, is of particular interest with regard to Ca^{2+} transport in mitochondria, part of which could be accounted for by this phospholipid mediate transport. This model also suggests that phospholipids could be transported across the membrane in association with calcium. Such a Ca-phospholipid displacement within the membrane may be relevant for the activation of membrane-linked phospholipase A_2 (32). Normally the activity of mitochondrial phospholipase A_2 is silent because it is inaccessible to Ca^{2+}, owing to the organization of the mitochondrial membrane and the sequestration of calcium within the matrix space. However, when the ternary complex "phospholipase A_2–Ca^{2+}–phospholipids" becomes possible, phospholipase A_2 is activated and the phospholipid organization within the membrane is more or less profoundly perturbed (32).

These recent findings in regard to the possibility of a nonbilayer configuration of biomembranes may change the current concept of transmembrane transport and open new perspectives for the elucidation of the relative molecular mechanism.

TRANSLOCATION OF PHOSPHOLIPIDS ACROSS AND BETWEEN MEMBRANES AND THEIR RENEWAL

Within the membranes, phospholipids are in a state of motion. This is attributed to two types of diffusion: the so-called "flip-flop" translocation and lateral diffusion

(12). The flip-flop motion consists in the passage of phospholipids from one to another monolayer, and although it is a rather slow process a physiological role cannot be ruled out (27). Lateral diffusion, on the other hand, occurs very rapidly within a single monolayer (25). There is a physiological exchange between membranes as well and this has been shown to occur between microsomes, wherein the synthesis of phospholipids is very active, and mitochondria, which are dependent on microsomes for their phospholipid provision (37). Transfer of phospholipids also occurs between hepatic plasma membranes and microsomes or mitochondria (24). This type of exchange of phospholipids is carried out by a series of phospholipid-exchange specific proteins, now being identified in a variety of animal and plant tissues (41). These proteins are useful for the study of membrane structure. For instance, when unilamellar vesicles of isotopically labeled phosphatidylcholine are incubated with nonlabeled mitochondria in the presence of phospholipid-exchange protein, only the outer portion of the phosphatidylcholine bilayer is exchangeable, whereas, the translocation of lipids between the inner and outer part of the bilayer (flip-flop) is exceedingly slow (41).

As recently reported by Van Deenen (36) in mature mammal erythrocytes two mechanisms appear to play a major role in phospholipid renewal:

1. Exchange of phospholipids between serum lipoproteins and cell membranes.
2. Enzymatic incorporation of fatty acids into lysophospholipids, either formed in the membrane or supplied by the serum.

Evidence has been provided that the exchange process, mediated by phospholipid-exchange proteins, between erythrocytes and ambiance mainly involves the phospholipid molecules of the outer membrane layer (41).

The renewal of the inner membrane layer is ensured by the transacylation process between acyl-CoA and lysolecithins, catalyzed by the transacylases located at the cytoplasmic side. According to Van Deenen (36) it is likely that a slow translocation between the two layers links the exchange reactions occurring at the outer region with the transacylations of lysophosphatidylcholine at the inner side.

These processes are relevant in clarifying how exogenous phospholipids circulating in blood could be incorporated into blood cells and equilibrated with endogenously formed phospholipids. The concerted action of phospholipid-exchange proteins and phospholipases is crucial, not only for the renewal of membrane phospholipids but also for the adaptation of the physicochemical properties of biomembranes to the changeable physiological conditions.

UTILIZATION OF EXOGENOUS PHOSPHOLIPIDS AND THEIR EFFECTS

Exogenous phospholipids introduced into the bloodstream as liposomes do not undergo relevant changes in their physical state. While in circulation they retain their typical lamellar structure (16). This relative stability is further increased if cholesterol is also present in the liposome structure (8). However, the amount of circulating exogenous phospholipids decreases rapidly as a consequence of their accumulation into liver and spleen phagocytic cells (35) and of their interaction with plasma lipoproteins.

This interaction is of particular interest in relation with the postulated protective or preventive action of unsaturated phospholipids against atherosclerosis (13). As recently reported (22), saturation of bovine high-density lipoproteins (HDL) with small vesicles of egg phosphatidylcholine and cholesterol (2:1 mole/mole) gave final lipoprotein particles with essentially unchanged protein content and composition, unchanged cholesteryl esters and nonpolar lipid content, but with markedly increased phospholipid content and moderately increased free cholesterol content. These results indicate the possibility of a direct transfer of lipids from liposomes to HDL and also suggest a structural flexibility of HDL allowing the addition of significant amounts of surface components with consequent changes in the fluidity of the lipid domains of blood lipoproteins.

The transfer of liposomal phospholipids to HDL is mediated by HDL apoproteins. These apoproteins are able to associate with lipid bilayers and transfer phospholipids to, or exchange phospholipids with, HDL. The insertion of apolipoproteins into bilayers is more easily accomplished at lipid phase transition, at phase boundaries, and in liquid-crystalline lipid. Since only the outer layer phospholipids are available for exchange, relatively little exchange would be expected for multilayer liposomes as compared with that of unilamellar liposomes. Those factors which tighten the bilayer, such as cholesterol, prevent liposome-HDL interaction and increase the stability of liposome in blood (1).

Conceivably this exchange between exogenous phospholipids and HDL, together with the fluidity of blood lipoproteins, may modify the activity of lecithin-cholesterol acyltransferase (LCAT) and the nature of the acyl moiety of esterified cholesterol. In this regard only those lecithins bearing a polyunsaturated fatty acid in the 2-position could serve as effective substrate for LCAT in producing polyunsaturated cholesteryl esters (2,15). Moreover, since HDL interacts with other plasma lipoproteins, all blood lipoproteins could be, to some extent, modified by exogenous phospholipids.

These *in vitro* results have been confirmed *in vivo* by Rosseneu et al. (29). These authors found that administration of polyunsaturated lecithin to male chimpanzees induces an increase in cholesteryl esters and lysolecithins in HDL_3, presumably via activation of LCAT. These modified HDL particles have a more fluid surface and a denser core, and are susceptible to act as better cholesterol carriers. A complementary effect of this treatment was a decrease of plasma triglyceride and very low-density lipoprotein (VLDL) concentration, and an increase in the unsaturated ratio of the triglycerides which might take place via activation of lipoprotein lipase.

Considering that whatever the pathogenetic mechanism, the interaction of plasma lipoproteins with arterial walls is certainly involved in atherosclerosis, the above-reported data are of some significance in postulating a potentially beneficial effect of exogenous phospholipids in the prevention of atherosclerotic lesions. In this regard it is notable that individuals with familial LCAT deficiency, which is associated with abnormal plasma lipoproteins and increased levels of unesterified cholesterol and lecithin, are more susceptible to the development of premature atherosclerotic disease (15).

POSSIBLE EFFECTS OF EXOGENOUS PHOSPHOLIPIDS ON THE NERVOUS SYSTEM

Neurologists and nutritionists were taken aback a few years ago by the communication of Bari Kolata (4) that the activity of some brain neurons varies in response to fluctuations in the diet. Previously, Cohen and Wurtman (10) had reported that the synthesis of acetylcholine in the brain can be enhanced by increasing the amount of choline in the blood. Shortly after, Wurtman et al. demonstrated that lecithin consumption elevates serum free-choline levels (39), as well as acetylcholine concentration in rat brain and adrenal gland (19).

On the basis of these and other similar results, a symposium was held (in Tucson) to discuss evidence that choline or lecithin, one of the best dietary sources of choline, might be useful in treating a number of neurological disorders (5). An unquestionable success so far obtained with lecithin administration is the alleviation of the symptoms of tardive dyskinesia (5). More recently, Barbeau (3) has presented observations that confirm and extend these results to other neurological disorders with presumed cholinergic deficiencies, such as Huntington's chorea and Friedreich's ataxia. Therefore, exogenous lecithin, either as a precursor of brain acetylcholine or by promoting exchange of fatty acids with membrane components, might be a useful nutritional or pharmacological tool for the control of presumed central cholinergic deficiency states. This possibility has been strengthened by Pauling (28) who has defined as "orthomolecular psychiatry" the treatment of mental disease by the provision of the optimum concentrations of substances normally present in human blood.

Also phosphatidylserine appears to be active in modifying some brain metabolic parameters. As reported by Toffano and Bruni (35) phosphatidylserine administration to rats increases catecholamine turnover and glucose accumulation in the brain and enhances acetylcholine output from the cerebral cortex. Such biological activity might be rationalized by the role of phosphatidylserine as a specific activator of some enzymatic activities (38).

Taken as a whole the above-reported results should be considered with some caution. In fact, as outlined by Juliano (23) there are a number of anatomical sites from which phospholipidic liposomes are essentially excluded; thus, liposomes appear unable to cross the blood-brain barrier and appear to penetrate poorly into the myocardium and skeletal muscle, presumably because of the characteristics of the capillary endothelium of these tissues.

INTESTINAL ABSORPTION OF PHOSPHOLIPIDS

Another incompletely solved problem is the intestinal absorption of dietary phospholipids. Although a portion of orally administered phospholipids can be absorbed as such (13,20), the major part is hydrolyzed by pancreatic phospholipases with the hydrolysis products taken up by mucosal cells. According to Beil and Grundy (6) the subsequent fates of lysolecithins and accompanying fatty acids are not well understood. Fatty acids could be a source of chylomicron triglycerides or could be reesterified with lysolecithins to produce lecithins. In turn, lysolecithins might be deacylated to glycerophosphorylcholine or secreted into the portal circulation. Indeed an enterohepatic circulation for lecithin has been postulated by Boucrot (7). This enterohepatic cycle of lecithin has been recently confirmed by Garguly et al. (13) by administering double-labeled lecithin to rats. Dietary lecithin was absorbed intact, transported to the liver, and secreted with the bile. The enrichment of bile in exogenous phospholipids induces physicochemical modification whereby cholesterol seems to be more efficiently packed in the matrix of polyunsaturated phospholipids. Such a modification might be beneficial in preventing the formation of cholesterol stones in the gallbladder.

CONCLUSION

The advanced knowledge of the physicochemical properties of phospholipid in biomembranes, as well as of their role as activators of membrane-bound (40) and soluble enzymes (38), permits a more rational interpretation of their role in a number of physiological processes. Some effects of administered phospholipids might be foreseen and explained in the light of their physiological role. However, a valuable appreciation of their authentic significance needs further and careful investigation.

As pointed out by Gregoriadis (17) a promising field for explaining phospholipidic liposome development will derive from tailoring liposome structure to the particular biological milieu in which it acts. Success in this field will most likely complement the attempts to modify the blood lipoproteins with exogenous phospholipids or those to introduce phospholipids into the brain across the blood-brain barrier.

Finally, the idea that drugs entrapped in phospholipid vesicles may provide a better means of delivery to specific sites within the body opens new perspectives in pharmacology and therapy (18).

ACKNOWLEDGMENT

I am indebted to Dr. I. A. Bartlett for the revision of the English text.

REFERENCES

1. Allen, T. M. (1981): A study of phospholipid interactions between high-density lipoproteins and small unilamellar vesicles. Biochim. Biophys. Acta, 640:385–397.
2. Assmann, G. (1976): Lecithin-cholesterol-Acyl-transferase. In: Phosphatidylcholine, edited by H. Peeters, pp. 34–46. Springer-Verlag, Berlin.
3. Barbeau, A. (1978): Lecithin in neurologic disorders. N. Engl. J. Med., 299:200–201.
4. Bari Kolata, G. (1976): Brain biochemistry: Effects of diet. Science, 192:41–42.
5. Bari Kolata, G. (1979): Mental disorders: A new approach to treatment? Science, 203:36–38.
6. Beil, F. U., and Grundy, S. M. (1980): Studies on plasma lipoproteins during absorption of exogenous lecithin in man. J. Lipid Res., 21:525–536.

7. Boucrot, P. (1972): Is there an entero-hepatic circulation on the bile phospholipids? *Lipids*, 7:282–288.
8. Breisblatt, W., and Ohki, S. (1976): Fusion in phospholipid spherical membranes. II. Effect of cholesterol, divalent ions and pH. *J. Membr. Biol.*, 29:127–146.
9. Chapman, D. (1973): Some recent studies of lipids, lipid-cholesterol and membrane systems. In: *Biological Membranes*, Vol. 2, edited by D. Chapman and D. F. A. Wallach, pp. 91–144. Academic Press, London.
10. Cohen, E., and Wurtman, R. J. (1975): Brain acetylcholine: Increase after systematic choline administration. *Life Sci.*, 16:1095–1102.
11. Cullis, P. R., and De Kruijff, B. (1979): Lipid polymorphism and the functional roles of lipids in biological membranes. *Biochim. Biophys. Acta*, 559:399–420.
12. Cullis, P. R., De Kruijff, B., Hope, M. J., Nayar, R., and Schmid, S. L. (1980): Phospholipids and membrane transport. *Can. J. Biochem.*, 58:1091–1100.
13. Ganguly, J., Paul, R., Ramesha, C. S., and Balaram, P. (1979): Mechanism of cholesterol-lowering effects of polyunsaturated fats. In: *Biochemical Aspects of Nutrition*, edited by K. Yagi, pp. 105–113. Japan Scientific Societies Press, Tokyo.
14. Gerritsen, W. J., Henricks, P. A. J., De Kruijff, B., and Van Deenen, L. L. M. (1980): The transbilayer movement of phosphatidylcholine in vesicles reconstituted with intrinsic proteins from the human erythrocyte membrane. *Biochim. Biophys. Acta*, 600:607–619.
15. Glomset, J. A. (1972): Plasma lecithin:cholesterol acyltransferase. In: *Blood Lipids and Lipoproteins*, edited by G. J. Nelson, pp. 745–787. Wiley-Interscience, New York.
16. Gregoriadis, G., Siliprandi, N., and Turchetto, E. (1977): Possible implications in the use of exogenous phospholipids. *Life Sci.*, 20:1773–1786.
17. Gregoriadis, G. (1980): Tailoring liposome structure. *Nature*, 283:814–815.
18. Gregoriadis, G., and Allison, D. C. (1980): *Liposomes in Biological Systems*. John Wiley, New York.
19. Hirsch, M. J., and Wurtman, R. J. (1978): Lecithin consumption increases acetylcholine concentrations in rat brain and adrenal gland. *Science*, 202:223–225.
20. Holzl, J. (1976): Pharmacokinetic studies on phosphatidylcholine and phosphatidylinositol. In: *Phosphatidylcholine*, edited by H. Peeters, pp. 66–79. Springer-Verlag, Berlin.
21. Janardana Sarma, M. K. (1980): New insights into the biochemical criteria for the integrity of synaptosomal membranes. *Abstracts of the Second Congress of the Federation of Asian and Oceanian Biochemists*, p. 60, Bangalore, India.
22. Jonas, A. (1979): Interaction of bovine serum high density lipoprotein with mixed vesicles of phosphatidylcholine and cholesterol. *J. Lipid Res.*, 20:817–824.
23. Juliano, R. L. (1981): Liposomes as a drug delivery system. *Trends Pharm. Sci.*, 2:39–42.
24. Kamath, S. A., and Rubin, E. (1973): The exchange of phospholipids between subcellular organelles of the liver. *Arch. Biochem. Biophys.*, 158:312–322.
25. Kornberg, R. D., and McConnell, H. M. (1971): Lateral diffusion of phospholipids in a vesicle membrane (spin-labeled phosphatidylcholine/nuclear resonance). *Proc. Natl. Acad. Sci. USA*, 68:2564–2568.
26. Lenaz, G. (1979): The role of lipids in the structure and function of membranes. In: *Subcellular Biochemistry*, Vol. 6, edited by D. B. Roodyn, pp. 233–343. Plenum Press, New York.
27. McNamee, M. G., and McConnell, H. M. (1973): Transmembrane potentials and Phospholipid flip-flop in excitable membrane vesicles. *Biochemistry*, 12:2951–2958.
28. Pauling, L. (1979): Treating mental disorders. *Science*, 206:404.
29. Rosseneu, M., Declercq, B., Vandamme, D., Vercaemst, R., Soetewey, F., Peeters, H., and Blaton, V. (1979): Influence of oral polyunsaturated phospholipid treatment on the lipid composition and fatty acid profile of chimpanzee lipoproteins. *Atherosclerosis*, 32:141–153.
30. Sambasiva Rao, D. (1980): Entry of sucrose into mitochondrial matrix space: An experimental evaluation. *Abstracts of the Second Congress of the Federation of Asian and Oceanian Biochemists*, p. 60, Bangalore, India.
31. Shimshick, E. J., and McConnell, H. M. (1973): Lateral phase separation in phospholipid membranes. *Biochemistry*, 12:2351–2360.
32. Siliprandi, D., Rugolo, M., Zoccarato, F., Toninello, A., and Siliprandi, N. (1979): Involvement of endogenous phospholipase A_2 in Ca^{2+} and Mg^{2+} movements induced by inorganic phosphate and diamide in rat liver mitochondria. *Biochim. Biophys. Res. Commun.*, 88:388–394.
33. Singer, S. J., and Nicolson, G. L. (1972): The fluid mosaic model of the structure of cell membranes. *Science*, 175:720–731.

34. Sitaramam, V. (1980): A pulsatile model for energized membranes. *Abstracts of Second Congress of the Federation of Asian and Oceanian Biochemists*, p. 61. Bangalore, India.
35. Toffano, G., and Bruni, A. (1980): Pharmacological properties of phospholipid liposomes. *Pharmacol. Res. Commun.*, 12:829–845.
36. van Deenen, L. L. M. (1981): Topology and dynamics of phospholipids in membranes. *FEBS Lett.*, 123:3–15.
37. Wirtz, K. W. A., and Zilversmit, D. B. (1969): The use of phenobarbital and carbon tetrachloride to examine liver phospholipid exchange in intact rats. *Biochim. Biophys. Acta*, 187:468–476.
38. Wrenn, R. W., Katoh, N., Wise, B. C., and Kuo, J. F. (1980): Stimulation by phosphatidylserine and calmodulin of calcium-dependent phosphorylation of endogenous proteins from cerebral cortex. *J. Biol. Chem.*, 255:12042–12046.
39. Wurtman, R. J., Hirsch, M. J., and Growodon, J. H. (1977): Lecithin consumption elevates serum free choline levels. *Lancet*, ii:68–69.
40. Zakim, D., and Vessey, D. A. (1980): The importance of phospholipid-protein interactions for regulation of the activities of membrane-bound enzymes. In: *Principles of Metabolic Control in Mammalian Systems*, edited by R. H. Herman, D. Zakim, and D. A. Vessey, pp. 337–371. Plenum Press, New York.
41. Zilversmit, D. B. (1978): Phospholipid-exchange proteins as membrane probes. In: *Liposomes and Their Uses in Biology and Medicine*, Vol. 308, edited by D. Papahadjopoulos, pp. 149–163. New York Academy of Science, New York.

Phospholipids and Atherosclerosis, edited by
P. Avogaro, M. Mancini, G. Ricci, and
R. Paoletti. Raven Press, New York © 1983.

Role of Lecithin in the Absorption of Dietary Fat

Martin C. Carey

*Department of Medicine, Harvard Medical School, and Division of Gastroenterology,
Brigham and Women's Hospital, Boston, Massachusetts 02115*

The purpose of this chapter is to summarize recent advances in the understanding of dietary fat (triacylglycerol) digestion and absorption with particular emphasis on the role played by phospholipids, especially dietary and biliary lecithins (phosphatidylcholine).[1] This chapter will also emphasize several aspects of the biochemistry and biophysics of lipid digestion that have received little attention in previous accounts. The general theme will profess the belief that an understanding of the physical-chemical state of dietary lipids in model systems offers profound insights into their pathophysiological behavior within the gastrointestinal tract.

DIETARY LECITHIN AND TRIGLYCERIDE: SOURCE, PHYSICOCHEMICAL PROPERTIES, AND INTERACTIONS

Long-chain triglycerides constitute the major biological form of lipids. In both animals and plants they provide an economic storage source of reserve chemical energy, yielding 9 kcal/g, compared with 4 kcal/g for carbohydrates and 5.5 kcal/g for protein. On a typical Western diet, the average healthy adult consumes about 150 g of fat each day, of which two-thirds is animal fat and one-third is vegetable fat (126). The extremes of human intake vary widely and are generally low (<50 g/day) in underdeveloped countries where starchy tubers and seeds constitute major food staples (34). The triglyceride stores in living organisms occur intracellularly as liquid oil droplets surrounded by a monomolecular layer of phospholipid and protein. Such cells also contain membranous intracellular organelles and plasma membranes composed principally of phospholipids (160). Hence, about 2 to 4 g of membrane phospholipids are ingested daily (14). The predominant phospholipid is lecithin (phosphatidylcholine), with smaller amounts of sphingomyelin, cephalin (phosphatidylethanolamine), and traces of minor phospholipids. Quantitatively more

---

[1]For convenience, the words *fat* and *lecithin* are used in their restricted meanings to denote natural triglycerides (triacylglycerols) and the major natural phospholipid (phosphatidylcholine) respectively.

important is endogenous phospholipid of hepatic origin, which is secreted into the intestinal lumen via bile. The quantity of biliary phospholipid (essentially pure lecithin) varies from 7 g to about 22 g/day (99). This secretion rate principally depends on the enterohepatic cycling rate of the bile salt pool (27). A vast array of other lipids (106) are ingested as minor components of dietary fats, but these will not be discussed here.

Dietary triglycerides and phospholipids contain a variety of fatty acid species in their molecular structures and occur in nature as highly complex mixtures (151). Vegetable fats are distinct from animal fats by containing a much higher proportion of unsaturated fatty acids. In most dietary fats, as in lecithins, there is a higher proportion of unsaturated fatty acids in the sn-2 position of the molecules than in the other ester positions. Milk lipids are an exception to this rule. Triglycerides and lecithins are chemically inert and their ester bonds are generally stable during food processing and cooking. During digestion these bonds become remarkably susceptible to specific hydrolytic enzymes.

In the solid crystalline state, the triglyceride molecule (Fig. 1) adopts a tuning-fork conformation (38,50,162) with the sn-2 fatty acid pointing in the opposite direction to the sn-1 and sn-3 fatty acids. Solid triglycerides are polymorphic; by means of X-ray diffraction, three distinct crystallization patterns have been identified: α, β, and β' (151). In the liquid state, there is free rotation of atoms around all but double bonds. Further, the individual molecules are not oriented randomly

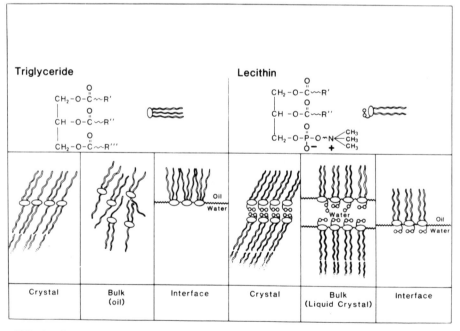

FIG. 1. Possible physicochemical states of major dietary lipids. **Left:** Long-chain triglyceride (triacylglycerol). **Right:** Long-chain lecithin (3-sn-phosphatidylcholine). See text for description.

in space (Fig. 1): Recent evidence suggests that in the oil state, molecules of saturated triglyceride are quasi-crystalline, forming closely packed swarms of molecules (50), with nearest-neighbor interactions of ~200Å (26).

Because natural fats are complex blends of triglycerides, melting occurs over a wide temperature range. With pure synthetic triglyceride mixtures, complex composition- and temperature-dependent physicochemical behavior is observed (128). Taking the lowest temperature at which all fat is "liquid," human fat melts a few degrees below the ambient temperature for the organ of origin, at about 30 to 35°C for visceral fat and 0 to 10°C for peripheral subcutaneous fat (135). Some animal fats, particularly lard and tallow, do not melt completely until ~50 to 60°C (162); at 37°C these present as either mixtures of liquid and solid fats or supercooled melts.

The interfacial orientation of triglycerides, whether medium (C_8–C_{12})- or long (> C_{14})-chain with saturated or unsaturated fatty acids, is shown in Fig. 1. Medium-chain triglycerides generally form more expanded surface films (~100Å²/molecule) than do long-chain saturated triglycerides, which form condensed or solid monomolecular films (~60Å²/molecule). In each case (Fig. 1) the three fatty acid chains are oriented toward the hydrophobic side of the interface (52). Synthetic short-chain triglycerides (triacetin and tripropionin) adopt a tuning-fork arrangement at interfaces with the sn-2 fatty acid projecting into the aqueous phase. For this reason, these triglycerides give the smallest interfacial areas (~40–50Å²/molecule) (52).

Crystal, bulk, and interfacial configurations of natural lecithins (Fig. 1) show that in the solid state, the molecules form bilayer lamellae, tilted in relation to the interface to allow close packing between the long fatty acid chains. A number of polymorphic forms of crystalline lecithins have been described. The approximate average orientation of the phosphorylcholine head group is *in* the bilayer plane (133), i.e., parallel to the surface. This arrangement is maintained when the phospholipid swells in water to form lamellar liquid crystals (23) (Fig. 1). Admixture with cholesterol forces the hydrocarbon regions to become normal to the interface and their molecular motions adopt "intermediate fluid" properties, that is, trans conformations in the proximal parts of the chains and gauche conformations at the terminal ends are increased. Cholesterol appears to have no influence on the polar head group conformation of lecithin (22,48,164). A similar head group orientation (Fig. 1) also appears to be typical of monomolecular films at an air-water interface (25). Fully expanded lecithin monolayers occupy an interfacial area of 60 to 70Å²/molecule, with condensed films occupying ~40 to 45Å²/molecule or about two-thirds of the corresponding areas for long-chain triglyceride molecules (113). The predominant physical state of natural lecithins in aqueous systems at 37°C is that of liquid crystalline bilayers (60–70Å²/molecule).

Long-chain triglycerides and lecithins are insoluble in water. A crude estimate based on the solubilities of short-chain homologs (52) suggests that the monomeric solubility of tripalmitin (C_{16}) lies in the vicinity of 10^{-25} M. The solubility of dipalmitoyl lecithin has been estimated to be 5×10^{-10} M (146). A useful classification based on bulk aqueous behavior is that long-chain triglycerides are insoluble, nonswelling amphiphiles and that lecithins are soluble, swelling amphiphiles (145). Hence, both molecules spread to form stable monomolecular surface films. Dietary triglyceride "oils" out of water to form a separate bulk phase and lecithin swells with water to form lamellar liquid crystals. Water can slightly hydrate the triester head group of triglycerides via dipole–dipole interactions (114), whereas the strong zwitterionic head groups of lecithins bind water tightly via ion–dipole interactions. Natural lecithin can solubilize 40% of its weight as water (145), and even more so if lipids with negative or positive charges are incorporated within the bilayers.

When shaken in excess water, triglyceride forms crude emulsion droplets and hydrated lecithin disperses to form concentric lamellar structures called liposomes (Fig. 2). For these reasons, the major digestive lipases (in contrast to esterases) have been designed by evolutionary pressure to function at oil-water interfaces and have little or no activity on water-soluble substrates (21). Accordingly, the interfacial area/volume ratio ("interfacial concentration") of the lipid becomes a major determinant of hydrolytic rates. Emulsification increases the oil-water interfacial area (and surface/volume ratio) by the dispersion of large oil masses into fine oil–water emulsion particles. The interfacial tension between pure triglyceride and water is ~15–20 mN/m. Therefore, energy expenditure is required to break up bulk oil into fine emulsion droplets. For example, when emulsified into droplets of 1 μm in diameter, a 1-cm oil drop increases its surface area 1,000 times (78), requiring 20 kergs of energy. Surface active materials dramatically lessen this energy requirement by lowering the oil-water interfacial tension. Emulsifiers also stabilize the emulsion droplets by preventing coalescence and breakup of the emulsion.

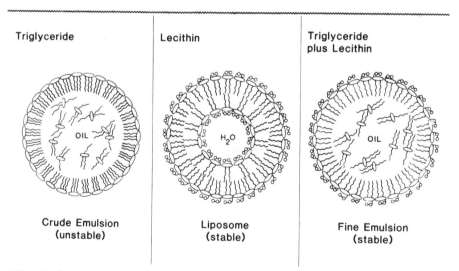

Triglyceride

Lecithin

Triglyceride plus Lecithin

OIL

H₂O

OIL

Crude Emulsion (unstable)

Liposome (stable)

Fine Emulsion (stable)

FIG. 2. Dispersed states of major dietary lipids in water. In the triglyceride plus lecithin emulsion particles, some triglyceride is solubilized in the surface coat.

A number of dietary fats occur naturally or are processed for eating in an emulsified state (as in milk, ice cream, salad dressings, sauces, baked goods, and so on). Food emulsifiers, in general, are phospholipids, diglycerides, monoglycerides, nonionic detergents, and a variety of polysaccharide gums and gels—all of which are degradable. The diameter of triglyceride droplets in food may range from several microns, as in milk, to several hundred microns, as in adipose tissue (106). Before food is eaten, cells are broken and are mixed with secretions and membrane fragments by partial germination, autolysis, refining, blending, marinating, and, especially, cooking. During cell rupture, intracellular fat droplets, which are surrounded by a monolayer of phospholipids, may acquire an additional envelope of phospholipids from the plasma membrane. One of the best studied examples is the secretion of milk droplets by the mammary gland (109). During rupture of the acinar cells, the extruded fat globules become enveloped by the plasma membrane; the final milk fat globule membrane consists of a trimolecular layer of phospholipids (and protein). With most unprocessed food, emulsification is initiated during mastication and deglutition in the oropharyngeal region, and by peristalic activity together with endogenous emulsifiers throughout the upper gastrointestinal tract (78).

The desirable characteristics (55) of a good emulsifier are several: (a) It should reduce interfacial tension to about 0.5 to 1 mN/m, i.e., for emulsification without intense agitation. (b) It should form a condensed (closely packed) film around the dispersed oil droplets to prevent thinning out when they collide by Brownian movement. (c) It should be an amphiphile so that the polar groups of the molecule are attracted to water and the nonpolar groups are attracted to oil. (d) It should be in a suitable physical state so as to quickly adsorb around the dispersed droplets. (e) It should impart an electrical potential to the droplets. (f) It should be sparingly soluble in both oil and water phases so that the system can be emulsified with small concentrations of emulsifier. Dietary lecithin fulfills most of these conditions and is an excellent emulsifier of triglycerides. Emulsification occurs with low shear forces (as occur in the stomach) and with low concentrations (as occur in the diet). Ninety grams of triglyceride divided into 1 μm emulsion particles (surface area of 600 m^2) can be covered by 1 g of lecithin as a closely packed monomolecular film (60Å^2 per head group). It has been suggested (130) that a monomolecular layer may be insufficient, since the minimum amount of a mixed phospholipid emulsifier required to stabilize soybean oil-water emulsions corresponds to a multilayered interfacial film of ~80Å in thickness. However, like Intralipid®, these may be conventional emulsion particles in equilibrium with excess liquid-crystalline lecithin. Not only is the interfacial concentration of triglyceride dramatically increased for promoting lipolysis, but also the lecithin coat of the emulsion particles is in a suitable physical state for hydrolysis by pancreatic phospholipase A$_2$ (15).

A simple working model for droplets of long-chain triglyceride emulsified with dietary lecithin is shown in Fig. 2. Nuclear magnetic resonance spectroscopic studies and enzymatic assays (24) of mixed micelles formed by short-chain triglycerides (tributyrin, trihexanoin) solubilized by short-chain (di-C$_6$ to di-C$_8$) lecithins are consistent with a model in which the majority of the triglyceride is solubilized in an hydrophobic core by an enveloping monolayer of lecithin. The core lipid is not constrained and its molecular motion is similar to that of neat triglycerides. Also, the molecular motion of the solubilizer (lecithin) is not detectably perturbed by the presence of the triglyceride. As will be discussed below, some core lipid must be solubilized in the surface coat since triglyceride in the mixed micelles can be hydrolyzed with pancreatic lipase. The corresponding long-chain analogs in emulsified form are not readily hydrolyzed by pancreatic lipase, and a long "latent phase" is observed before triglyceride hydrolysis commences (10,15,108). A similar "latent period" occurs when endogenous biliary lecithin adsorbs to dietary fat globules in the duodenum (108) (see section on digestion in the duodenum-jejunum).

LIPID DIGESTION IN THE STOMACH

Gastrointestinal lipid digestion consists of three sequential steps: (a) the dispersion of bulk fat globules into finely divided emulsion particles, (b) the enzymatic hydrolysis of fatty acid esters at the emulsion-water interface, and (c) the desorption and dispersion of the hydrolyzed products into an absorbable form. Although it has long been known that muscle contractions of the stomach and pylorus are responsible for promoting emulsification by mixing and grinding the stomach contents, it has now become clear that enzymatic hydrolysis of triglycerides also begins in the stomach (62,64). In man, up to 30% of dietary triglyceride may be digested during the 2 to 3 hr period that fat remains in the stomach. However, quantitative hydrolysis and absorption require less acidic conditions, appropriate lipases and detergents (bile salts), and the specialized absorptive cells of the upper small intestine.

Lingual Lipase Hydrolysis

The major source of gastric lipolytic activity has been unambiguously identified as originating in a group of lingual serous glands (Ebner) which lie beneath the V-shaped circumvallate papillae of the tongue (60,61). The fine structure of these glands is reminiscent of pancreatic acinar cells. Each acinus terminates in a short duct which opens onto the papillary troughs. Basal secretion occurs continuously, but can be stimulated by sympathetic agonists, a high fat diet, suckling, and deglutition (59). Although unrecognized as such, the calf, kid goat, and lamb lipases have been utilized by Mediterranean cheesemakers for hundreds of years, since lingual lipase is an important component of the rennet pastes used to curdle milk (74). Before the role of stomach hydrolysis in human fat digestion was recognized (62), lingual lipases (usually called pregastric esterase, or pharyngeal or salivary lipases) had received much attention in the dairy and veterinary literature (94). Despite their discovery in 1924 (94), no lingual lipase has yet been purified to homogeneity; therefore, molecular weights, pH optima, and cofactor requirements have not been established with any certainty (94).

Both lingual lipase and the classic pancreatic lipase are true lipases (in contrast to esterases) and act only on insoluble aggregated substrates. In addition, both enzymes are stereospecific for the primary ester bonds of triglycerides; fatty acid linkages of phospholipids and cholesterol esters are resistant to hydrolysis (106). Lingual lipase exhibits much higher activity on triglycerides with short- and medium-chain fatty acids than on those with long-chain fatty acids (41,45,149), whereas pancreatic lipase demonstrates no preference between medium- and long-chain fatty acids (Fig. 3). In contrast to pancreatic lipase, lingual lipase has a stereospecific preference for the fatty acid at the sn-3 ester linkage rather than the sn-1 position (45,105,149). Crude lingual lipase is acid resistant, apparently requires no cofactor, and displays a broad pH-activity range (2.6–7.0) (60,94). The major products formed in the stomach and *in vitro*, even after prolonged incubation, are diglycerides and fatty acids (41,45,63,149). In contrast, monoglycerides and fatty acids are the final products of pancreatic lipase hydrolysis (Fig. 4).

Physical State and Fate of Hydrolytic Products

Since lingual lipase preferentially hydrolyzes sn-3 linkages and short- and medium-chain fatty acid esters much faster than their long-chain homologs, the products of digestion differ depending on whether the source of triglyceride is milk (41) or common animal or vegetable fat (94). The major products of lingual lipase hydrolysis of milk fat are short- and medium-chain fatty acids (esterified predominantly at the sn-3 position) and sn-1,2 diglycerides, which contain the long-chain fatty acids. The released short- and medium-chain fatty acids have pK_a values in water in the vicinity of 4.8 (1). On account of their hydrophilicity, they are soluble in both ionized and protonated form in the postprandial stomach. As indicated in Fig. 5, there is now good evidence (3,45,149) that, by virtue of their solubility in the acid-aqueous phase, the free fatty acids leave the surface of the fat droplets and

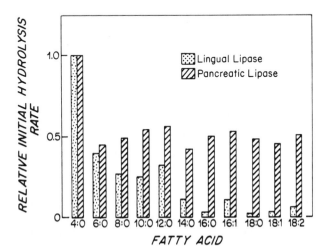

FIG. 3. Relative initial hydrolysis rates by lingual and pancreatic lipases for individual fatty acids of cow's milk fat. Values are fractions of initial rate (1.0) for butyrate (C_4). (From Edwards-Webb and Thompson, ref. 41, with permission.)

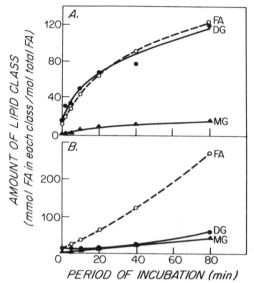

FIG. 4. Rates of release of different lipid classes during hydrolysis of cow's milk fat by **(A)** calf lingual lipase and **(B)** calf pancreatic lipase. ○, free fatty acid (FA), ●, diglyceride (DG), ▲, monoglyceride (MG). (From Edwards-Webb and Thompson, ref. 41, with permission.)

are absorbed by the stomach mucosa, to be transported to the liver, bound to albumin, in the portal blood. The aqueous pK_a values of long-chain fatty acids are, in general, well above neutrality (76,81,87) so that they are protonated at stomach pH values and form hydrogen-bonded liquid fatty acid oils and crystals (43,51). Such protonated long-chain fatty acids have high solubilities within fat droplets (Fig. 5).

Crude Emulsification

Very little experimental work on stomach emulsification has been done (34, 49,78,89). Despite claims to the contrary (34,49,78), stable emulsions have been observed in the stomach of normal subjects within minutes of feeding test meals (89,106). Provided a suitable emulsifier is available, the classic "kneading, churning, and squirting" action (138) of the body and antral regions of the stomach against a closed pylorus (Fig. 6) supplies mechanical energy (30) to facilitate emulsification. Since long-chain fatty acids are unionized in the stomach, the only available luminal amphiphiles that could act as emulsifiers are membrane-derived phospholipids (78) and peptic digests of dietary proteins (89). Phospholipid-coated emulsions are extremely stable (78,130). Further, in the presence of small concentrations (~1 mM) of calcium ions, the phospholipids gain a net charge by binding divalent cations to their zwitterionic head groups (79,80). Since lingual lipase is not inhibited by phospholipids (41,45,60,149), hydrolysis of the triglyceride molecules in the emulsion particles takes place. As will be discussed below, such

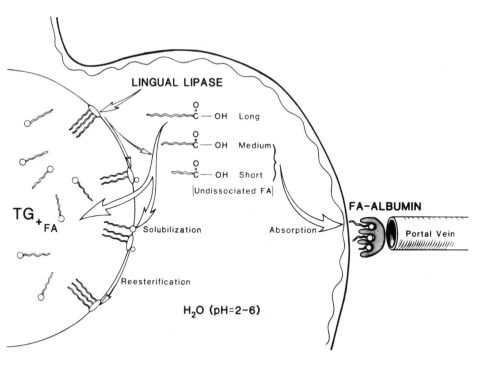

FIG. 5. Physical state and fate of hydrolyzed cow's milk fatty acids during lingual lipase hydrolysis in the stomach. Short- and medium-chain fatty acids are absorbed. Long-chain fatty acids are solubilized within the fat droplets. TG, triglycerides; FA, fatty acids.

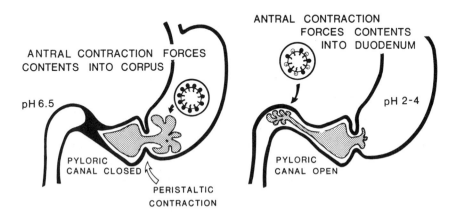

FIG. 6. Role of the stomach and pyloric canal in the emulsification of dietary fat. See text for description.

emulsions cannot easily be hydrolyzed by the pancreatic enzyme (10,15,24,108) without the presence of a cofactor (phospholipase A_2, colipase, bile salts).

DIGESTION IN THE DUODENUM-JEJUNUM

Lingual lipase hydrolysis of dietary fat in the stomach is crucial for efficient and continued fat digestion in the small intestine. In rats (129) diversion of lingual lipase decreased fat absorption by ~30%, and substitution of a fine emulsion corrected the malabsorption. This strongly suggests that partial ionization of long-chain fatty acids (released by lingual lipase) is important in promoting fine emulsification in the duodenum (Fig. 6). In other studies, preincubation of cow's milk (41,115) with lingual lipase *in vitro* enhanced subsequent pancreatic lipolysis. Since emulsification is not a factor here, the most likely explanation is that the affinity of colipase (an essential cofactor for pancreatic lipase action) for the emulsion interface is increased. Small amounts of partially ionized long-chain fatty acids apparently increase not only the binding of colipase to the emulsion interface, but also the binding of colipase to lipase (110,111,121). Nevertheless, the ability of lingual lipase to "prime" the substrate for pancreatic lipase may have other explanations. Diglycerides may diffuse preferentially to the emulsion-water interface where they can be hydrolyzed more quickly by pancreatic lipase (123). Further, partially ionized long-chain fatty acids in the duodenal bulb initiate the complex hormonal control of small intestinal digestion (54). In particular, long-chain fatty acids on the surface of triglyceride emulsions are far more potent stimuli than are fatty acids dispersed in liposomes or micelles. These promote the release of cholecystokinin from intestinal endocrine cells into the portal circulation. Cholecystokinin in turn induces gallbladder contraction and bile secretion and is the major stimulus for pancreatic enzyme secretion (54).

Fine Emulsification

At all levels of the upper small intestine, dietary fat is found in a very finely divided state; the particle sizes are generally less than 0.5 μm in diameter and they are extremely stable (42,47). Forceful gastric propulsion through the antral-pyloric regions of the stomach into the upper small intestine produces mechanical energy sufficient for dispersion of stomach emulsions into smaller and smaller particles (138). The corresponding increase in total surface area is of key importance for subsequent digestion (9). While the intestinal emulsifiers responsible have not yet been fully elucidated experimentally, dietary lecithin, partially ionized long-chain fatty acids ("acid soaps"), biliary lipids, and the products of triglyceride hydrolysis all appear to be involved (Fig. 7).

Donnan (37) was aware that partially ionized fatty acids caused a marked decrease in interfacial tension and induced emulsion stability. He also noted that fatty acids were good emulsifiers only when presented in the oil phase with alkali in the water phase. Frazer and associates (42,49) confirmed these findings using physiological systems and observed such rapid and stable emulsification that they termed it

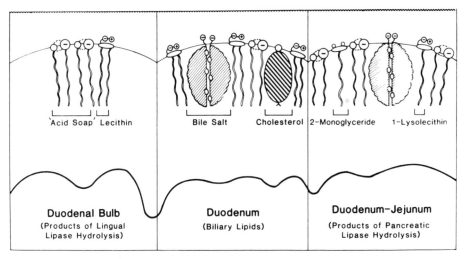

FIG. 7. Possible physiological emulsifiers in the upper small intestine. Hypothetical molecular arrangement at a triglyceride-water interface.

"spontaneous." They found that emulsion stability with oleic acid was maximal at pH 8.5 and became progressively poorer at lower pH. Emulsification occurred only at a typical duodenal pH (6.5) when ionized bile salts and monoglycerides were also present. The superior results in preparing emulsions with long-chain fatty acids dissolved in the oil phase (often called the "nascent soap" in contrast to the "agent in water" method) (55) are explained by the fact that "acid soaps" form immediately at the interface of the fat droplets. In the latter ("agent in water") system, diffusional processes are not as rapid in bringing the emulsifier to the interface. Thus, coalescence of droplets may occur before the emulsifier is distributed homogeneously. Emulsification can never be truly "spontaneous," i.e., without the aid of mechanical energy. Although external agitation may be totally absent, there are *internal* physicochemical processes occurring near the interface that lead to a breakup of the bulk oil phase. In the presence of very low interfacial tensions, these arise from the nonuniform distribution of the amphiphilic molecules at the interface, inducing surface shearing forces, turbulence, and interfacial agitation.

When stomach chyme is propelled through a partially opened pyloric canal into the duodenum (see Fig. 6), the strong shear forces tear the liquid interfaces apart. These forces are analogous to those found in a commercial "colloid mill" (55). The solubilized long-chain fatty acids diffuse from the bulk of the triglyceride droplets, become partially ionized, and, together with lecithin, further stabilize the emulsion particles (Figs. 6 and 7). However, as noted above, fatty acids induce a minimum interfacial tension and maximum emulsion stability only when they are partially ionized to form 1:1 "acid soap" (132). Using hydrocarbons emulsified with laurate, Saleeb and colleagues (132) found that maximum emulsion stability occurred at a bulk pH 8.0. Similarly, the bulk pH at which long-chain fatty acids are 50% ionized is pH 8 to 11 (40,53,112), much higher than the pH prevailing in the upper small intestine. "Acid soaps" are insoluble in water [less soluble than their analogous undissociated fatty acids (69)] and swell in water to form lamellar liquid crystals (liposomes) (28,53). Several important intestinal amphiphiles and ions are known to increase the ionization of the interface, and thereby lower the bulk pH at which long-chain fatty acids form interfacial 1:1 "acid soap" complexes. Principal among these are bile salts (139), lecithin (5), and calcium (7), and perhaps other amphiphiles.

Within the duodenum, peristaltic and segmental contractions continue to supply mechanical energy (shearing/compression forces) to increase the interfacial area of fat droplets and, as a consequence, reduce the size of the particles. For triglyceride emulsification to occur under these low shear forces, emulsifiers which can lower the interfacial tension to very small values must be available. It is important to emphasize that bile salts alone (49,78,127) are extremely poor emulsifiers of dietary fat. However, in dilute combinations with other lipid amphiphiles of bile and triglyceride digestive products, bile salts play important roles in fat emulsification (Fig. 7). Recent work on the phase equilibria and structure of biliary mixed micelles (29,88) and upper intestinal contents after a fatty meal (147) suggests that the biliary micellar phase becomes saturated with lecithin when diluted within the intestinal lumen. Similarly, during established fat digestion the micellar phase is saturated with the products of lipolysis. Figure 7 displays how the emulsion droplets within the upper small intestine could be enveloped with a mono- or even multilayer of biliary lipids or mixed with the products of hydrolysis. Lairon et al. (77) demonstrated that the composition of an adsorbed monomolecular film of porcine biliary lipids around siliconized glass beads was 1:2:3 cholesterol/phospholipid/bile salt molecules; Nalbone et al. (93) found that most biliary phospholipid associated initially with the emulsion phase during fat digestion in the rat. Table 1 surveys the oil-water interfacial tensions generated by a number of potential physiological emulsifiers (8,32,33,49,65,66,71,78).

Pancreatic Lipase-Colipase and Phospholipase A_2 Hydrolysis

Both pancreatic colipase and phospholipase A_2 are secreted in a pro-coenzyme and proenzyme form, respectively, and they require tryptic catalyzed hydrolysis of an Arg-Gly and Arg-Ala bond, respectively, in their N-terminal chains (20,58) to unmask their functions. Pancreatic phospholipase A_2 catalyzes the specific hydrolysis of fatty acids esterified at the sn-2 position of a variety of phosphoglycerides (phosphatidylcholine, phosphatidylethanolamine, phosphatidylglycerol, phosphatidylserine, phosphatidylinositol, cardiolipin); it is without effect on sphingolipids (sphingomyelin, cerebrosides, and gangliosides) (157). This enzyme has an absolute requirement for Ca^{2+} ions which bind in a 1:1 stoichiometry to substrate and enzyme (35), thereby ensuring fixation and stabilization of the enzyme-substrate complex. Aggregation of the substrate appears to ensure the nonequivalent interaction of the sn-2 fatty acid ester with the catalytic site of the enzyme (36). Hydrolytic rates are also dependent on the type of aggregation, which presumably influences the packing

TABLE 1. *Physiological emulsifiers: Interfacial tensions at oil-water interface*

Oil	Emulsifier(s)	T(°C)	pH	[Na⁺]	γ(mN/m)	Reference
Olive oil	None	RT[a]	ns[b]	ns	15–16	Harvey (65)
Castor oil	None	RT	ns	ns	15–16	Harvey (65)
Cottonseed oil	None	37	6.0	0.15 M	18	Dasher (33)
Mackerel oil	None (FA impurities?)[c]	RT	ns	Seawater	7	Danielli and Harvey (32)
Mackerel oil	None (FA impurities?)	RT	6.8	0.15 M	9	Harvey and Shapiro (66)
"Egg Oil"	Crude lecithin + membrane proteins	RT	ns	ns	0.8	Danielli and Harvey (32)
Cyclohexane	Egg lecithin	25	ns	0	2–3	Johnson and Saunders (71)
Benzene	Egg lecithin	25	ns	0	1–2	Johnson and Saunders (71)
Olive oil	Na Taurocholate	RT	ns	0.15 M	5	Linthorst et al. (78)
Cottonseed oil	Na Glycocholate	37	ns	0.15 M	7–9	Dasher (33)
Cottonseed oil	1-Monoolein	37	ns	0.15 M	8–10	Dasher (33)
Cottonseed oil	2-Monopalmitin	37	ns	0.15 M	9	Dasher (33)
Cottonseed oil	1-Monopalmitin	37	ns	0.15 M	9	Dasher (33)
Cyclohexane	Lauric acid-laurate "acid soap"	RT	8.0	0.01 M	8	Saleeb et al. (132)
Vaseline oil	Oleic acid-oleate "acid soap"	25	9.0	0.1 M	6.5	Benzonana and Baret (8)
Cottonseed oil	Oleic acid-oleate "acid soap"	37	8.0	0.15 M	2–3	Dasher (33)
Cottonseed oil	Monoolein + oleic/oleate "acid soap"	37	8.0	0.15 M	1.5	Dasher (33)
Cottonseed oil	Monoolein + oleic/oleate "acid soap" + bile salts	37	8.0	0.15 M	0.5	Dasher (33)
Cottonseed oil	Monoolein + oleic/oleate "acid soap" + bile salts	37	7.0	0.15 M	3.5	Dasher (33)
Cottonseed oil	Monoolein + oleic/oleate "acid soap" + bile salts	37	6.0	0.15 M	0.5–2	Dasher (33)

[a]RT, room temperature.
[b]ns, not stated.
[c]FA, fatty acid.

of the fatty acid chains and head group area (104). For example, lecithin liposomes are hydrolyzed more slowly than lecithin contained in mixed micelles or emulsions (15,104).

Colipase appears to be essential for the hydrolysis of artificial and natural triglyceride emulsions in the presence of micellar concentrations of bile salts (18). Bile salts, like other detergents, appear to induce the interfacial desorption of pancreatic lipase, which is only weakly surface active (17). However, colipase can bind to a bile salt-covered triglyceride-water interface and provide a high affinity "anchor" for lipase attachment. With physiological triglyceride emulsions carrying an envelope of phospholipids and free fatty acids from lingual lipase hydrolysis (19), the interactions of pancreatic lipase, phospholipase A_2, colipase, and bile salts are much more complex, as shown in Figs. 8 and 9. Pancreatic lipase alone (in contrast to lingual lipase) cannot readily hydrolyze triglycerides when covered with phospholipids, nor can it hydrolyze phospholipids (58). Hence, triglycerides in this physical state are hydrolyzed to fatty acids either extremely slowly (Fig. 8A) or not at all (Fig. 8B) (10,15,73,108). The long "latent phase" (Fig. 8) can be counteracted by colipase (Fig. 8B, D) (10,15,108) which penetrates lecithin mono- and bilayers (134). As shown in Fig. 9, colipase can, in turn, bring lipase into juxtaposition with its substrate. The perturbation of the packing of lecithin molecules by colipase (134) may also increase the transfer of bulk triglyceride into the surface mono- or multilayers of lecithin and render the substrate available to hydrolysis by pancreatic lipase. Bile salts enhance the binding of colipase (Fig. 8B, D) by forming

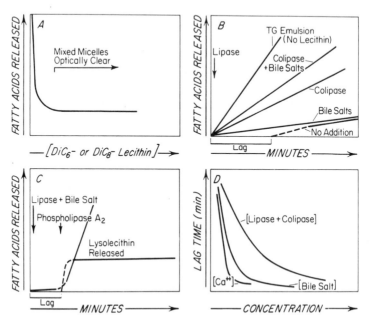

FIG. 8. Factors influencing pancreatic lipase hydrolysis of triglyceride (TG)-lecithin emulsions (see text).

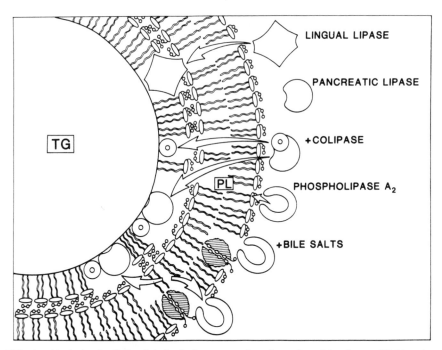

FIG. 9. Lipolysis of milk fat globules in the mammalian stomach and duodenum. Highly schematized representation of the action of lipolytic enzymes on emulsions of triglycerides (TG) coated with a trilayer of phospholipid (PL) molecules. Some triglyceride molecules are solubilized in the surface coat (not shown).

colipase-bile salt aggregates (31), and also enhance the binding of phospholipase A_2 (Fig. 9). Physiologically, phospholipase A_2 hydrolysis of the emulsifier (Fig. 8C) is probably the dominant mechanism for facilitating triglyceride hydrolysis (10,15,108). The exact role of calcium ions (Fig. 8D) and bile salts in promoting this schema (Figs. 8 and 9) has not yet been determined. They may act by promoting enzyme binding through perturbation of the physical state of the lecithin molecules (Fig. 9) (161) or facilitating the desorption of the lipolytic products from the interfaces (11). Cholesterol and proteins may modify the physical structure of the emulsifier even after hydrolysis of the phospholipid, but no studies analogous to those on cell membranes (159) have been carried out. In summary, the available evidence suggests that several intraluminal factors, i.e., pancreatic lipase, colipase, pancreatic phospholipase A_2, and intraduodenal bile salts and calcium, all act synergistically (Fig. 9) in a dilute, slightly acid milieu to promote the rapid hydrolysis of emulsified triglycerides and phospholipids.

Chemical Composition of Substrates and Hydrolytic Products

In the upper small intestine, fat digestion and absorption take place in a remarkably constant physicochemical environment. Between 1 and $1\frac{1}{2}$ hr after a meal, the

mean pH of the upper intestinal contents falls from pH ∼6.8 to ∼5.3 (39,82) (Fig.
10). A comparable pH value is typically found in the lumen of the stomach about
30 min after a meal (Fig. 10). While osmolality of stomach contents generally
reflects that of the diet (>600 mOsm/kg), dilution occurs in the duodenum and
lowers the osmolality to 300–350 mOsm/kg (82). Fasting bile salt levels lie in
the 3 to 7 mM range, but gallbladder emptying causes a rise in total bile salt
concentration to 13–46 mM within 30 min (144). Thereafter, bile salt concentrations decrease to values between 2.5 and 10 mM and remain constant for 1 to 4
hr, i.e., during two to three enterohepatic cycles of the bile salt pool (144). The
triglyceride concentration is also fairly constant, generally ∼10 to 40 mM (15,107),
but the total phospholipid concentration (2,85,116–118) is somewhat more variable
(0.3–5.5 mM). Because of the contribution of biliary lecithin, the molar ratio of
lecithin/triglyceride in duodenal content is about 1:10, in contrast to ∼1:40 in the
diet. Calcium concentrations vary from 5 to 15 mM (85), and sodium and potassium
concentrations are ∼100 and ∼25 mM, respectively. Lipase and colipase concentrations are found in equimolar proportions [1–2 × 10^{-7} M (16)]. This is equivalent
to the release of 150 to 300 μmoles of sn-1 and sn-2 long-chain fatty acids per
minute per milliliter of intestinal fluid (106) (Fig. 11). The corresponding activity
of intestinal phospholipase A_2 is 0.5 to 1.5 μmoles of sn-2 long-chain fatty acids
released per minute per milliliter of intestinal fluid (2) (Fig. 11). Pancreatic lipase
has a high turnover number (250,000 to 500,000 long-chain triglyceride molecules
per minute) so that its activity in intestinal contents is 100- to 1,000-fold in excess

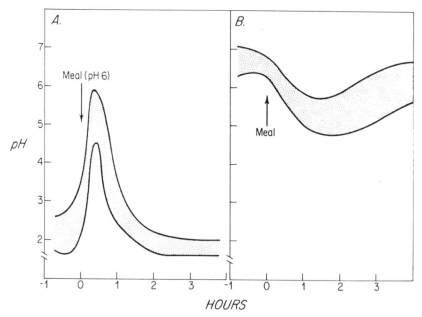

FIG. 10. Variations in **(A)** gastric and **(B)** duodenal pH of man as functions of time after both
solid and liquid meals. (From Malagelada et al., ref. 82, with permission.)

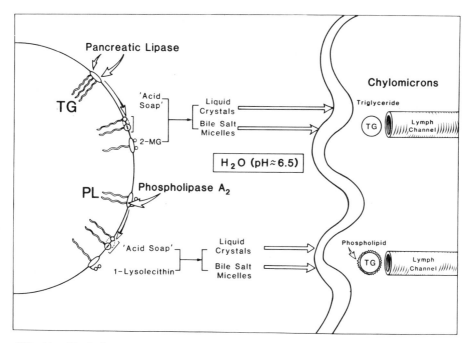

FIG. 11. Physical state and fate of long-chain fatty acids in the duodenum-jejunum. Note that the products of pancreatic lipase and phospholipase A_2 hydrolysis are mixed in the same mixed micelles and liquid crystals. TG, triglycerides; MG, monoglycerides; PL, phospholipids.

of that required for complete intraduodenal hydrolysis of dietary triglycerides. In contrast, phospholipase A_2 hydrolysis of dietary and endogenous phospholipids is slower and continues in the jejunum and even in the ileum (2).

PHYSICOCHEMICAL STATE OF AQUEOUS LIPIDS DURING FAT DIGESTION

The work of Hofmann and Borgström (67,68) and a large number of subsequent studies (4,75,85,90–92,116–118,122,124,125,136,137,158) showed that the lipids in postprandial intestinal content constituted a two-phase system composed of oil and an aqueous micellar phase. Attempts to isolate the micellar phase from human intestinal contents have relied on either prolonged ultracentrifugation (4,67,68,75,90–92,117,118,122,124,125,136,137,158) or mild centrifugation followed by multiple ultrafiltrations (85,116). In the former method, the aspirated intestinal contents were heated to 70°C for 10 min to inactivate pancreatic lipase. With the multiple ultrafiltration technique, no attempt was made to inactivate pancreatic lipase before filtration. All of these manipulations induce artifacts which influence subsequent physicochemical observations. For example, heat treatment, filtration, and centrifugation are commonly employed to achieve demulsification (55). In addition, heating, by stimulating lipase and phospholipase A_2 activities, markedly increases fatty acid production and also alters phospholipid composition (116). Further, phase disequilibrium is induced and phase boundaries are altered (29). Several investigators (85,116,153) have suggested that the Hofmann-Borgström hypothesis is an oversimplification. Ultracentrifugation produces a marked bile salt-fatty acid gradient in the aqueous portion of distal duodenal fluid; even with prolonged contrifugation, only a small portion of intestinal content becomes clear (116). Other authors have noted that an insoluble pellet phase is produced (153) and that ultrafiltration generally results in an opalescent, rather than a clear, filtrate (85,116).

Patton and Carey (107) examined fat digestion by light microscopy *in vitro* and, with stomach emulsions of purified olive oil, observed the sequential appearance of a number of visible product phases (Fig. 12). The remaining oil was largely triglyceride and diglyceride; the birefringent phase was an insoluble calcium soap; and the fatty acids and monoglycerides formed a nonbirefringent "viscous isotropic" phase. In an attempt to reconcile these findings with the Hoffman-Borgström hypothesis, Stafford and Carey (147,148) defined the phase equilibria of model systems of the aqueous intestinal lipids (Fig. 13) and also elucidated the compositions of the aqueous phases of postprandial distal-duodenal content after chemical inhibition of pancreatic lipase activity. After low-speed centrifugation, the total aspirates separated into an oily emulsion "phase" and a cloudy aqueous "phase." Upon

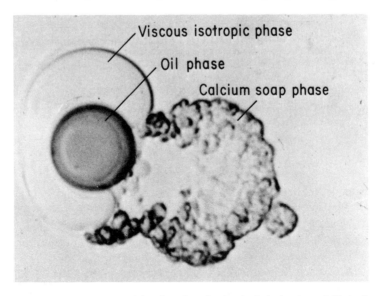

FIG. 12. The light microscopy of fat digestion. *In vitro* hydrolysis of emulsified olive oil by pancreatic lipase-colipase in the presence of physiological concentrations of calcium, bile salts, H+ concentration, and enzyme-coenzyme. (From Patton and Carey, ref. 107, with permission.)

FIG. 13. Phase relations of gallbladder bile and aqueous intestinal lipids during fat digestion in the duodenum. Mixed micelles are small in the gallbladder, but become markedly enlarged and coexist with a liquid crystalline phase during established fat digestion. The relative lipid composition of each phase is indicated *(small arrows and open circles)*. An emulsion particle with a monomolecular layer of emulsifier is shown (upper right).

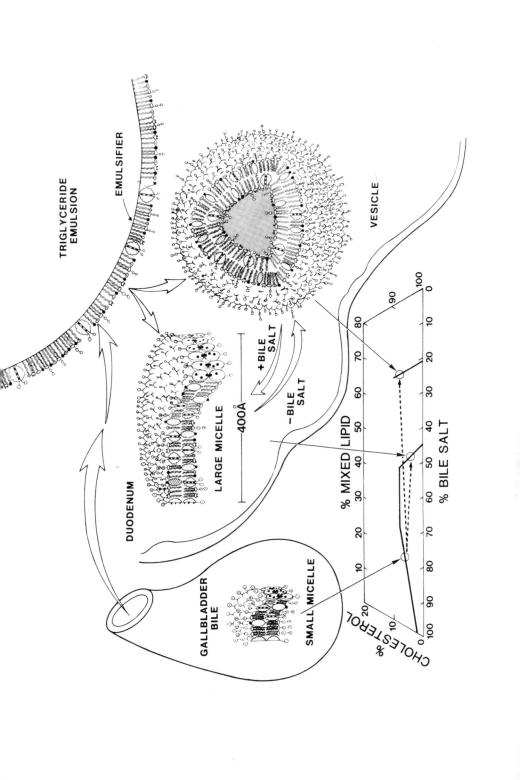

ultracentrifugation of the cloudy aqueous "phase", a bile salt micellar phase, saturated with the products of lipolysis, *and* a liquid-crystalline phase, saturated with bile salts, were obtained (Fig. 13).

Emulsion Particles

The chemical composition and physical properties of emulsion particles from human intestinal contents can be inferred from three studies (68,90,124). Hofmann and Borgström (68) fed 22.3 g of corn oil in a formula meal to adults and separated the *duodenal* oil particles by ultracentrifugation for 18 hr. Ricour and Rey (124) separated the *jejunal* oil particles in a similar manner in children, whereas Miettinen and Siurala (90) gave 176 g of olive oil intragastrically to adults and also separated the *jejunal* oil particles by ultracentrifugation. A phase diagram can be constructed by plotting free cholesterol, fatty acids plus monoglycerides and phospholipids, and higher glycerides plus cholesterol esters as single components (Fig. 14). It is apparent that free cholesterol is a minor component of the emulsion particles, and that in all three studies, the particles are highly enriched in emulsifiers (fatty acids, monoglycerides, and phospholipids). A simple calculation shows that this is greatly in excess of what would be needed to coat emulsion particles of ~0.5 μm. The most likely possibilities are that the oil particles are contaminated with "acid soap"-monoglyceride liquid crystals; the emulsion particles are much smaller than assumed, i.e., in the size range of "micro-emulsions," or the oil droplets are covered with multilayers of emulsifying amphiphiles.

Micellar Solubilization of Lipids

Since studies (see Fig. 13) suggest that liquid crystalline vesicles and micelles coexist during human fat digestion, the aqueous phase analyses in earlier studies probably represent a mixture of both particles. Since earlier analyses (4,67,68, 75,85,90–92,116–118,122,124,125,136,137,153,158) showed that the molar ratio

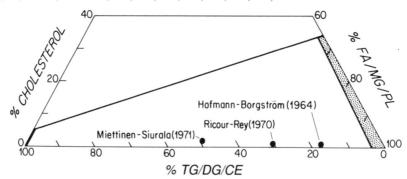

FIG. 14. Relative lipid compositions of the "oil" phase in human duodenal-jejunal content after a fat-containing meal. Fatty acids (FA) plus monoglycerides (MG) and phospholipids (PL), tri- and diglycerides (TG, DG) plus cholesteryl ester (CE) and free cholesterol are shown as separate components (68,90,124).

of fatty acids to monoglycerides in the aqueous phase invariably exceeds 2:1, being usually in the range of 5:1 to 20:1, phase equilibria studies of Stafford et al. (147) were carried out with fatty acid/monoglyceride/diglyceride/lecithin ratios of 5:2:0.2:1 or 5:1:0.2:1 or 20:1:0.2:1 to encompass this physiological variable. The phase boundaries (Fig. 13) varied with pH (range 4.5–7.5), temperature (4°–70°C), total lipid concentration (0.25–5 g/dl), and fatty acid/monoglyceride ratio (2.5:1 to 20:1). Using laser light scattering, the hydrodynamic radii of the micelles in the micellar phase were found to vary from ~30Å for conjugated bile salts alone to ~200Å at the mixed lipid/bile salt phase boundary. Similarly sized particles (~200Å) were found in separated aspirates of the human postprandial duodenum whose relative composition corresponds to the micellar phase boundary (Fig. 13). The most probable structure of the mixed micelles is shown in Fig. 13. These are similar in structure to, but much larger than, the "mixed disc" bile salt-lecithin micelles in bile (88).

Mesophase Dispersion of Lipids

Although Patton and Carey (107) and two groups of investigators in the past (85,116) have alluded to the possibility, Stafford et al. (147,148) have directly verified that a portion of the aqueous lipids of the postprandial intestine is dispersed as liquid crystalline liposomes (nonmicellar particles). It has been estimated from model systems that these particles have hydrodynamic radii of 400 to 600 Å. These liposomes appear to be mainly unilamellar; and their probable structure is shown in Fig. 13.

This discovery has important pathophysiological relevance: It is well known that fat malabsorption may be minimal in many patients with low intraluminal bile salt concentrations (86). In patients with biliary fistulas, triglycerides are hydrolyzed normally. The resulting free fatty acids are poorly solubilized in a "clear" aqueous phase (< 0.05 mM), yet fat absorption occurs efficiently in the upper small intestine as visualized by electron microscopy of intestinal biopsies (117). Phase analyses of the relative compositions of the *total* aqueous phase lipids from such subjects (86,91) suggest that free fatty acids and monoglycerides are present as a liquid crystalline phase whose relative lipid compositions fall on or close to the right-hand phase boundary in Fig. 13. It is to be noted that previous investigators (86,91) interpreted their findings to imply a "defective transfer of hydrolysed dietary fat products to the micellar phase." In contrast to patients with pancreatic insufficiency (140), where the intraluminal concentration of solubilized free fatty acid can be 50-fold greater, the high index of the fat absorption in bile-salt deficient patients highlights the physiological importance of liposomal particles.

Interrelationships Between Dispersed Lipid Particles

A possible dynamic scheme for digestion and absorption in the upper small intestine is as follows. On dilution of the total lipid concentration in the intestine, biliary mixed micelles from the gallbladder enlarge dramatically as a result of the altered micelle-monomer equilibrium (88). A portion of these lipids then adsorb to the surface of the emulsions en masse or via a monomer phase (77,93). The emulsion particles become reduced in size and are stabilized. Upon pancreatic lipase-colipase and phospholipase A_2 hydrolysis of the surface lipids the mass of products formed, plus part of the emulsion coat, pinch off as unilamellar liposomal vesicles and large micelles. The process is continuously repeated with adsorption of reserve biliary lipids from the bulk, interfacial hydrolysis and desorption. Lipid exchange may progressively enrich both micellar and liposomal particles with hydrolytic products. Other mechanisms may induce the transformation of enlarged mixed micelles into liposomes, and vice versa (88). For example, diffusion barriers provided by unstirred water layers and mucin gels may result in the transformation of mixed micelles into vesicles, or vesicles into mixed micelles. This is likely to occur near the absorptive membranes where the interparticle bile salt concentration may be higher or lower than in bulk water.

ABSORPTION AND FATE OF LIPOLYTIC PRODUCTS WITHIN MUCOSAL CELLS

It is not known how the dispersed lipid molecules in the intestinal lumen gain entrance into the absorptive enterocytes (154). It is generally agreed that this is a wholly passive and extremely efficient process. It could occur via a hydrocarbon continuum (106), micelle-membrane fusion, liposome-membrane fusion, or the monomers in the intermicellar/intervesicular aqueous phase. Whatever the mechanism, a large number of perplexing physiological interrelationships require explanation. These include the obligatory requirement of bile salts for cholesterol absorption (143), the differential uptake of sterols with slight structural differences (154), the marked inhibition of cholesterol and fatty acid absorption by unhydrolyzed phospholipid (119,120), the decrease in cholesterol uptake with progressive unsaturation of the micellar phase (152,154), and the absorption of hydrocarbons coincident with dietary triglyceride digestion and absorption (106). Further, it now appears that some phospholipids and perhaps sphingolipids need not be hydrolyzed completely prior to their absorption (12,13,141). Sphingolipids are resistant to pancreatic phospholipase A_2 hydrolysis and may be hydrolyzed on the brush border or absorbed intact to be degraded within the enterocyte (96–98). It has also been suggested that small amounts of unsplit di- and triglycerides may be absorbed (44).

Triglyceride Resynthesis and Chylomicron Formation

Short- and medium-chain fatty acids (57), and perhaps a portion of polyunsaturated long-chain fatty acids (150), diffuse through enterocytes without metabolism (120) and enter tributaries of the portal vein (Fig. 15). Most long-chain fatty acids and their monoglycerides are processed within the enterocyte in a specific manner (Fig. 15). Possibly at the inner monolayer of the apical membranes, long-chain fatty acids are bound to a low molecular weight protein (MW ~ 12,000), called "fatty acid binding protein" or Z-protein (101,102). This protein apparently prevents

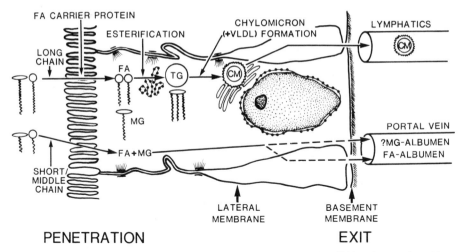

FA CARRIER PROTEIN
ESTERIFICATION
LONG CHAIN
FA
TG
CHYLOMICRON (+VLDL) FORMATION
CM
LYMPHATICS
CM
MG
PORTAL VEIN
FA+MG
?MG-ALBUMEN
FA-ALBUMEN
SHORT/ MIDDLE CHAIN
LATERAL MEMBRANE
BASEMENT MEMBRANE
PENETRATION
EXIT

FIG. 15. Fate of absorbed long- and short/medium- chain fatty acids (FA) and monoglycerides (MG) within intestinal absorptive cells. CM, chylomicron; VLDL, very low-density lipoprotein.

the intracellular accumulation of unbound fatty acids, facilitates the desorption of fatty acids from the inner part of the plasma membrane, and may be a carrier protein for transport to the endoplasmic reticulum. Triglycerides are resynthesized in the endoplasmic reticulum (70,100) by specific pathways which involve coenzyme A activation of the fatty acids, followed by esterification of the fatty acids to 2-monoglyceride. If the acyl receptor is in short supply, a scavenger pathway generates glycerol from glucose metabolism with the subsequent formation of phosphatidic acid and diglyceride, which is then acylated to form triglyceride. The newly formed "fat" mixes with resynthesized cholesteryl ester and receives an emulsifying coat of phospholipid (mainly lecithin), unesterified cholesterol, and several apolipoproteins, apo B (which is distinct from hepatic apo B) (165), apo A-I, A-IV, and small amounts of Apo A-II (56). The composition of these nascent "chylomicrons" is (by weight) triglyceride 86 to 92%, cholesteryl ester 0.8 to 1.4%, free cholesterol 0.6 to 1.6%, phospholipid 6 to 8%, and apolipoprotein 1 to 1.5%. The particles are heterogenous in size, ranging from 750 to 6,000Å with a mean diameter of ~1200Å. Their size is dependent upon many factors, including the rate of lipid absorption, the site of intestinal absorption, and the availability of surface constituents (56). Chylomicrons exit the intestinal cells via the basilateral membrane to enter lymphatic channels and thereby reach the systemic circulation (131). Their subsequent physicochemical and metabolic fate is beyond the scope of this chapter.

Fate of Dietary and Biliary Lysolecithin

In the endoplasmic reticulum of the absorptive cells, absorbed lysolecithin is both deacylated by tissue lysophospholipases, and resynthesized into triglyceride and lecithin molecules. The function of the intracellular lecithin pool is to coat the oily core of chylomicrons as a monomolecular layer. Accordingly, chylomicron phospholipids are mainly lecithin (70–100%) with smaller amounts of sphingo-myelin and phosphatidylethanolamine. Although the fatty acids of chylomicron triglycerides reflect the fatty acid composition of ingested triglycerides (72), the fatty acids of the chylomicron phospholipids differ from those present in the diet and remain relatively constant despite large variations in dietary fatty acid composition (163). Evidence from a number of studies (83,84,95,103,155,156) suggests that biliary lecithin (as lysolecithin) may be preferentially incorporated into the surface coat of chylomicra. After absorbed lysolecithin (from bile lecithin) is dea-cylated intracellularly to a fatty acid and glycerophosphorylcholine, most of the released fatty acids enter chylomicron triglycerides (6,46); the remainder enter phospholipids for the surface coat (84,163). This occurs after acyl exchange, since 80% of biliary lecithin has palmitic acid in the 1-position, whereas up to 40% of chylomicron lecithin has stearic acid in the 1-position (142). In the absence of biliary lecithin, the contribution of dietary lecithin to chylomicron synthesis increases in proportion to the dietary supply (84). When luminal lecithin is totally unavailable, circulatory lecithins are utilized to maintain the phospholipid composition of chylomicra and very low-density lipoprotein (VLDL) (84,95,103,155,156). *De novo* synthesized intestinal lecithins do not appear to be a major source of intestinal chylomicron phospholipid; however, their role in the formation of intestinal high-density lipoprotein (HDL) remains to be elucidated (56).

CONCLUSIONS

Dietary and biliary lecithin, and perhaps other phospholipids, play pivotal roles in: the emulsification of dietary triglycerides; the hydrolysis of triglycerides by lingual and pancreatic lipases; the formation of intestinal mixed micelles and li-posomal vesicles; and the assembly of chylomicra and other lipoproteins within absorptive cells. The manipulation of exogenous, and perhaps endogenous, lecithin by dietary and pharmacological means may influence lipid absorption, metabolism and disposition.

ACKNOWLEDGMENTS

This work was supported by National Institutes of Health (U.S. Public Health Service) Research Grant AM 18559 and Research Career Development Award AM 00195. Figures 3 and 4 are reproduced with permission of Cambridge University Press and Figure 12 is reproduced with permission of the American Association for the Advancement of Science.

REFERENCES

1. Albert, A., and Sergeant, E. P. (1971): *The Determination of Ionization Constants*, p. 84. Chapman & Hall, London, 2nd ed.
2. Arnesjö, B., Nilsson, A., Barrowman, J., and Borgström, B. (1969): Intestinal digestion and absorption of cholesterol and lecithin in the human. *Scand. J. Gastroenterol.*, 4:653–665.
3. Aw, T. Y., and Grigor, M. R. (1980): Digestion and absorption of milk triacylglycerols in 14-day-old suckling rats. *J. Nutr.*, 110:2133–2140.

4. Badley, B. W. D., Murphy, G. M., Bouchier, I. A. D., and Sherlock, S. (1970): Diminished micellar phase lipid in patients with chronic non-alcoholic liver disease and steatorrhea. *Gastroenterology*, 58:781–789.
5. Barton, P. G., and Jevons, S. (1970): Interactions of phosphatides with some paraffin-chain salts. *Chem. Phys. Lipids*, 4:289–310.
6. Beil, F. U., and Grundy, S. M. (1980): Studies on plasma lipoproteins during absorption of exogenous lecithin in man. *J. Lipid Res.*, 21:525–536.
7. Benzonana, G. (1968): Sür le rôle des ions calcium durant l'hydrolyze des triglycerides insolubles par le lipase pancréatique en presence de sels biliaires. *Biochim. Biophys. Acta.*, 151:137–146.
8. Benzonana, G., and Baret, J. F. (1968): Interactions between bile acids and fatty acids. Behavior of mixed solutions at air-water and oil-water interfaces. In: *Chemistry, Physics and Practical Application of Surface Active Substances*, Vol. 2, edited by P. Desnuelle, pp. 595–603. Ediciones Unidas, Barcelona.
9. Benzonana, G., and Desnuelle, P. (1965): Etude cinétique de l'action de la lipase pancréatique sur des triglycerides en emulsion. Essai d'une emzymologie en milieu hétérogène. *Biochim. Biophys. Acta.*, 115:121–136.
10. Bläckberg, L., Hernell, O., and Olivecrona, T. (1981): Hydrolysis of human milk fat globules by pancreatic lipase. *J. Clin. Invest.*, 67:1748–1752.
11. Bläckberg, L., Hernell, O., Bengtsson, G., and Olivecrona, T. (1979): Colipase enhances hydrolysis in the absence of bile salts. *J. Clin. Invest.*, 64:1303–1308.
12. Blomstrand, R. (1955): The intestinal absorption of phospholipids in the rat. *Acta Physiol. Scand.*, 34:147–157.
13. Bloom, B., Kiyasu, J. Y., Reinhardt, W. O., and Chaikoff, I. L. (1954): Absorption of phospholipids: Manner of transport from intestinal lumen to lacteals. *Am. J. Physiol.*, 177:84–86.
14. Borgström, B. (1976): Phospholipid absorption. In: *Lipid Absorption: Biochemical and Clinical Aspects*, edited by K. Rommel, H. Goebell, and R. Böhmer, pp. 65–70. MTP Press, Lancaster, England.
15. Borgström, B. (1980): Importance of phospholipids, pancreatic phospholipase A_2 and fatty acid for the digestion of dietary fat. *Gastroenterology*, 78:954–962.
16. Borgström, B., and Hildebrand, H. (1975): Lipase and colipase activity of human small intestinal contents after a liquid test meal. *Scand. J. Gastroenterol.*, 10:585–591.
17. Borgström, B., and Erlanson, C. (1978): Interaction of serum albumin and other proteins with porcine pancreatic lipase. *Gastroenterology*, 75:382–386.
18. Borgström, B., Erlanson-Albertsson, C., and Wieloch, T. (1979): Pancreatic colipase: Chemistry and physiology. *J. Lipid Res.*, 20:805–816.
19. Borgström, B., Lundh, G., Dahlquist, A., and Sjövall, J. (1957): Studies of intestinal digestion and absorption in the human. *J. Clin. Invest.*, 36:1521–1536.
20. Borgström, B., Weiloch, T., and Erlanson-Albertsson, C. (1979): Evidence for a pancreatic procolipase and its activation by trypsin. *FEBS Lett.*, 108:407–410.
21. Brockerhoff, H., and Jensen, R. G. (1976): *Lipolytic Enzymes*. Academic Press, New York.
22. Brown, M. F., and Seelig, J. (1978): Influence of cholesterol on the polar regions of phosphatidylcholine and phosphatidylethanolamine bilayers. *Biochemistry*, 17:381–384.
23. Buldt, G., Gally, H. U., Seelig, J., and Zaccai, G. (1979): Neutron diffraction studies on phosphatidylcholine model membranes. I. Head group conformation. *J. Mol. Biol.*, 134:673–691.
24. Burns, R. A., Jr., and Roberts, M. F. (1981): Physical characterization and lipase susceptibility of short chain lecithin/triglyceride mixed micelles. *J. Biol. Chem.*, 256:2716–2722.
25. Cadenhead, D. A., Demchak, R. J., and Phillips, M. C. (1967): Monolayer characteristics of 1,2-dimyristin, 1-2-dimyristoyl-3-cephalin and 1,2-dimyristoyl-3-lecithin at the air-water interface. *Kolloid Z.Z. Polym.*, 220:59–64.
26. Callahan, P. T. (1979): The use of ^{13}C spin relaxation to investigate molecular motion in liquid tristearin. *Chem. Phys. Lipids*,19:56–73.
27. Carey, M. C. (1982): The enterohepatic circulation. In: *The Liver: Biology and Pathobiology*, edited by I. M. Arias, H. Popper, D. Schachter, and D. Shafritz, pp. 429–465. Raven Press, New York.
28. Carey, M. C., and Small, D. M. (1970): The characteristics of mixed micellar solutions with particular reference to bile. *Am. J. Med.*, 49:590–608.
29. Carey, M. C., and Small, D. M. (1978): Physical chemistry of cholesterol solubility in bile: Relationship to gallstone formation and dissolution in man. *J. Clin. Invest.*, 61:998–1026.

30. Carlson, H. C., Code, C. F., and Nelson, R. A. (1966): Motor action of the canine gastroduodenal junction; a cineradiographic, pressure and electrical study. *Am. J. Dig. Dis.*, 11:155–172.
31. Cozzone, P. J., Canioni, P., Sarda, L., and Kaptein, R. (1981): 360-MHz Nuclear magnetic resonance and laser photochemically induced dynamic nuclear polarization studies of bile salt interaction with porcine colipase A. *Eur. J. Biochem.*, 114:119–126.
32. Danielli, J. F., and Harvey, E. N. (1935): The tension at the surface of mackerel egg oil, with remarks on the nature of the cell surface. *J. Cell. Comp. Physiol.*, 5:483–496.
33. Dasher, G. F. (1952): Surface activity of naturally occurring emulsifiers. *Science (Wash. DC)*, 116:660–663.
34. Davenport, H. W. (1971): *Physiology of the Digestive Tract*, p. 147. Year Book Medical Publishers, Chicago.
35. Deenan, L. L. M. van, and deHaas, G. H. (1964): The synthesis of phosphoglycerides and some biochemical applications. *Adv. Lipid Res.*, 2:167–234.
36. Dijkska, B. W., Drenth, J., and Kalk, K. H. (1981): Active site and catalytic mechanism of phospholipase A_2. *Nature (Lond.)*, 289:604–606.
37. Donnan, F. G. (1899): Uber die Natur der Seifenemulsionen. *Z. Phys. Chem.*, 31:42–49.
38. Dorset, D. L., Pangborn, W. A., Hancock, A. J., Van Soest, T. C., and Greenwald, S. M. (1978): Glycerol conformation and the crystal structure of lipids. *Z. Naturforsch.*, 33:50–55.
39. Dutta, S. K., Russell, R. M., and Iber, F. L. (1979): Influence of exocrine pancreatic insufficiency on the intraluminal pH of the proximal small intestine. *Dig. Dis. Sci.*, 24:529–534.
40. Eagland, D., and Franks, F. (1965): Association equilibria in dilute aqueous solutions of carboxylic acid soaps. *Trans. Faraday Soc.*, 61:2468–2477.
41. Edwards-Webb, J. D., and Thompson, S. Y. (1977): Studies on lipid digestion in the preruminant calf. 2. A comparison of the products of lipolysis of milk fat by salivary and pancreatic lipases *in vitro*. *Br. J. Nutr.*, 34:431–440.
42. Elkes, J. J., Frazer, A. C., Shulman, J. H., and Stewart, H. C. (1944): The mechanism of emulsification of triglyceride in the small intestine. *Proc. Physiol. Soc.*, 103:318(Abstr).
43. Ernst, J., Sheldrick, W. S., and Fuhhop, J. H. (1979): The structures of the essential unsaturated fatty acids. Crystal structures of linolenic acid and evidence for the crystal structures of α-linolenic acid and arachidonic acid. *Z. Naturforsch.*, 34b:706–711.
44. Feldman, E. B., and Borgström, B. (1966): Absorption of di- and triglycerides by intestinal slices in vitro. *Lipids*, 1:128–131.
45. Fernando-Warnakulasuriya, G. J. P., Staggers, J. E., Frost, S. C., and Wells, M. A. (1981): Studies on fat digestion, absorption and transport in the suckling rat. I. Fatty acid composition and concentrations of major lipid components. *J. Lipid Res.*, 22:668–674.
46. Fox, J. M., Betzing, H., and Lekim, D. (1979): Pharmacokinetics or orally ingested phosphatidylcholine. In: *Nutrition and the Brain*, Vol. 5, edited by A. Barbeau, J. H. Growdon, and R. J. Wurtman, pp. 95–108. Raven Press, New York.
47. Frazer, A. C. (1946): The absorption of triglyceride fat from the intestine. *Physiol. Rev.*, 26:103–119.
48. Franks, N. P. (1976): Structural analysis of hydrated egg lecithin and cholesterol bilayers. I. X-ray diffraction. *J. Mol. Biol.*, 100:359–375.
49. Frazer, A. C., Schulman, J. H., and Stewart, H. C. (1964): Emulsification of fat in the intestine of the rat and its relationship to absorption. *J. Physiol. (Lond.)*, 103:306–316.
50. Frede, E. Von, and Precht, D. (1977): Mokekülanordnungen in Fetten mit trikliner Kristallstruktur. *Fette Seifen Anstrichm.*, 79:69–75.
51. Friberg, S., Gezelius, L-H., and Wilton, I. (1971): Influence of acid-soap interactions on the solubility of soaps in triglycerides. *Chem. Phys. Lipids*, 6:364–372.
52. Funasaki, N., Hada, S., and Suzuki, K. (1976): The dissolution state of a triglyceride molecule in water and its orientation state at the air-water interface. *Chem. Pharm. Bull. (Tokyo)*, 24:731–735.
53. Gebicki, J. M., and Hicks, M. (1976): Preparation and properties of vesicles enclosed by fatty acid membranes. *Chem. Phys. Lipids*, 16:142–160.
54. Go, V. L. M. (1973): Coordination of the digestive sequence. *Mayo Clin. Proc.*, 48:613–616.
55. Gopal, E. S. R. (1968): Principles of emulsion formation. In: *Emulsion Science*, edited by P. Sherman, pp. 2–75. Academic Press, New York.
56. Green, P. H. R., and Glickman, R. M. (1981): Intestinal lipoprotein metabolism. *J. Lipid Res.*, 22:1153–1173.

57. Greenberger, N. J., Rogers, J. B., and Isselbacher, K. J. (1966): Absorption of medium and long chain triglycerides: Factors influencing their hydrolysis and transport. *J. Clin. Invest.*, 45:217–227.
58. Haas, G. H. de, Postema, N. M., Nieuwenhuizen, W., and Deenen, L. L. M. van (1968): Purification and propeties of an anionic zymogen of pholpholipase A from porcine pancreas. *Biochim. Biophys. Acta.*, 159:118–129.
59. Hamosh, M. (1978): Rat lingual lipase. Factors affecting enzyme activity and secretion. *Am. J. Physiol.*, 235:E416–E421.
60. Hamosh, M. (1979): A Review. Fat digestion in the newborn: Role of lingual lipase and preduodenal digestion. *Pediatr. Res.*, 13:615–622.
61. Hamosh, M., and Burns, W. A. (1977): Lipolytic activity of human lingual glands (Ebner). *Lab. Invest.*, 37:603–608.
62. Hamosh, M., and Scow, R. O. (1973): Lingual lipase and its role in the digestion of dietary lipid. *J. Clin. Invest.*, 52:88–95.
63. Hamosh, M., Ganot, D., and Hamosh, P. (1979): Rat lingual lipase: Characteristics of enzyme activity. *J. Biol. Chem.*, 254:12121–12125.
64. Hamosh, M., Klaeneman, H. L., Wolf, R. O., and Scow, R. O. (1975): Pharyngeal lipase and digestion of dietary triglyceride in man. *J. Clin. Invest.*, 55:908–913.
65. Harvey, E. N. (1954): Tension at the cell surface. *Protoplasmatologia 2*, E5:1–30.
66. Harvey, E. N., and Shapiro, H. (1934): The interfacial tension between oil and protoplasm within the living cells. *J. Cell. Comp. Physiol.*, 5:255–267.
67. Hofmann, A. F., and Borgström, B. (1962): Physical-chemical state of lipids in intestinal content during their digestion and absorption. *Fed. Proc.*, 21:43–50.
68. Hofmann, A. F., and Borgström, B. (1964): The intraluminal phase of fat digestion in man: The lipid content of the micellar and oil phases of intestinal content obtained during fat digestion and absorption. *J. Clin. Invest.*, 43:247–257.
69. Hofmann, A. F., and Mekhjian, H. S. (1973): Bile acids and the intestinal absorption of fat and electrolytes in health and disease. In: *The Bile Acids*, Vol. 2, edited by P. P. Nair and D. Kritchevsky, pp. 103–152. Plenum, New York.
70. Johnson, J. M. (1978): Triglyceride biosynthesis in the intestinal mucosa. In: *Lipid Absorption: Biochemical and Clinical Aspects*, edited by K. Rommel, M. Goebell, and R. Bohmer, pp. 85–98. MTP Press, Lancester, England.
71. Johnson, M. C. R., and Saunders, L. (1973): Time dependent interfacial tensions of a series of phospholipids. *Chem. Phys. Lipids*, 10:318–327.
72. Kayden, H. J., Karmen, A., and Dumont, A. (1963): Alterations in the fatty acid composition of human lymph and serum lipoprotein by single feedings. *J. Clin. Invest.*, 42:1373–1381.
73. Klein, E., Lyman, R. B., Petersen, L., and Berger, R. I. (1967): The effect of lecithin on the activity of pancreatic lipase. *Life Sci.*, 6:1305–1307.
74. Kosikowski, F. (1977): *Cheese and Fermented Milk Foods*, pp. 213–227. Edwards, Ann Arbor, 2nd ed.
75. Krone, C. L., Theodor, E., Sleisenger, M. H., and Jeffries, G. H. (1968): Studies on the pathogenesis of malabsorption: Lipid hydrolysis and micelle formation in the intestinal lumen. *Medicine (Baltimore)*, 47:89–106.
76. Lachampt, F., and Perron, R. (1953): *Savons et Products Similaires. Extract du trâite de Chimie orgánique*, Vol. 22, edited by V. Grignard, C. Dupont, and R. Locquin. Masson et Cie, Paris.
77. Lairon, D., Nalbone, G., Lafont, H., Leonardi, J., Domingo, N., Hauton, J. C., and Verger, R. (1978): Possible roles of bile lipids and colipase in lipase adsorption. *Biochemistry*, 17:5263–5269.
78. Linthorst, J. M., Bennett-Clark, S., and Holt, P. R. (1977): Triglyceride emulsification by amphipaths present in the intestinal lumen during digestion of fat. *J. Colloid Interface Sci.*, 60:1–10.
79. Lis, L. J., Parsegian, V. A., and Rand, R. P. (1981): Detection of the binding of divalent cations to dipalmitoyl phosphatidylcholine bilayers by its effect on bilayer interaction. *Biochemistry*, 25:1761–1770.
80. Lis, L. J., Lis, W. T., Parsegian, V. A., and Rand, R. P. (1981): Adsorption of divalent cations to a variety of phosphatidylcholine bilayers. *Biochemistry*, 20:1771–1777.
81. Lucassen, J. (1966): Hydrolysis and precipitates in carboxylate soap solutions. *J. Phys. Chem.*, 70:1824–1830.

82. Malagelada, J-R., Go, V. L. W., and Summerskill, W. H. J. (1979): Different gastric, pancreatic and biliary responses to solid, liquid or homogenized meals. *Dig. Dis. Sci.*, 24:101–110.
83. Mansbach, C. M. (1963): Complex lipid synthesis in hamster intestine. *Biochim. Biophys. Acta*, 296:386–400.
84. Mansbach, C. M. (1977): The origin of chylomicron phosphatidycholine in the rat. *J. Clin. Invest.*, 60:411–420.
85. Mansbach, C. M., Cohen, R. S., and Leff, P. B. (1975): Isolation and properties of the mixed lipid micelles present in intestinal content during fat digestion in man. *J. Clin. Invest.*, 56:781–791.
86. Mansbach, C. M., Newton, D., and Stevens, R. D. (1980): Fat digestion in patients with bile acid malabsorption but minimal steatorrhea. *Dig. Dis. Sci.*, 25:353–362.
87. McBain, J. W., and Stewart, A. (1927): Acid soaps: A crystalline potassium hydrogen dioleate. *J. Chem. Soc.*, 130:1392–1395.
88. Mazer, N. A., Benedek, G. B., and Carey, M. C. (1980): Quasielastic light scattering studies of aqueous biliary lipid systems: Mixed micelle formation in bile salt-lecithin solutions. *Biochemistry*, 19:601–615.
89. Meyer, J. H., Stevenson, E. A., and Watts, H. D. (1976): The potential role of proteins in the absorption of fat. *Gastroenterology*, 70:232–239.
90. Miettinen, T. A., and Siurala, M. (1971): Bile salts, sterols, sterol esters, glycerides and fatty acids in micellar and oil phases of intestinal contents during fat digestion in man. *Z. Klin. Chem. Klin. Biochem.*, 9:47–52.
91. Miettinen, T. A., and Siurala, M. (1971): Micellar solubilization of intestinal lipids and sterols in gluten enteropathy and liver cirrhosis. *Scand. J. Gastroenterol.*, 6:527–535.
92. Modai, M., Theodor, E. (1970): Intestinal contents in patients with viral hepatitis after a lipid meal. *Gastroenterology*, 58:379–387.
93. Nalbone, G., Lairon, D., Lafont, H., Domingo, N., and Hauton, J. C. (1974): Behavior of biliary phospholipids in intestinal lumen during fat digestion in rat. *Lipids*, 9:765–770.
94. Nelson, J. H., Jensen, R. G., and Pitas, R. E. (1976): Pregastric esterase and other oral lipases— A review. *J. Dairy Sci.*, 60:327–362.
95. Ng, P. Y., Bennett-Clark, S., and Holt, P. R. (1977): Intestinal phospholipid absorption and utilization for chylomicron formation in the rat. *Gastroenterology*, 72:A85.
96. Nilsson, A. (1968): Metabolism of sphingomyelin in the intestinal tract of the rat. *Biochim. Biophys. Acta.*, 164:575–584.
97. Nilsson, A. (1969): Metabolism of cerebroside in the intestinal tract of the rat. *Biochim. Biophys. Acta.*, 187:113–121.
98. Nilsson, A. (1970): Conversion of dihydrosphingosine to palmitic acid and palmitaldehyde with cell-free preparations of guinea-pig intestinal mucosa. *Acta Chem. Scand.*, 24:598–604.
99. Northfield, T. C., and Hofmann, A. F. (1975): Biliary lipid output during three meals and an overnight fast. I. Relationship to bile acid pool size and cholesterol saturation of bile in gallstone and control subjects. *Gut*, 16:1–17.
100. Ockner, R. K., and Isselbacher, K. J. (1974): Recent concepts of intestinal fat absorption. *Rev. Physiol. Biochem. Pharmacol.*, 71:107–146.
101. Ockner, R. K., and Manning, J. A. (1974): Intestinal fatty acid binding protein (FABP): Studies on physiological function. *J. Clin. Invest.*, 53:57a.
102. Ockner, R. F., and Manning, J. A. (1974): Fatty acid binding protein in small intestine. Identification, isolation and evidence for its role in cellular fatty acid transport. *J. Clin. Invest.*, 54:326–338.
103. O'Doherty, P. J. A., Kakis, G., and Kuksis, A. (1973): Role of luminal lecithin in intestinal fat absorption. *Lipids*, 8:249–255.
104. Olive, J., and Dervichian, D. G. (1968): Action d'une phospholipase sur la lecithine a l'etat micellaire. *Bull. Soc. Chim. Biol.*, 50:1409–1418.
105. Paltauf, F., Esfandi, F., and Holasek, A. (1974): Stereospecificity of lipases. Enzymatic hydrolysis of enantiomeric alkyl diglycerides by lipoprotein lipase, lingual lipase and pancreatic lipase. *FEBS Lett.*, 40:119–123.
106. Patton, J. S. (1981): Gastrointestinal lipid digestion. In: *Physiology of the Gastrointestinal Tract*, edited by L. R. Johnston, pp. 1123–1146. Raven Press, New York.
107. Patton, J. S., and Carey, M. C. (1979): Watching fat digestion. *Science (Wash. DC)*, 204:145–148.

108. Patton, J. S., and Carey, M. C. (1981): The inhibition of lipase-colipase activity by phospholipid-bile salt mixed micelles. *Am. J. Physiol.*, 241:G328–336.
109. Patton, S., and Keenan, T. W. (1975): The milk fat globule membrane. *Biochim. Biophys. Acta.*, 415:273–309.
110. Patton, J. S., Donnér, J., and Borgström, B. (1978): Lipase-colipase interactions during gel filtration: High and low affinity binding situations. *Biochim. Biophys. Acta.*, 529:67–78.
111. Patton, J. S., Albertsson, P. A., Erlanson, C., and Borgström, B. (1978): Binding of porcine pancreatic lipase and colipase in the absence of substrate studied by two-phase partition and affinity chromatography. *J. Biol. Chem.*, 253:4195–4202.
112. Peters, R. A. (1931): Interfacial tension and hydrogen ion concentration. *Proc. R. Soc.*, 133A:140–154.
113. Phillips, M. C. (1972): The physical state of phospholipids and cholesterol in monolayers, bilayers and membranes. *Prog. Surf. Membr. Sci.*, 5:139–221.
114. Platford, R. F. (1979): Glyceryl trioleate-water partition coefficients for three simple organic compounds. *Bull. Environ. Contam. Toxicol.*, 21:68–73.
115. Plucinski, T. M., Hamosh, M., and Hamosh, P. (1979): Fat digestion in rats: Role of lingual lipase. *Am. J. Physiol.*, 237:E541–E547.
116. Porter, H. P., and Saunders, D. R. (1971): Isolation of the aqueous phase of human intestinal contents during the digestion of a fatty meal. *Gastroenterology*, 60:997–1007.
117. Porter, H. P., Saunders, D. R., Tytgat, G., Brunster, O., and Rubin, C. E. (1971): Fat absorption in bile fistula man. A morphological and biochemical study. *Gastroenterology*, 60:1008–1019.
118. Poley, J. R., Smith, J. D., Thompson, J. B., and Seely, J. R. (1977): Improved micellar dispersal of dietary lipid by bile acids during replacement therapy in growth hormone-deficient children. *Pediatr. Res.*,12:1186–1191.
119. Rampone, A. J. (1973): The effect of lecithin on intestinal cholesterol uptake by rat intestine in vitro. *J. Physiol. (Lond.)*, 229:505–514.
120. Rampone, A. J., and Lang, L. R. (1977): The effect of phosphatidylcholine and lysophosphatidylcholine on the absorption and mucosal metabolism of oleic acid and cholesterol in vitro. *Biochim. Biophys. Acta*, 486:500–510.
121. Rathelot, J., Julien, R., Bosc-Bierne, I., Gargouri, Y., Canioni, P., and Sarda, L. (1981): Horse pancreatic lipase. Interaction with colipase from various species. *Biochimie (Paris)*, 63:227–234.
122. Rautureau, M., Bisalli, A., and Rambaud, J-C. (1981): Bile salts and lipids in aqueous intraluminal phase during the digestion of a standard meal in normal man. *Gastroenterol. Clin. Biol.*, 5:417–425.
123. Richardson, G. H., and Nelson, J. H. (1967): Assay and characterization of pregratric esterase. *J. Dairy Sci.*, 50:1061–1065.
124. Ricour, C., and Rey, J. (1970): Study of the oil and micellar phases during fat digestion in the normal child. *Eur. J. Clin. Biol. Res.*, 15:287–293.
125. Ricour, C., and Rey, J. (1972): Study on the hydrolysis and micellar solubilization of fats during intestinal perfusion. I. Results in the normal child. *Eur. J. Clin. Biol. Res.*, 17:172–178.
126. Rizek, R. L., Friend, B., and Page, L. (1974): Fat in today's food supply-level of use and source. *J. Am. Oil Chem. Soc.*, 51:244–250.
127. Rochford, B. K. (1981): The influence of bile on the fat-splitting properties of pancreatic juice. *J. Physiol. (Lond.)*, 12:72–92.
128. Rossell, J. B. (1973): Interactions of triglycerides and of fats containing them. *Chem. Ind. (Lond.)*, September 1, 1973, pp. 832–835.
129. Roy, C. C., Roulet, M., Lefebure, D., Chartrand, L., Lepage, G., and Fournier, L. A. (1979): The role of gastric lipolysis on fat absorption and bile acid metabolism in the rat. *Lipids*, 14:811–815.
130. Rydhag, L., and Wilton, I. (1981): The function of phospholipids of soybean lecithin in emulsions. *J. Am. Oil Chem. Soc.*, 58:830–837.
131. Sabesin, S. M., and Frase, S. (1977): Electron microscopic studies of the assembly, intracellular transport and secretion of chylomicrons by rat intestine. *J. Lipid Res.*, 18:496–511.
132. Saleeb, F. Z., Cante, C. J., Streckfus, T. K., Frost, J. R., and Rosano, H. L. (1975): Surface pH and stability of oil-water emulsions derived from laurate solutions. *J. Am. Oil Chem. Soc.*, 52:208–212.
133. Sakurai, I., Iwayanagi, S., Sakurai, T., and Seto, T. (1977): X-ray study of egg-yolk lecithin: Unit cell data and electron density profile. *J. Mol. Biol.*, 117:285–291.

134. Sari, H., Dukes, J-P., Tachoire, H., Entressangles, B., and Desnuelle, P. (1981): Effet de l'addition de la colipase pancréatique de porc sur la pérmeabilité au glucose et le transition de phase de liposome de phosphatidylcholine. *Biochimie (Paris)*, 63:389–395.
135. Schmidt-Nielsen, K. (1946): Melting points of human fats as related to their location in the body. *Acta Physiol. Scand.*, 12 (Suppl. 37):123–129.
136. Schneider, R. E., and Viteri, F. E. (1974): Luminal events of lipid absorption in protein-calorie malnourished children: Relationship with nutritional recovery and diarrhea. II. Alterations in bile acid content of duodenal aspirates. *Am. J. Clin. Nutr.*, 27:788–796.
137. Schneider, R. E., and Viteri, F. E. (1974): Luminal events of lipid absorption in protein-calorie malnourished children: Relationship with nutritional recovery and diarrhea. I. Capacity of the duodenal content to achieve micellar solubilization of lipids. *Am. J. Clin. Nutr.*, 27:777–787.
138. Senior, J. R. (1964): Intestinal absorption of fats. *J. Lipid Res.*, 5:495–521.
139. Shankland, W. (1970): The ionic behavior of fatty acids solubilized by bile salts. *J. Colloid Interface Sci.*, 34:9–25.
140. Shimoda, S. S., Saunders, D. R., Schuffler, M. D., and Leinbach, G. L. (1974): Electron microscopy of small intestinal mucosa in pancreatic insufficiency. *Gastroenterology*, 67:19–24.
141. Sklar, D., and Budowski, P. (1978): Hydrolysis of biliary phospholipids in the upper small intestine of the chick. *Lipids*, 13:158–160.
142. Simmonds, W. J. (1972): Fat absorption and chylomicron formation. In: *Blood Lipids and Lipoproteins: Quantitation, Composition, and Metabolism*, edited by G. J. Nelson, pp. 705–743. Wiley-Interscience, New York.
143. Siperstein, M. D., Chaikoff, I. L., and Reinhardt, W. O. (1952): ^{14}C-cholesterol V. obligatory function of bile in intestinal absorption of cholesterol. *J. Biol. Chem.*, 198:111–114.
144. Sjövall, J. (1959): On the concentration of bile acids in the human intestine. *Acta Physiol. Scand.*, 46:339–345.
145. Small, D. M. (1968): A classification of biologic lipids based upon their interaction in aqueous systems. *J. Am. Oil Chem. Soc.*, 45:108–119.
146. Smith, R., and Tanford, C. (1972): The critical micelle concentration L-α dipalmitoyl phosphatidylcholine in water, and water/methanol solutions. *J. Mol. Biol.*, 67:75–83.
147. Stafford, R. J., and Carey, M. C. (1981): Physical-chemical nature of the aqueous lipids in intestinal content after a fatty meal: Revision of the Hofmann-Borgström Hypothesis. *Clin. Res.*, 28:511A.
148. Stafford, R. J., Donovan, J. M., Benedek, G. B., and Carey, M. C. (1980): Physical-chemical characteristics of aqueous duodenal content after a fatty meal. *Gastroenterology*, 80:1291 (Abstr).
149. Staggers, J. E., Fernando-Warnakulasuriya, G. J. P., and Wells, M. A. (1981): Studies on fat digestion, absorption, and transport in the suckling rat. II. Triacylglycerol molecular species, stereospecific analysis and specificity of hydrolysis by lingual lipase. *J. Lipid Res.*, 22:675–679.
150. Surawicz, C. M., Saunders, D. R., Sillery, J., and Rubin, C. E. (1981): Linoleate transport by human jejunum: presumptive evidence for portal transport at low absorption rates. *Am. J. Physiol.*, 240:G157–162.
151. Taylor, R. J. (1965): *The Chemistry of Glycerides*, pp. 1–31. Blackfriars, London.
152. Thompson, A. B. R. (1980): Influence of site and unstirred layers on the rate of uptake of cholesterol and fatty acids into rabbit intestine. *J. Lipid Res.*, 21:1097–1107.
153. Thompson, G. R., Barrowman, J., Gutierrez, L., and Dowling, R. H. (1971): Action of neomycin on the intraluminal phase of lipid absorption. *J. Clin. Invest.*, 50:319–323.
154. Thompson, A. B. R., and Dietschy, J. M. (1981): Intestinal Lipid Absorption: Major extracellular and intracellular events. In: *Physiology of the Gastrointestinal Tract*, edited by L. R. Johnson, pp. 1147–1220. Raven Press, New York.
155. Tso, P., Balint, J. A., and Simmonds, W. J. (1976): Role of biliary lecithin in lymphatic transport of fat. *Gastroenterology*, 13:1362–1367.
156. Tso, P., Lam, J., and Simmonds, W. J. (1978): The importance of the lysophosphatidylcholine and choline moiety of bile phosphatidylcholine in lymphatic transport of fat. *Biochim. Biophys. Acta*, 538:364–372.
157. Van Deenen, L. L. M., deHaas, G. H., and Heemskerk, C. H. Th. (1963): Hydrolysis of synthetic mixed phosphatides by pholpholipase A from human pancreas. *Biochim. Biophys. Acta*, 67:295–306.
158. Van Deest, B. W., Fortran, J. S., Morawski, S. G., and Wilson, J. D. (1968): Bile salt and micellar fat concentration in proximal small bowel contents of ileectomy patients. *J. Clin. Invest.*, 47:1314–1324.

159. Van Meer, G., Kruijiff, B. de, Op den kamp, J. A. F., and Van Deenen, L. L. M. (1980): Preservation of bilayer structure in human erythrocytes and erythrocyte ghosts after phospholipase treatment. A ^{31}P NMR study. *Biochim. Biophys. Acta*, 596:1–9.
160. Vaughan, J. G., ed. (1979): *Food Microscopy*. Academic Press, New York.
161. Verger, R., Rietsch, J., Van Dam-Mieras, M. C. E., and deHaas, G. H. (1976): Comparative studies of lipase and phospholipase A$_2$ acting on substrate monolayers. *J. Biol. Chem.*, 251:3128–3133.
162. Wawra, H. (1978): Investigation of crystalline structures of fats of animals by x-ray scattering. *Z. Naturforsch.*, 33:28–38.
163. Whyte, M., Karmen, A., and Goodman, D. W. S. (1963): Fatty acid esterification and chylomicron formation during fat absorption. 2. Phospholipids. *J. Lipid Res.*, 4:322–329.
164. Worcester, D. L., and Franks, N. P. (1976): Structural analysis of hydrated egg lecithin and cholesterol bilayers. II. Neutron diffraction. *J. Mol. Biol.*, 100:359–378.
165. Wu, A-L., and Windmueller, H. G. (1981)): Variant forms of plasma apolipoprotein B: Hepatic and intestinal biosynthesis and heterogeneous metabolism in the rat. *J. Biol. Chem.*, 256:3615–3618.

Phospholipids and Atherosclerosis, edited by
P. Avogaro, M. Mancini, G. Ricci, and
R. Paoletti. Raven Press, New York © 1983.

Polyene Phosphatidylcholine: Pharmacokinetics After Oral Administration—A Review

J. M. Fox

*Faculty of Medicine, University of Saarland, D-6650 Homburg/Saar, and
Nattermann Research Laboratories, D-5000 Köln 30, West Germany*

Polyene phosphatidylcholine (PPC) constitutes a subgroup of special phosphatidylcholines (or lecithins) having polyunsaturated fatty acids in the side chains of the molecule (7). The prototype is 1,2-dilinoleoyl phosphatidylcholine (dilinoleoyl-PC). Polyene phospatidylcholine occurs naturally in plants (e.g., soybeans, safflower), or can be obtained by synthetic or semisynthetic processes. Investigation of the pharmacokinetics of PPC especially has to provide evidence on the preservation of the integrity of this particular molecule (among the "animal" phosphatidylcholines) during absorption and organ distribution—particularly if therapeutic aims, such as the treatment of atherosclerosis, require the use of this special phosphatidylcholine.

The present review is based on experiments mainly using synthetic radiolabeled dilinoleoyl-PC. The evidence accumulated thus far has been gained mostly from experiments in animals (mainly rats, but also dogs and monkeys). Only recently a study using radiolabeled dilinoleoyl-PC provided reliable human data (31).

METHODOLOGICAL REMARKS

Phosphatidylcholine is found ubiquitously in mammals. Polyene phosphatidylcholine, if orally administered, therefore, has to be distinguished from endogenous lecithins when investigating its absorption and metabolic fate. Quantitative conclusions thus may be drawn only from experiments using radiolabels in the fatty acids and choline moieties of the molecule. A further restriction has to be taken into account since label exchange may occur, particularly if a tritium label is used in the fatty acid moiety. It was observed (6) that a considerable amount of tritium from the fatty acids exchanges for nonradioactive hydrogen with body water. It appears, therefore, desirable for most experiments that a ^{14}C label be used in the fatty acid moiety and a tritium label in the methyl groups of the choline, if double labeling is required. For positional analysis, single-label PPC molecules were synthesized carrying a ^{14}C label either in the 1-, 2-, or 3-position (13). Detailed descriptions of the individual techniques are in the below cited reports. Synthesis of radiolabeled PPC was described by Lekim and Betzing and Stoffel et al. (14,15,27).

ABSORPTION OF POLYENE PHOSPHATIDYLCHOLINE

Total Absorption from the Gut

Polyene phosphatidylcholine (orally administered to rats, rhesus monkeys, or humans as a single dose) was more than 90% absorbed, since there was only little excretion with the feces during the first 5 or 7 days (Table 1). Similar results were obtained in males as well as in females (5,6,31). In rats the absorption as measured by the disappearance of radiolabel from the gut showed a rapid initial phase (65% during the first 4 hr) and a slow final phase (approximately a further 25% from 4 to 24 hr). The time course of disappearance from the gut and the total amount of absorption was similar for the fatty acids and for the choline moieties (8).

Integrity of the Absorbed PPC

The pharmacokinetics of orally ingested PPC involve the question of bioavailability of the intact molecule. Therefore, the primary step, the mechanism of intestinal absorption, has been of particular research interest (1–3,8,11–13,17–21, 25,28). It has been established that a major portion of phosphatidylcholine is hydrolyzed to 1-acyl-lysophosphatidylcholine and is reacylated by the mucosal cells to phosphatidylcholine after absorption. However, some evidence is available that a minor portion of the molecule might be absorbed intact (1,2). This view was supported in particular by recent investigations in humans (31).

TABLE 1. *Fecal excretion of radioactivity accumulated during a period of 5 or 7 days[a]*

	% administered dose		
	Rats	Rhesus monkey	Human
PPC-FA moiety	6.1[b]	8.0[b]	5.7
PPC-choline moiety	3.2	3.6	2.2
N (males/females)	4/4	3/3	4/1
Reference	(5)	(6)	(32)

[a]After a single oral dose of 1,2-^{3}H-dilinoleoylphosphatidyl-^{14}C-choline (rat, rhesus) or 1,2-^{14}C-dilinoleoylphosphatidyl-^{3}H-choline. Mean values of N animals or patients. PPC, polyene phosphatidylcholine; FA, fatty acid.
[b]Values for nonvolatile ^{3}H, i.e., non-[3]H$_2$O (see methods section).

Lymph cannulation experiments were performed in rats to avoid interchange of exogenous PPC with endogenous PC (4,13). The lymph was collected immediately after production from the thoracic duct for different periods after giving doses of dilinoleoyl-PC, labeled with ³H in the fatty acids and with ¹⁴C in the choline moiety. (Under these circumstances ³H-label exchange with body water did not occur considerably.)

Table 2 displays the recovery of the radiolabel in the lymph. More than 88% of the tritium but only 50% of the carbon label were recovered in the lymph chylomicrons. A small amount of tritium (fatty acids) and almost half of the carbon (choline moiety) could bypass the lymph. Apparently, a certain portion of the molecules was degraded, and the degradation products (mainly nonlipids) entered the liver directly via the portal vein. The other portion (the lipids) was recovered with the lymph. These percentages of recovery were independent of time after dose administration (13). They represent, therefore, the average absorption process.

A further step was to investigate where in the lipid fractions of the lymph the labels were located. No labeled free fatty acids (FFA) and no labeled lysophosphatidylcholine were detected. The ¹⁴C radioactivity (the choline label) was 100% in phosphatidylcholine; the fatty acid label (tritium) was 25% in phosphatidylcholine and 75% in triglycerides (TG) (Table 3). The tritium/carbon ratio was almost half of the original ratio. All these figures were independent of time, again representing the average absorption process.

Phospholipase A is present in the intestinal lumen. The data suggest that the following might happen:

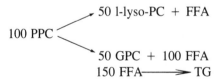

The free fatty acids are incorporated into triglycerides in the mucosa and the glycerylphosphatidylcholine (GPC) bypasses the lymph and is found in the liver

TABLE 2. *Distribution of radioactivity in the intestinal tract, in the liver and in the lymph chylomicrons of the rat[a]*

	³H Radioactivity		¹⁴C Radioactivity	
	% Dose	% Absorption	% Dose	% Absorption
Lymph chylomicrons	24.8	88.2	17.4	51.6
Liver	0.8	2.9	12.5	36.3
Other organs (difference)	2.5	8.9	4.3	12.3
Total absorption	28.1	100.0	34.2	100.0
Intestinal tract	71.9	0	65.8	0

[a]At 6.5 hr after oral administration of 1,2-(9,10,12,13-³H₄)-dilinoleoyl-*sn*-glycero-phospho-(N-¹⁴CH₃)-choline.

TABLE 3. *Distributions of ^{3}H and ^{14}C radioactivities[a]*

| Time after dose (hr) | Phosphatidylcholine | | Neutral lipids |
	% ^{3}H	^{3}H/^{14}C	% ^{3}H
1.5	23.5	24.3	77.5
2.5	24.0	17.2	76.0
3.5	24.5	20.4	75.5
4.5	25.0	19.7	75.0
5.5	24.0	17.9	76.0
6.5	24.5	20.9	75.5

[a]Radioactivities in lipid fractions of the lymph chylomicrons in lymph-cannulated male rats ($N = 7$) after a single oral dose of 70 mg/kg polyunsaturated phosphatidylcholine labeled as in Table 1 (^{3}H/^{14}C = 58:1). After 0.5 hr the lymph was collected for periods of 1 hr. The only labeled lipid fractions were phosphatidylcholine and triglycerides. No labeled lysophosphatidylcholine and no labeled free fatty acids were detected; 100% of the ^{14}C radioactivity was located in the phosphatidylcholine fraction, and practically none was found in the triglyceride fraction.

and in the other organs. According to this scheme the ^{3}H-label distribution (fatty acids) in the lymph is expected to be 25% in the PC fraction and 75% in the TG fraction. The values observed were 23.5 to 25.0 and 75.0 to 76.5, respectively. The ^{14}C-label distribution between the lymph and the liver plus other organs should be equal. The actual values were 52% and 48% (see Table 2). Further, in this scheme the ^{3}H/^{14}C ratio in the PC fraction should be half of the original ratio, i.e., 26. The observed values were 17.2 to 24.3.

Apparently, phosphatidylcholine was absorbed after hydrolyzation as lysophosphatidylcholine and was reacylated in the mucosa again to phosphatidylcholine since no radioactive lyso-PC has been detected. These data confirm on a quantitative basis the view of the absorption of PC, as it was derived from earlier investigations (2,15,20). There are reports that PC may also be absorbed to a certain extent as intact molecules (1,2). Although this possibility has not been ruled out completely, the present data show that intact PPC absorption (in rats) accounts only for a minor portion.

Identity of the Absorbed PPC

After absorption, approximately 50% of the orally administered PPC was available in the lymph (and blood stream) intact or via reacylation. Positional analysis of the fatty acids had to clarify if the identity of the PPC, in contrast to the body-owned PC, was preserved. The lymph phosphatidylcholine was cleaved by using phospholipase A_2. Only 10% of the ^{3}H label (linoleic acid) was found in the 2-position, but 90% was found in the 1-position (13).

A further experiment was performed using single-carbon labels separately in each of the three positions of the PC molecule and then collecting the CO_2 of the expired air (Fig. 1). Cleaving of PC in only the 2-position should result in the occurrence

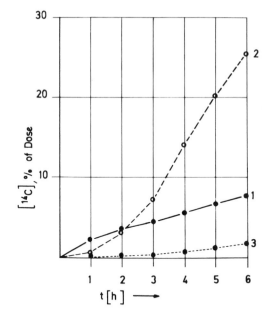

FIG. 1. Cumulative amounts of respiratory $^{14}CO_2$ collected after a single oral dose of 70 mg/kg labeled with ^{14}C in the acyl-1 position **(1)**, the acyl-2 position **(2)**, and the 3-position (choline) **(3)**. Mean values in percent of the administered dose measured in two male plus two female animals for each labeled phosphatidylcholine species. The standard deviations for the cumulated values after 6 hr were ± 4% **(1)**, ± 7% **(2)**, and ± 11% **(3)** of the mean. The exact labeling was as follows:

1. 1-(1-^{14}C)-linoleoyl-2-(9,10,12,13-$^3H_4$)-linoleoyl-*sn*-glycero-3-phosphorylcholine: 37,300,000 dpm ^3H and 620,000 dpm ^{14}C
2. 1-(9,10,12,13-$^3H_4$)-linoleoyl-2-(1-^{14}C)-linoleoyl-*sn*-glycero-3-phosphorylcholine: 66,900,000 dpm ^3H and 1,730,000 dpm ^{14}C
3. 1,2-(9,10,12,13-$^3H_4$)-dilinoleoyl-*sn*-glycero-3-phosphoryl-(N-$^{14}CH_3$)-choline: 186,000,000 dpm ^3H and 5,500,000 dpm ^{14}C.

(Data according to Lekim, ref. 13.)

of ^{14}C in the expired CO_2 if the label was introduced in the 2–position. By far, the highest amount of ^{14}C label in the expired CO_2 was found in this case.

Obviously, in rats, hydrolyzation of PPC during absorption took place mostly at the 2-position resulting in 1-lyso-PC, which is reacylated predominantly with an unsaturated fatty acid because of the specificity of lyso-PC-acyltransferase (EC 2.3.1.2.3). Consequently, a polyene phosphatidylcholine was made available to the organism. This is particularly important since the mammalian endogenous PC contains practically 100% palmitic acid in the 1-position. According to Whyte et al. (29) this cannot be changed by ingesting unsaturated free fatty acids. As during absorption of PC the 1-position of phosphatidylcholine is usually not attacked; the unsaturated type of a polyunsaturated phosphatidylcholine will not be changed and can thus be introduced into the organism by oral administration of PPC.

This was further proved by a study of Rosseneau and co-workers (23) in chimpanzees. The experimental setup was as follows. The chimpanzees received by mouth PPC, then a control diet, and finally saturated lecithin for three 1-month periods. The fatty acid distribution in the lipoprotein fractions was determined by gas chromatography. The result is shown in Table 4, where for the three dietary regimens the ratio of oleic/linoleic acid (i.e., the $C_{18:1}/C_{18:2}$ ratio) is presented as it is found in the phospholipids, cholesteryl esters, and triglycerides of the three lipoprotein classes. The data show that after a PPC diet the ratio of oleic/linoleic acids in the phospholipids was significantly decreased; whereas, an increase was seen for saturated lecithin. This is also true for the cholesteryl esters in all three lipoprotein classes and, of course, for the triglycerides since part of the fatty acids of the ingested polyene phosphatidylcholine is transferred to triglycerides.

The results of recent pharmacokinetic studies in humans (31) using radiolabeled PPC are completely in line with these findings with one exception: the specificity of hydrolyzation of PPC at the 2-position appears to be less marked in humans, meaning that 1-lyso-PC and 2-lyso-PC are formed during absorption in almost equal amounts; both entities however are reacylated as in other animals. Nevertheless, these authors emphasize that oral administration of PPC allows the introduction of the special PPC type of PC into the human organism, particularly since the absorption rate of intact (reacylated) PPC appears to be higher in humans than in other animals (see below).

Influence of Media on PPC Absorption

The medium in which PPC is dissolved or suspended may influence its absorption. Therefore, comparative studies in dogs were performed applying radiolabeled PPC

TABLE 4. *Changes in fatty acid compositions of phospholipids, cholesteryl esters, and triglycerides in the lipoprotein classes VLDL, LDL, and HDL₃ of chimpanzees[a]*

Lipid	Lipoprotein class	$C_{18:1}/C_{18:2}$[b]		
		PPC	Saturated lecithin[c]	Control diet
Phospholipids	VLDL	0.5	1.0	0.8
	LDL	0.3	0.8	0.4
	HDL₃	0.3	0.8	0.4
Cholesteryl esters	VLDL	0.3	1.1	0.4
	LDL	0.2	0.8	0.3
	HDL₃	0.2	0.8	0.3
Triglycerides	VLDL	0.4	2.5	1.5
	LDL	0.7	2.9	1.5
	HDL₃	0.7	2.4	1.4

[a]After 4 weeks of oral treatment with polyenephosphatidylcholine (PPC), saturated lecithin (20 g/day), or a control diet. VLDL, very low-density lipoprotein; LDL, low-density lipoprotein; HDL, high-density lipoprotein.

[b]Ratio of oleic/linoleic acid ($C_{18:1}/C_{18:2}$), as derived from data of Rosseneau et al. (23).

[c]The saturated lecithin was obtained by hydrogenation of PPC, so that the chain length distribution was identical.

dissolved either in oil/monoglyceride/diglyceride, in 11% ethanol, or suspended in mannitol/water (8). The label was ^{14}C in the fatty acids (to avoid label-exchange with body water) and tritium in the choline moiety. Figure 2 shows the plasma radioactivity originating from the choline moiety as given in percent of the administered oral dose. The time course (i.e., the kinetics) as well as the radioactivity levels did not differ significantly from each other for the different media. The same is true for the tritium label (Fig. 3) originating from the fatty acids. Thus, there is no great influence on absorption by the media in which the phosphatidylcholine is offered.

Stein and Stein (26) reported a higher absorption of phosphatidylcholine if it is ingested together with large amounts of oil. Whether this is an effect of an accelerated rate of absorption, because of the higher need of phosphatidylcholine to build up more chylomicrons, or whether the reacylated portion is increased is not clear at present.

KINETIC DATA: TIME COURSE OF BLOOD LEVELS

Figure 4 presents comparative data of total plasma levels of radioactivity (percent of ingested dose) originating from the choline moiety after absorption of orally

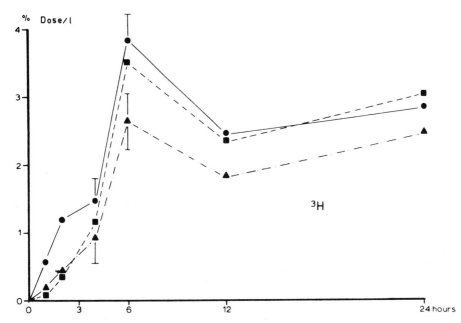

FIG. 2. Time course of blood ^{3}H radioactivity (choline moiety) in dogs after a single oral dose of polyunsaturated phosphatidylcholine (150 mg/kg) dissolved in either oil/monoglyceride/diglyceride, 11% ethanol or suspended in mannitol/H$_2$O. Blood levels calculated as percentage of dose/liter whole blood (mean ± SD; noninserted error bars are of the same magnitude as the inserted ones). Label: 1,2-(^{14}C)-dilinoleoyl-3sn-phosphatidyl(N-^{14}CH$_3$)choline. ●, ethanol/H$_2$O solution; ■, mannitol/H$_2$O suspension; ▲, mono/diglyceride solution; $N = 6$. (Data according to Fox et al., ref. 8.)

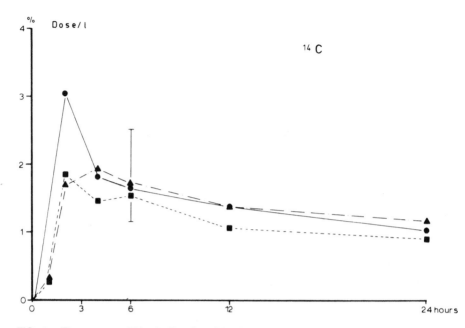

FIG. 3. Time course of blood ^{14}C radioactivity (fatty acid moieties) in dogs after a single oral dose of polyunsaturated phosphatidylcholine (150 mg/kg) in different media (see Fig. 2). ●, ethanol/H$_2$O solution; ■, mannitol/H$_2$O suspension; ▲, mono/diglyceride solution; N = 6. (Data according to Fox et al., ref. 8.)

administered PPC in dogs, rats, and monkeys. The peak levels of absorbed PPC in plasma were approximately 5% of the oral dose in rhesus monkeys and rats, and approximately 1.8% in dogs. A recent investigation in humans (31) revealed peak values in total blood 19.9 ± 3.9% of the administered ^{3}H label (choline moiety) and of 27.9 ± 4.4% of the administered ^{14}C label (fatty acid moiety). Since approximately three-fourths of the radioactivity was detected in the plasma and only one-fourth in the erythrocytes, these data suggest that the absorption rate of PPC (intact or reacylated) is approximately three times higher than in rats or rhesus monkeys.

The time course of plasma radioactivity was found to be similar in all species (see Fig. 4) as well as in humans. The peak radioactivity was observed at 6 hr after dose administration; whereas, there was an indication for a lag time of 1 or 2 hr in dogs. (Early data for rhesus monkeys or rats are not available.) In humans the ^{3}H label (choline moiety) peaked between 6 and 24 hr, whereas the ^{14}C label (fatty acid moiety) peaked between 4 and 12 hr. A lag time of 2 hr was observed in the beginning. The half-life of decay of PC radioactivity between 24 and 96 hr averaged 64.7 hr for ^{3}H and 37.8 hr for [14]C. Similar values were obtained in rats (6,17) and in rhesus monkeys (5). It has to be emphasized that the decay is overlapped by reformation of PC from GPC in the liver originating from the portion of PPC being disintegrated during absorption (see above).

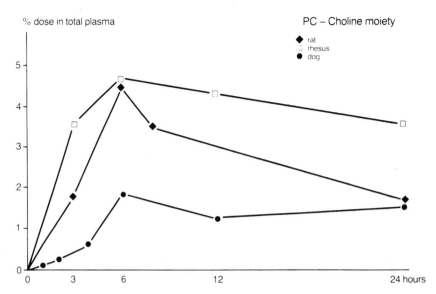

FIG. 4. Absorption in different species of polyunsaturated phosphatidylcholine (PC) suspended in H_2O as measured by the time course of plasma radioactivity originating from the label of the choline moiety after a single oral dose. Monkeys and rats: 1,2-(^{3}H)-dilinoleoyl-3sn-phosphatidyl(N-C^{3}H$_3$) choline; dog: as in Fig. 2. (Data according to Fox et al., ref. 8.)

ORGAN DISTRIBUTION

Tissue Concentrations

Experiments in rats (6) were performed using 1,2-^{3}H-dilinoleoyl-3sn-phosphatidyl-^{14}C-choline. Because of exchange of the tritium label with body water, only the values of the ^{14}C-radioactivity (choline moiety of PPC) gave representative results.

After a single oral dose of radiolabeled PPC, ^{14}C radioactivity was accumulated in the liver, with maximal concentrations occurring at 24 hr after dose administration (24.5% dose); these declined slowly during 8 days (4.0% dose). Significant amounts of radioactivity were detected in the striated muscle (5.8% dose during 6 hr), which increased during 8 days after dose administration (up to 25.0% dose). Limited amounts of ^{14}C radioactivity were detected in the kidneys after 24 hr (2.7% dose). Radioactivity was detected in the lungs (maximal 0.9% dose at 24 hr) and myocardium (0.3% dose at 24 hr, which was retained during the 8 days).

Concentrations of radioactivity (expressed in terms of tissue weight) were highest in the liver (1,196 μg/g) and ^{14}C radioactivity was detected in the brain (0.20% dose/g, 101 μg/g, after 4 hr). ^{14}C Radioactivity associated with the blood after a single oral dose of radiolabeled PPC was associated almost entirely with the plasma for 48 hr. At 96 hr, some ^{14}C radioactivity (approximately 22%) was associated with the cells; after 8 days up to 54% was located in the cells. [In humans three-fourths of the blood radioactivity was associated with the plasma during the first period (31).]

Radioactivity in the tissues of rats after five daily oral doses of $^3H/^{14}C$-PPC was calculated in terms of the estimated cumulative dose retained (Table 5). These values were estimated from the rates of excretion in the single-dose study (see below). Concentrations of ^{14}C radioactivity in the tissues of rats after the first four daily oral doses of $^3H/^{14}C$-PPC showed that liver, depot fat, striated muscle, and bone had accumulated significant amounts of ^{14}C radioactivity (18.6, 7.0, 31.4, and 5.6%, respectively, of the estimated dose retained). Limited amounts of ^{14}C radioactivity were detected in the lungs, kidneys, testes, small and large intestine, blood, and plasma (1.3, 3.0, 1.3, 1.9, 1.6, 2.7, and 1.4% dose, respectively).

After the fifth dose of radiolabeled PPC, some ^{14}C radioactivity had accumulated in the liver at 6 hr (22.9% dose, 3718 μg/g), and this declined during the next 16 days (2.3% dose; 245 μg/g). The total ^{14}C radioactivity in the striated muscle increased after the fifth dose to a maximum after 4 days (36.9%, 545 μg/g). Some ^{14}C radioactivity was associated with the bone (up to 4.7% dose; 653 μg/g) and depot fat (up to 5.6% dose; 560 μg/g) at 24 hrs after the fifth dose. ^{14}C Radioactivity (expressed in terms of tissue weight) showed that radioactivity was concentrated into the adrenals at 6 hr after the fifth dose (1.75% dose/g). ^{14}C Radioactivity associated with the liver was maximal at 6 hr after fifth dose (2.0% dose/g) and that associated with the kidneys was also maximal (1.33% dose/g) at this time. The ^{14}C radioactivity in the blood was approximately equally distributed between cells and plasma immediately before and during 4 days after the fifth daily dose, and was concentrated (up to 65% of the total blood radioactivity) into the cells at 8 days after the fifth daily dose. After 16 days ^{14}C radioactivity in the blood was located mainly in the cells (76%). Rather similar results after a single dose, as well as after repeated doses, were obtained in rhesus monkeys using identical methods and radiolabeled PPC as in rats (5).

TABLE 5. *Estimated cumulative retention of ^{14}C-radioactivity (choline moiety) during five daily oral doses of $^3H/^{14}C$-PPC to rats and rhesus monkeys[a,b]*

Day	Male rat	Female rat	Male rhesus monkey	Female rhesus monkey
			Percent of cumulative dose retained	
1	63.0	55.0	53.9	57.8
2	64.3	56.5	54.2	58.0
3	65.8	58.2	54.9	58.4
4	67.5	60.4	57.4	59.9
5	74.0	68.3	65.9	67.9

[a]References 5 and 6.
[b]Estimation was based on single-dose excretion rates. Four rats of each sex and three rhesus monkeys of each sex were used.

The situation in rhesus monkeys was comparable to that in rats (5). Hours after the last daily dose, radiolabeled PPC in the liver and depot fat contained 11 and 7% dose, respectively; this declined to 1.7 and 4.5% dose during the next 16 days. The total ^{14}C radioactivity in striated muscle was between 16.2 and 20.3% dose at 6 hr after five repeated daily oral doses. This value was observed between 10 and 14% after the next 5 days and between 17 and 19% after the next 16 days. The ^{14}C radioactivity in the blood at 6 hr after the last dose was associated mainly with the plasma (74–85%). After 5 days, between 69 and 72% was present in the plasma, and this had declined further after 17 days to 46 to 48%.

Whole-Body Autoradiography

Whole-body autoradiography was performed in rats using 1,2-^{3}H-dilinoleoyl-3*sn*-phosphatidyl-^{14}C-choline (6,13). In both experiments, essentially the same results were obtained.

During 6 hr after a single oral dose of ^{14}C-PPC, radioactivity was located mainly in the liver, kidneys, and the intestinal mucosa. At this time, small amounts of radioactivity were present in the secretory glands (thymus, thyroid, and salivary glands) and the lymph nodes. Only limited amounts of radioactivity were present in the gut contents.

After 12 hr, the distribution of radioactivity was more general, but was mainly located in the liver, kidneys, and intestinal mucosa. Some radioactivity was associated with the secretory glands, especially in the salivary glands and in the testes and epididymis. Limited amounts were present in the gut contents, and some was associated with a fur or skin (possibly with sebaceous glands).

After 24 hr, radioactivity was still mainly associated with the liver, kidneys, and intestinal mucosa. Radioactivity was associated with the bone marrow, lungs, spleen, testes, epididymis, secretory glands, and fur or skin (sebaceous glands) in limited amounts. Higher concentrations were associated with the seminal vesicles and the preputial glands.

The autoradiographs after 6 hr showed part of the intestinal radioactivity in the gut contents and part in the intestinal wall. After 12, 24, and 48 hr practically no radioactivity was observed in the lumen, but quite high concentrations (still after 48 hr) were associated with the intestinal mucosa. These findings are in line with (a) the human data suggesting a protracted absorption (31) and (b) animal results (22) of PPC secretion into the bile, thus undergoing enterohepatic circulation.

After 48 hr, radioactivity was generally distributed but remained mainly associated with the liver and intestinal mucosa. High concentrations were located in the kidneys, testes, and epididymis, together with the secretory glands, notably the salivary, thyroid, and thymus glands. Radioactivity was associated in limited amounts in the bone marrow, lachrymal glands, and lymph nodes of the head region. A general distribution of radioactivity into the striated muscle was evident at this time.

After 96 hr, the concentration of radioactivity had declined generally, with no major concentrations present in any particular organ. Some radioactivity was located in the liver, kidneys, and gastric mucosa with local concentrations in the thymus, lachrymal glands, lymph nodes of the head region, epididymis, coagulating glands, and preputial glands. A general distribution of low concentrations of radioactivity was evident in the other tissues.

After 8 days, the concentrations of radioactivity were low but generally distributed. Local concentrations were evident in the gastric mucosa, epididymis, testes, and seminal vesicles with some radioactivity present in the thymus and lachrymal glands.

Whole-body autoradiographs taken immediately before the fifth and final daily dose of ^{14}C-PPC indicated general distribution of radioactivity throughout the tissues. Major concentrations were located in the liver, spleen, kidneys, adrenal glands, gastric and intestinal mucosae, and the salivary glands. High concentrations were evident in the lachrymal glands, thymus, lymph nodes, seminal vesicles, epididymis, preputial glands, and bone marrow. Low concentrations of radioactivity were located in the striated muscle and brain. At 12 hr after the fifth daily dose, the radioactivity was mainly concentrated into the liver, kidneys, spleen, and intestinal and gastric mucosae with local high concentrations in the lymph nodes, thymus, bone marrow, epididymis, seminal vesicles, and testes. Some radioactivity was present in the brown fat, and there was a general distribution of radioactivity at low concentrations in the striated muscle.

At 48 hr after the fifth dose, higher concentrations of radioactivity were evident in the lymph nodes, gastric mucosa, epididymis, seminal vesicles, and testes with lower concentrations in the brain, spinal cord, and striated muscle. Ninety-six hours after the last dose the pattern of distribution remained similar, with local concentrations in the secretory glands (lachrymal, salivary, and Harderian), adrenal gland, seminal vesicles, epididymis, and testes. Generally lower concentrations were present in the brain, spinal cord, and striated muscle.

After 8 days, the concentration of radioactivity in most tissues was low with higher concentrations occurring in the secretory glands (salivary and lachrymal). Radioactivity was distributed generally in the central nervous system and striated muscle.

METABOLIC FATE OF PPC: INCORPORATION INTO SERUM LIPOPROTEINS, RED BLOOD CELLS, AND HEPATOCYTES

Figure 5 represents a schematic, tentative view of the present knowledge of the pathways for absorption of PPC and for metabolization of the disintegrated portions of the molecule based on the recent absorption studies as described above. In rats around 52% of PPC are available (after intact absorption or reacylated lyso-PC) in the chylomicrons. This percentage may be even higher in humans (31). The disintegrated portion (GPC and the polyunsaturated fatty acids) undergoes partial resynthesis to PC and triglyceride. The remaining components are transported to the liver. Here again resynthesis takes place with incorporation into hepatocytes (10,16).

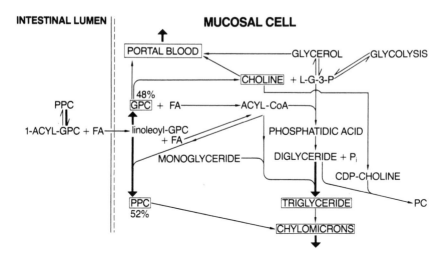

FIG. 5. Schematic, tentative view of the metabolic pathways of polyenephosphatidylcholine (PPC) in the mucosal cell after absorption. Major portion of PPC is absorbed as 1-lyso-PC, part of which (in rats, ~48%) is further disintegrated and bypasses the lymph to the liver (via portal vein); the other part is reacylated to PPC and incorporated in the lymph chylomicrons. The liberated fatty acids (FA) and part of GPC and choline are resynthesized to triglycerides and phosphatidylcholine (PC), respectively. L-G-3-P, glucose 3-phosphate; CoA, coenzyme A; P_i, inorganic phosphate; CDP, cytidine diphosphate; GPC, glycerylphosphatidylcholine.

A matter of great importance are the observations of a special uptake of PPC from the chylomicrons by high-density lipoprotein (HDL). These recent investigations are reported elsewhere (O. Zierenberg, *this volume* and ref. 30). They indicate that body-owned saturated PC is exchanged by PPC particularly in HDL, thus increasing the cholesterol-transporting capacity of the HDL particles. These studies were performed in rats and dogs after oral and intravenous PPC administration. The incorporation of PPC was further investigated *in vitro* using human HDL, as well as HDL from animal source. The results were basically confirmed by a recent human pharmacokinetic study (31); it appears to put forth a better understanding of the antiatherogenic effect of PPC (in contrast to saturated lecithin) as derived from animal experiments (9).

As seen from the organ distribution studies, increasing amounts of PPC with time after oral administration were detected in the blood cells. Six hours after dose administration of radiolabeled PPC in animals and in humans, approximately 75% of the radioactivity of total blood were found in the lipoproteins (particularly in HDL) and only about 25% in blood corpuscles. This ratio reverses during the next 6 days. Incorporation of polyunsaturated phosphatidylcholine into the membranes of erythrocytes enlarges the flexibility and fluidity of the red blood cells as shown by Salvioli et al. (24).

No particular investigations on the metabolization of the PPC molecules have been undertaken so far. One has to assume that PPC undergoes the same metabolic pathways as endogenous PC.

EXCRETION AND RETENTION OF PPC

The knowledge on excretion and retention of PPC is almost entirely based on radioactivity measurements after single or repeated doses of radiolabeled PPC. Since a considerable portion of PPC is already disintegrated during the absorption process, excretion and retention of radioactivity comprises the intact PPC as well as both its metabolites and the metabolites of other resynthesized material, such as triglycerides. Excretion with the feces is very low (see Table 1). Considerable radioactivity is excreted with the expired air, approximately 15% after a single oral dose in rats and rhesus monkeys (5,6) (see also Fig. 1). This almost entirely has to be attributed to the metabolization of fatty acids that are liberated during absorption and incorporated into triglycerides (19).

The renal excretion of ^{14}C radioactivity after a single dose of ^{3}H/^{14}C-PPC was 17.4% dose in rats and 17.7% in rhesus monkeys during 5 days after a single dose (5,6). From bile duct cannulation experiments (22) it is known that a considerable amount of PPC appears in the bile. Since the fecal excretion is low, PPC must undergo an effective enterohepatic recirculation.

Retention of PPC was estimated from the single-dose excretion rates in rats and rhesus monkeys (5,6) (see Table 5). These retention values again comprise intact and disintegrated PPC. Retention as such is not an important factor, since PPC and its metabolites are considered to be nontoxic.

CONCLUSION

The knowledge of the pharmacokinetics of polyene phosphatidylcholine accumulated thus far provides evidence that more than 50% of orally administered PPC is made biologically available for the organism either by intact absorption (lesser extent) or by reacylation of absorbed lyso-PC (greater extent). This is true for several animal species (rats, dogs, rhesus monkeys, chimpanzees) and for humans. Obviously, there are some differences in the specificity of hydrolyzing PPC to lyso-PC. In rats hydrolyzation takes place mainly in the 2-position of the molecule (90%); in humans the 1- and the 2-position are almost equally attacked. Nevertheless, it is possible to exchange body-owned (endogenous) PC for the special PPC, particularly since the absorption in humans appears to be higher than in other animals. PPC is particularly incorporated into HDL particles, into the membranes of hepatocytes, and into red blood cells. These results have a specific implication for the beneficial effects of PPC in atherosclerosis and hepatic diseases.

REFERENCES

1. Artom, C., and Swanson, M. A. (1948): Absorption of phospholipids. *J. Biol. Chem.*, 75:871–881.
2. Blomstrand, R. (1955): The intestinal absorption of phospholipids in the rat. *Acta Physiol. Scand.*, 34:147–175.
3. Bloom, B., Kiyasu, J. Y., Reinhard, W. O., and Chaikoff, I. L. (1954): Absorption of phospholipids—Manner of transport from intestinal lumen to lacteals. *Am. J. Physiol.*, 177:84–88.
4. Bollmann, J. L., Cain, J. C., and Grindlay, J. H. (1943): Techniques for the collection of lymph from the liver, small intestine or thoradic duct of the rat. *J. Lab. Clin. Invest.*, 33:1344–1352.

5. Chasseaud, L. F., Down, W. H., and Sacharin, R. M. (1975): The metabolic fate of ^{3}H:^{14}C-essential phospholipid (EPL) in the rhesus monkey. Research Report NTN 5/75497. Huntingdon Research Centre, Huntingdon, Cambridgeshire, England *(unpublished)*.

6. Chasseaud, L. F., Down, W. H., Williams, J. M., Sacharin, R. M., and Franklin, E. R. (1975): The metabolic fate of ^{3}H:^{14}C-essential phospholipid (EPL) in the rat. Research Report NTN 4/75379. Huntingdon Research Centre, Huntingdon, Cambridgeshire, England *(unpublished)*.

7. Fox, J. M. (1976): A glossary of essential phospholipids, lipids and lipoproteins. In: *Phosphatidylcholine—Biochemical and Clinical Aspects of Essential Phospholipids*, edited by H. Peeters, pp. 2–7. Springer Verlag, Berlin.

8. Fox, J. M., Betzing, H., and LeKim, D. (1979): Pharmacokinetics of orally ingested phosphatidylcholine. In: *Nutrition and the Brain*, Vol. 5, edited by A. Barbeau, J. M. Growdon, and R. J. Wurtman, pp. 95–108. Raven Press, New York.

9. Galli, C. (1981): Polyenoyl phosphatidylcholine (PPC) and lipid metabilism in experimental and clinical atherosclerosis—An introduction to the pharmacology of PPC. Proceedings of hearing on therapeutic selectivity and risk to benefit assessment of hypolipidemic drugs. Rome, June 3 1980.

10. Hegner, D., and Platt, D. (1975): Effect of essential phospholipids on the properties of ATP-ases of isolated rat liver plasma membranes of young and old animals. *Mech. Aging Dev.*, 4:191–200.

11. Hölzl, J. (1976): Pharmacokinetic studies on phosphatidylcholine and phosphatidylinositol. In: *Phosphatidylcholine—Biochemical and Clinical Aspects of Essential Phospholipids*, edited by H. Peeters, pp. 66–79. Springer-Verlag, Berlin.

12. Hölzl, J., and Wagener, H. (1971): Über den Einbau von intraduodenal appliziertem ^{14}C/^{32}P Polyen-Phosphatidylcholine in die Leber von Ratten und seine Ausscheidung durch die Galle. *Z. Naturforsch.*, 26b:1151–1158.

13. Lekim, D. (1976): On the pharmacokinetics of orally applied essential phospholipids (EPL). In: *Phosphatidylcholine—Biochemical and Clinical Aspects of Essential Phospholipids*, edited by H. Peeters, pp. 48–65. Springer-Verlag, Berlin.

14. Lekim, D., and Betzing, H. (1973): Synthesis of labelled phosphatidyl-choline, N-dimethylethanolamine and phosphatidylcholine. *Hoppe Seylers Z. Physiol. Chem.*, 354:1490–1492.

15. Lekim, D., and Betzing, H. (1976): Synthesis of labelled absorption of polyunsaturated phosphatidylcholine in the rat. *Hoppe Seylers Z. Physiol. Chem.*, 357:1321–1331.

16. Lekim, D., Betzing, H., and Stoffel, W. (1972): Incorporation of complete phospholipid molecules in cellular membranes of rat liver after uptake from blood serum. *Hoppe Seylers Z. Physiol. Chem.*, 353:949–964.

17. Lekim, D., and Graf, E. (1976): Tierexperimentelle Studien zur Pharmakokinetik der "essentiellen" Phospholipide (EPL). *Arzneim. Forsch.*, 26:1772–1782.

18. Mansbach, C. M. (1973): Complex lipid synthesis in hamster intestine. *Biochim. Biophys. Acta*, 296:386–402.

19. Nilsson, A. (1968): Intestinal absorption of lecithin and lysolecithin by lymph fistula in rats. *Biochim. Biophys. Acta*, 152:379–390.

20. Nilsson, A., and Borgström, B. (1967): Absorption and metabolism of lecithin and lysolecithin by intestinal slices. *Biochim. Biophys. Acta*, 137:240–254.

21. Parthasarathy, S., Subbaiah, P. V., and Ganguly, J. (1974): The mechanism of intestinal absorption of phosphatidylcholine in rats. *Biochem. J.*, 140:503–508.

22. Paul, R., and Ganguly, J. (1976): Effect of unsaturated lipids on the bile flow and biliary excretion of cholesterol and bile salts in rats. *Chem. Phys. Lipids*, 17:315–323.

23. Rosseneau, M., Declerq, B., Vandamme, D., Vercaemst, R., Soetewey, F., Peeters, H., and Blaton, V. (1979): Influence of oral polyunsaturated and saturated phospholipid treatment on the lipid composition and fatty acid profile of chimpanzee lipoproteins. *Atherosclerosis*, 32:141–152.

24. Salvioli, G. F., Mambrini, A., and Salati, R. (1980): Effect of polyunsaturated phosphatidylcholine infusion on deformability and lipid composition of erythrocytes. Proc. Symposium Arteriosclerosi: Fosfolipidi e Lipoproteine, Milan, June 26.

25. Scow, R. O., Stein, Y., and Stein, O. (1967): Incorporation of dietary lecithin and lysolecithin into lymph chylomicrons in the rat. *J. Biol. Chem.*, 242:4919–4924.

26. Stein, Y., and Stein, O. (1966): Metabolism of labeled lysolecithin, lysophosphatidyl-ethanolamine and lecithin in the rat. *Biochim. Biophys. Acta*, 116:95–107.

27. Stoffel, W., Lekim, D., and Tschung, T. S. (1971): A simple chemical method for labelling phosphatidylchline and sphingomyelin in the choline moiety. *Hoppe Seylers Z. Physiol. Chem.*, 352:1058–1064.

28. Wagener, H. (1972): Preparation, distribution and turnover of tritium-labelled "essential" phospholipids (EPL). In: *Phospholipids–Biochemistry, Experimentation, Clinical Application*, edited by G. Schettler, pp. 59–69. Georg Thieme Verlag, Stuttgart.
29. Whyte, M., Goodman, D. S., and Karmen, A. (1965): Fatty acid esterification and chylomicron formation during fat absorption in the rat: III. Positonal relation in triglycerides and lecithin. *J. Lipid Res.*, 6:233–240.
30. Zierenberg, O., Assmann, G., Schmitz, G., and Rosseneu, M. (1981): Effect of polyenephosphatidylcholine on cholesterol uptake by human high density lipoprotein. *Atherosclerosis (in press)*.
31. Zierenberg, O., and Grundy, S. M. (1981): Intestinal absorption of polyenephosphatidylcholine in man. *J. Lipid Res. (submitted for publication)*.

Phospholipids and Atherosclerosis, edited by
P. Avogaro, M. Mancini, G. Ricci, and
R. Paoletti. Raven Press, New York © 1983.

Relationships Between Lipid Composition of Erythrocytes and Their Deformability

Gianfranco Salvioli

Cattedra di Gerontologia e Geriatria, University of Modena, Italy

Blood's viscosity is low under high pressure and in small vessels; thus, it is a non-Newtonian liquid. This behavior depends on red blood cell (RBC) deformability, which is increasingly important as blood vessel diameter enlarges. The normal biconcave shape (discocyte) of erythrocytes, dependent on the high surface/volume ratio, allows either their deformability in the narrowest capillaries (1–3 μm wide) or an easy diffusion of gases (34). Membrane structure and resistance regulate RBC deformability. The components of RBC membrane are protein (skeleton is formed by contractile protein, like spectrin) in a fluid environment of lipids. Sheetz (33) reported a shell model for erythrocyte membrane in which the lipid bilayer is supported by a protein shell distinct from the bilayer (Fig. 1). The membrane shear elasticity of red blood cells arises largely from bilayer lipids, which help determine RBC shape; thus, abnormal erythrocytes with spicules over the surface (spur cells) occur in diseases with altered lipid metabolism, such as advanced liver cirrhosis and abetalipoproteinemia (7).

LIPID COMPOSITION OF ERYTHROCYTE MEMBRANES

As reported in Fig. 1 phosphatidylcholine and sphingomyelin are in the exterior half of the bilayer (2,37); phosphatidylethanolamine and phosphatidylserine are in the cytoplasmatic half. Cholesterol is in high concentration in the outer layer where it (a) decreases the interactions between adjacent paraffin side chains of phospholipids (a condensing effect, which is lower when phospholipid molecules contain polyunsaturated fatty acids) (9), and (b), serves as a wedge, bending the membrane into the biconcave shape (33). RBCs lack the ability to synthesize lipids *de novo*; the renewal of membrane lipids occurs largely with lipoprotein/cholesterol exchanges more rapidly and its partition between RBCs and lipoproteins depends on both the respective cholesterol/phospholipid molar ratio (7) and the unsaturation of fatty acids (3). For these reasons high-density lipoproteins (HDL) most effectively promote the efflux of cholesterol from cells (25). With regard to phospholipids only 60% of phosphatidylcholine and 30% of sphingomyelin are exchangeable

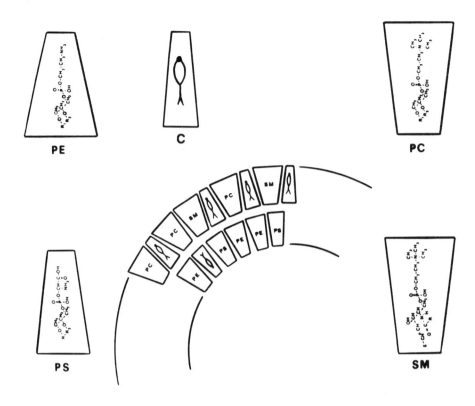

FIG. 1. Asymmetric distribution of phospholipids across erythrocyte membrane. The outer layer of the membrane contains neutral phospholipids having a large polar head group oriented at the interface (PC, phosphatidylcholine; SM sphingomyelin). Cholesterol prefers the outer layer because its shape is complementary to PC and SM. Phosphatidylethanolamine (PE), weakly acidic and with a small head group, and phosphatidylserine (PS), negatively charged at pH 7, are in the interior leaflet; they have anticomplementary shapes to cholesterol and low affinity for it. The organization of the bilayer depends on a balance owing to variations of lipid packing, which are caused by the shortening and broadening of the hydrophobic part of the molecules (acyl chains). The spectrin-actin complex is located exclusively on the cytoplasmatic side, adjacent to the inner lipid layer containing all the PS of erythrocytes; PS-spectrin binding may be an important factor in mantaining lipid asymmetry. (From Mombers et al., ref. 13.)

between RBCs and lipoproteins (26); however, lecithin may be formed inside the erythrocyte through the methylation of phosphatidylethanolamine (14). Both the cholesterol/phospholipid molar ratio and the unsaturation of fatty acids regulate the fluidity (i.e., resistance found on the particle to float freely at the interior of the lipid bilayer) and the permeability of RBC membrane. A shift from polyunsaturated to monounsaturated fatty acids seems a striking variable concerning lipids among animal species that is correlated with the ability of RBC to deform (35); the increase of cholesterol in RBC membranes leads to a reduction of oxygen diffusion (34).

The functions of the spectrin-actin cytoskeleton occur largely within the fluid environment created by lipids. There, Ca^{2+}-related activities (i.e., the regulation of spectrin contractility) are regulated by lipid fluidity (15); the activity of Ca^{2+}-ATPase is higher when fluidity increases. Low-density lipoproteins (LDL) determine a spherocyte transformation of red blood cells, probably inducing dephosphorylation of spectrin (16) and influencing the fluidity in critical regions of the membranes.

POSSIBILITY TO INFLUENCE ERYTHROCYTE SHAPE BY CHANGING ITS LIPID COMPOSITION

The shape of RBC may be influenced by (a) the amount of cholesterol, (b) the cholesterol/phospholipid molar ratio, (c) the lecithin/sphingomyelin ratio, and (d) the number of unsaturated double bonds within the phospholipid acyl chains (7). When RBC acquire cholesterol, their shape changes since the surface increases causing a spiculated contour (spur cells) and thus an impaired ability to pass through filters of small pores (36). Examples are the anemia of patients with advanced liver cirrhosis (17) and dogs receiving a cholesterol-rich diet (8). The appearance of spur cells is due to (a) increased free cholesterol/phospholipid ratio in circulating lipoproteins and in RBC membranes, and (b) decreased percentage of linoleic acid in lecithin of lipoprotein and RBCs (30). *In vitro* rate of cholesterol exchange between RBCs and lipid particles is affected greatly by the differences in the degree of phospholipid unsaturation, being faster *in vitro* when liposomes containing unsaturated lecithin are incubated with RBC (3). Moreover, *in vivo* erythrocytes of pig, fed with hydrogenated soybean oil, exchange cholesterol slower than do the RBC of the control animal (38). On the contrary, cholesterol-depleted RBCs are obtained *in vivo* by infusing animals with lecithin (29) or either incubating cholesterol-rich RBC with normal plasma or normal RBC with liposomes having a low cholesterol/phospholipid ratio (6).

The various lipoproteins may need to be in contact with the RBC surface in order to realize (a) the exchange of cholesterol and phospholipids (diffusion mechanism) and (b) the adsorption of lipoprotein onto RBC membranes with competition between HDL and LDL, with LDL adsorption inhibited by HDL (12,16).

Herewith it is possible that the variations of the lipid composition of the erythrocyte membrane influence RBC deformability and consequently the behavior of RBC in the micro-circulation. *In vivo* RBC cholesterol is maintained just below a critical level at which important organizational changes may occur; in type IIa hyperlipemia, the serum cholesterol/phospholipid ratio increases, influencing the lipid composition of platelets and erythrocytes (22). In patients with peripheral arterial disease the hyperlipemia is frequent and may be correlated with the observed reduction of RBC deformability and the increased viscosity of the blood (21).

ERYTHROCYTE DEFORMABILITY AND ITS MEASUREMENT IN DIFFERENT CLINICAL CONDITIONS

The factors regulating RBC deformability are (a) the geometry of the erythrocyte: the reduction of surface area leads to a spherical morphology and decreases RBC deformability; area increments, with respect to volume, induce spiculated contour (acanthocytes) and a reduced survival of RBCs (8); (b) the erythrocyte content (hemoglobin, Ca^{2+}, and so on): it is known that upon depletion of adenosine triphosphate (ATP), RBC become rigid echinocytes (burr cells) and intracellular Ca^{2+} increases. Human erythrocytes maintain a low intracellular Ca^{2+} concentration (0.1 μM versus 1 mM in plasma) by means of the low passive permeability of Ca^{2+} across the membrane and an outward-directed ATP-dependent Ca^{2+} pump; and (c) the structure of RBC membrane (the influence of the cholesterol/phospholipid molar ratio and of the other parameters was listed above). RBC deformability may be analyzed by means of (a) the aspiration of a portion of RBC membrane into a small hole (4), (b) a filtration technique using polycarbonate membranes with linear channels 3 to 5 μm in diameter (5,20,27), (c) a rheoscope where RBCs suspended in a constant shear are photographed through a microscope (31), and (d) the viscodiffractometric technique by which RBC deformability is studied in a shear field (13). Only (b) and (d) are suitable for measuring RBC deformability in clinical studies. Reduced deformability has been demonstrated in various hemoglobinopathies (where it is correlated with the severity of the anemia); however, in other common conditions, such as diabetes (22), myocardial infarction, peripheral arterial diseases (28), and liver cirrhosis (36), the deformability is reduced, thus indicating alterations of the physicochemical properties of the RBC membranes.

In vitro abnormal RBC of diabetic patients, i.e., poikilocytes, have the same flow pattern as normal cells. However, *in vivo* rigid erythrocytes do not enter small vessels because they are preferentially shunted to larger higher-velocity vessels (19), and at the bifurcations the less deformable cells may cause temporary occlusions. Moreover, a reduced deformability stimulates basement membrane thickening in proportion to the forces delivered by the erythrocytes to the endothelial cells (22).

CAN PHOSPHATIDYLCHOLINE INFLUENCE ERYTHROCYTE DEFORMABILITY?

Twelve patients (8 males and 4 females) with advanced liver cirrhosis and 12 patients (11 males and 1 female) with peripheral arterial disease were studied and compared with 12 normal subjects. RBC lipids were extracted as previously reported (30): neutral and acidic phospholipids were fractionated by two-dimensional thin-layer chromatography (TLC). After identification of the phospholipid classes, lipid phosphorous content of the spots was determined (1). Fatty acid composition of RBC lecithin was determined by gas-liquid chromatography. The lecithin fraction was isolated by one-dimensional TLC and submitted to transesterification using methanol-H_2SO_4 in order to obtain methyl esters of fatty acids. In Table 1 the values of RBC deformability and of the cholesterol/phospholipid molar ratio are reported. The deformability was reduced in both groups of patients with respect to the controls. The mean corpuscular volume in the three groups was 84.6 $\pm$ 3.9, 90.0 $\pm$ 7.0, and 91.9 $\pm$ 4.1 μm^3, respectively. Reticulocytes were higher ($p < 0.01$) only in

TABLE 1. *Deformability and cholesterol/phospholipid molar ratio (C/PL) of erythrocytes in different subjects*[a]

	N	Age (yr)	Deformability[b]	C/PL
Controls	12	45–70	0.36 ± 0.13 (0.23–0.66)	0.67 ± 0.11 (0.45–0.88)
Liver cirrhosis	12	45–63	0.08 ± 0.04[c] (0.02–0.29)	1.04 ± 0.17[c] (0.72–1.29)
Peripheral arterial disease	12	45–70	0.07 ± 0.04[c] (0.02–0.16)	0.93 ± 0.11[c] (0.68–1.08)

[a]Mean ± SD and range of the value; N = number of subjects studied.
[b]Deformability of RBC is expressed as milliliter of packed erythrocytes filtered per minute through 5 μm polycarbonate membrane according to Reed et al. (26).
[c]$p < 0.01$ with regard to normal subjects.

patients with liver cirrhosis (88,750 ± 13,840 mm³) with respect to the normal subjects (66,750 ± 12,840 mm³). The values of cholesterol/phospholipid ratio were higher in the patients than in the controls. An inverse correlation between RBC filterability and cholesterol/phospholipid ratio may be demonstrated ($r = -0.62$); the volume of RBCs filtered per minute was lower when the ratio was higher (Fig. 2). No correlations were found between RBC volume, fibrinogenemia, and RBC deformability. Eight patients with cirrhosis of the liver and eight with peripheral arterial disease were infused with polyunsaturated phosphatidylcholine [essential phospholipid (EPL), Natterman, Rome] containing 70% of linoliec acid, 2 g daily for 5 days; before and during the treatment the patients did not receive drugs or diets affecting lipid metabolism or RBC shape. Before and after the infusions the deformability and lipid composition of the RBCs were studied (Table 2). The treatment reduced the values of cholesterol/phospholipid ratio and increased the volume of erythrocyte filtered per minute in both groups of patients. The osmotic fragility of erythrocytes was little influenced by treatment and the mean corpuscular volume did not change in the patients with liver cirrhosis (from 92.0 ± 7.6 to 90.8 ± 6.4 μm³) and in patients with peripheral arterial disease (from 92.5 ± 4.7 to 91.2 ± 6.2 μm³). Both the hematocrit values and the number of reticulocytes did not change during treatment. These results demonstrate an increased filterability of RBC membranes when the cholesterol/phospholipid ratio is lowered by EPL infusions: the volume of erythrocytes filtered per minute increases without changes of other factors that are able to reduce RBC deformability (fibrinogenemia, mean corpuscular volume). The reticulocyte number was higher only in patients with liver cirrhosis and decreased after EPL infusion (from 90,180 ± 12,870 to 82,065 ± 13,680 mm³), but the change is not statistically significant. An inverse correlation between RBC deformability and the percentage of reticulocytes was found by

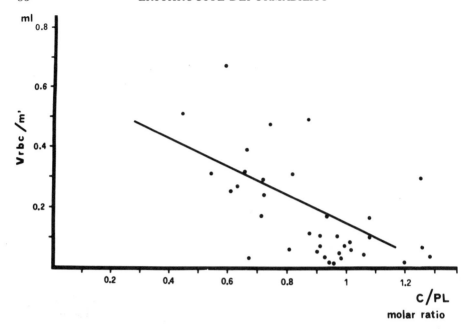

FIG. 2. Correlation between the volume of filtered RBC per minute and cholesterol/phospholipid (C/PL) molar ratio of RBC membrane. $N = 36$, $r = -0.62$.

TABLE 2. *Effect of polyunsaturated phosphatidylcholine infusion (2 g daily for 5 days) on erythrocyte deformability and cholesterol/phospholipid molar ratio (C/PL)[a]*

	Deformability		C/PL	
	Before	After	Before	After
Liver cirrhosis	0.05 ± 0.02 (0.02–0.10)	0.20 ± 0.14[b] (0.08–0.47)	1.09 ± 0.14 (0.91–1.29)	0.93 ± 0.12[b] (0.78–1.15)
Peripheral arterial disease	0.06 ± 0.03 (0.02–0.12)	0.21 ± 0.10[b] (0.09–0.35)	0.92 ± 0.11 (0.68–1.08)	0.80 ± 0.07[b] (0.72–0.91)

[a]Mean ± SD and range of the values; statistical analysis by means of paired Student's *t*-test.
[b]$p < 0.01$ between before and after treatment.

Leblond and Coulombe (20); however, the change after EPL is too low to explain the increased filterability of erythrocytes through polycarbonate membranes.

When RBC phospholipids were studied in detail, EPL infusion was found not to change phospholipid composition in patients with peripheral arterial disease, whereas the percentage of lecithin increased from 32.6 to 38.2% in patients with liver cirrhosis (Table 3). In those patients the fatty acid composition changed greatly after EPL infusion: the percentage of linoleic acid ($C_{18:2}$) rose from 15.2 to 19.1%.

TABLE 3. *Lipid composition of erythrocytes before and after essential phospholipid (EPL) infusion[a]*

		Cholesterol (mg/10^10 RBC)	Phospholipids (mg/10^10 RBC)	% of					
				PC	PE	SM	PS	LPC
PAD	Before	1.19 ± 0.12	2.62 ± 0.19	29.7 ± 2.4	29.2 ± 2.1	30.4 ± 1.8	8.7 ± 1.2	2.3 ± 0.2
	After	1.16 ± 0.15	2.95 ± 0.18	32.9 ± 2.1	28.6 ± 2.7	27.2 ± 2.5	8.8 ± 1.4	1.8 ± 0.1
LC	Before	1.48 ± 0.11	2.70 ± 0.21	32.6 ± 2.6	27.9 ± 1.4	29.1 ± 2.2	8.1 ± 1.1	1.8 ± 0.2
	After	1.40 ± 0.13	2.99 ± 0.27	38.2[b] ± 2.4	25.4 ± 1.7	27.0 ± 1.9	7.1 ± 1.4	1.6 ± 0.2

[a] Values are shown as mean ± SD. Eight patients of each group were studied (PAD, peripheral arterial disease; LC, liver cirrhosis) before and after EPL infusion (2 g daily for 5 days).
PC, phosphatidylcholine; PE, phosphatidylethanolamine; SM, sphingomyelin; PS, phosphatidylserine; LPC, lysophosphatidylcholine.
[b] $p < 0.01$.

These changes in patients with peripheral arterial disease were not statistically significant (Fig. 3).

The possibility of improving RBC morphology and of ameliorating hemolytic anemia has been demonstrated in patients with spur cell anemia receiving EPL infusions (30), in whom an increase of linoleic acid (low in the basal conditions) obtained with EPL infusions may increase membrane fluidity and prevent the effects of cholesterol excess in RBC membranes (24). With regard to the patients with peripheral arterial disease the cause of the high cholesterol/phospholipid ratio is not clear. Seven patients had hyperlipemia (five with type IV and three with type IIb) which influenced the composition of circulating membranes (32). EPL infusions reduced the ratio and increased RBC deformability. Recently, Ehrly and Blendin (10) found increased erythrocyte filtration through 8-μm filters after EPL administration in patients with peripheral arterial disease. They explained this observation

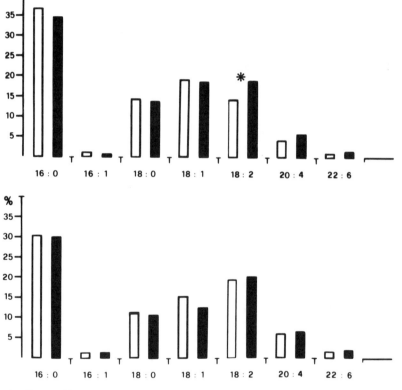

FIG. 3. Fatty acid composition of RBC lecithin in patients ($N = 8$) with liver cirrhosis **(top)** and peripheral arterial disease **(bottom)** before (□) and after (■) essential phospholipid infusion. $^{*}p < 0.01$.

by suggesting that RBC aggregation was inhibited by polyunsaturated phosphatidylcholine. In conclusion the metabolic effects of infused EPL are important in patients with liver cirrhosis and in those with peripheral arterial disease in whom HDL concentration is frequently low. Erythrocytes interact with lipoprotein via lipid exchange— above all with high-density lipoprotein (11,25), which take up and bind a high proportion of infused lecithin (18); a smaller amount is acquired by red blood cells. However, the uptake of EPL seems faster into lipoproteins (G. Salvioli, *unpublished data*) because the time course of the labeling of RBC lecithin is different with respect to lipoprotein. The specific activity of RBC lecithin is highest 9 hr after the intravenous injection of labeled EPL; whereas, the labeling of lipoprotein lecithin is greater after 1 to 2 hr. Apparently, the *in vivo* incorporation of infused lecithin in RBC membranes occurs preferentially after its incorporation in lipoproteins.

REFERENCES

1. Bartlett, G. R. (1959): Phosphorus assay in column chromatography. *J. Biol. Chem.*, 234:466–468.
2. Bloj, B., and Zilversmit, D. B. (1976): Asymmetry and transposition rates of phosphatidylcholine in rat erythrocyte ghosts. *Biochemistry*, 15:1277–1283.
3. Bloj, B., and Zilversmit, D. B. (1977): Complete exchangeability of cholesterol in phosphatidylcholine/cholesterol vesicles of different degrees of unsaturation. *Biochemistry*, 16:3943–3948.
4. Brailsford, J. D., Korpman, R. A., and Bull, B. S. (1977): The aspiration of red cell membrane into small holes: new data. *Blood Cells*, 3:25–38.
5. Chien, S., Luse, S. A., and Bryant, C. A. (1971): Hemolysis during filtration through micropores: A scanning electron microscopic and hemorheologic correlation. *Microvasc. Res.*, 3:183–203.
6. Cooper, R. A., Arner, E. C., Wiley, J. S., and Shattil, S. J. (1975): Modification of red cell membrane structure by cholesterol rich dispersions. A model for the primary spur-cell defect. *J. Clin. Invest.*, 55:115–126.
7. Cooper, R. A. (1977): Abnormalities of cell-membrane fluidity in the pathogenesis of disease. *N. Engl. J. Med.*, 297:371–377.
8. Cooper, R. A., Leslie, M. H., Knight, D., and Detweiler, D. K. (1980): Red cell cholesterol enrichment and spur cell anemia in dogs fed a cholesterol-enriched, atherogenic diet. *J. Lipid Res.*, 21:1082–1089.
9. Demel, R. A., and de Kruiff, B. (1976): The function of sterols in membranes. *Biochim. Biophys. Acta*, 457:109–132.
10. Ehrly, A. M., and Blendin, R. (1976): Influence of essential phospholipids on the flow properties of the blood. In: *Phosphatidylcholine*, edited by H. Peters, pp. 228–236. Springer-Verlag, Berlin.
11. Giraud, F., and Claret, M. (1979): A study of cholesterol transfer between erythrocytes and plasma lipoproteins. *FEBS Lett.*, 103:186–191.
12. Gottlieb, M. H. (1980): Rates of cholesterol exchange between human erythrocytes and plasma lipoproteins. *Biochim. Biophys. Acta*, 600:530–541.
13. Groner, W., Mohandas, N., and Bessis, M. (1980): New optical technique for measuring erythrocyte deformability with the ektacytometer. *Clin. Chem.*, 26:1435–1442.
14. Hirata, F., Viveros, H. O., Diliberto, E. J., Jr., and Axelrod, J. (1978): Identification and properties of two methyl transferases in conversion of phosphatidylethanolamine to phosphatidylcholine. *Proc. Natl. Acad. Sci. USA*, 75:1718–1721.
15. Hui, D. Y., and Harmony, J. A. K. (1979): Interaction of plasma lipoproteins with erythrocytes. I. Alteration of erythrocyte morphology. *Biochim. Biophys Acta*, 550:407–424.
16. Hui, D. Y., and Harmony, J. A. K. (1979): Interaction of plasma lipoproteins with erythroycytes. II. Modulation of membrane associated enzymes. *Biochim. Biophys. Acta*, 550:425–434.
17. Jandl, J. H. (1955): The anemia in liver disease: Observation on its mechanism. *J. Clin. Invest.*, 34:390–403.

18. Krupp, L., Chobanian, A. V., and Brecher, P. I. (1976): The in vivo transformation of phospholipid vesicles to a particle resembling HDL in rat. Biochim. Biophys. Res. Commun., 72:1251–1257.

19. La Celle, P. L. (1980): Behaviour of abnormal erythrocytes in capillaries. In: Erythrocytes Mechanics and Blood Flow, edited by G. R. Cokelet, H. J. Meiselman, and D. E. Brooks, pp. 195–209. Alan R. Liss, New York.

20. Leblond, P. F., and Coulombe, L. (1979): The measurement of erythrocyte deformability using micropore membranes. A sensitive technique with clinical applications. J. Lab. Clin. Invest., 94:133–143.

21. Leonhardt, N., Arntz, N. R., and Klemens, U. N. (1977): Studies of plasma viscosity in primary hyperlipoproteinemia. Atherosclerosis, 28:29–40.

22. McMillan, D. E. (1980): Reduced erythrocyte deformability and vascular pathology. In: Erythrocyte Mechanics and Blood Flow, edited by G. R. Cokelet, H. J. Meiselman, and D. E. Brooks, pp. 211–228. Alan R. Liss, New York.

23. Mombers, C., Verkleij, A. J., De Gier, J., and Van Deenen, L. L. M. (1979): The interaction of spectrin-actin and synthetic phospholipids. II. The interaction with phosphatidylserine. Biochim. Biophys. Acta, 551:271–281.

24. Papahadjoupoulos, D. (1974): Cholesterol and cell membrane function: A hypothesis concerning the ethiology of atherosclerosis. J. Theor. Biol., 43:329–337.

25. Quarfordt, S. H., and Hilderman, H. L. (1970): Quantitation of the in vitro free cholesterol exchange of human red cells and lipoproteins. J. Lipid Res., 11:528–535.

26. Reed, C. F. (1968): Phospholipid exchange between plasma and erythrocytes in man and in the dog. J. Clin. Invest., 47:749–760.

27. Reid, H. L., Barnes, A. J., Lock, P. J., and Dormandy, T. L. (1976): A simple method for measuring erythrocyte deformability. J. Clin. Pathol., 29:855–858.

28. Reid, H. L., Dormandy, J. A., Barnes, A. J., Lock, P. J., and Dormandy, T. L. (1976): Impaired red cell deformability in peripheral vascular disease. Lancet, i:666–668.

29. Robins, S. J., and Miller, A. (1974): Red cell cholesterol depletion and the formation of spiculated cells in vivo. J. Clin. Lab. Invest., 83:436–443.

30. Salvioli, G., Rioli, G., Lugli, R., and Salati, R. (1978): Membrane lipid composition of red blood cells in liver disease: regression of spur cell anemia after infusion of polyunsaturated phosphatidylcholine. Gut, 19:844–850.

31. Schmid-Schönbein, H., and Wells, R. (1969): Fluid drop-like transition of erythrocytes under shear. Science, 155:288–291.

32. Shattil, S. J., Bennet, J. S., Colman, R. W., and Cooper, R. A. (1977): Abnormalities of cholesterol-phospholipid composition in platelets and low density lipoproteins of human hyperbetalipoproteinemia. J. Lab. Clin. Invest., 89:341–353.

33. Sheetz, M. P. (1980): The bilayer and the shell model of the erythrocyte membrane. In: Erythrocyte Mechanics and Blood Flow, edited by G. R. Cokelet, H. J. Meiselman, and D. E. Brooks, pp. 1–13. Alan R. Liss, New York.

34. Shiga, T., Maeda, N., Suda, T., Korr, K., Sekiya, M., and Oka, S. (1979): Rheological and kinetic dysfunctions of the cholesterol-loaded human erythrocytes. Biorheology, 16:363–369.

35. Smith, J. E., Mohandas, N., and Shohet, S. B. (1979): Variability in erythrocyte deformability among various mammals. Am. J. Physiol., 236:H725–H730.

36. Teitel, P. (1967): Corrélations entre les caractéristique microrhéologiques (filterabilité) des globules rouges et leur séquestration splenique et hepatique. Nouv. Rev. Franc. Hématol., 7:321–338.

37. Verkleij, A. J., Zwaal, R. F. A., Roelofsen, B., Comfurius, P., Kastelijn, D., and Van Deenen, L. L. M. (1973): The asymmetric distribution of phospholipids in the human red cell: membrane. A combined study using phospholipase and freezy-etch electron microscopy. Biochim. Biophys. Acta, 323:178–193.

38. Yeh, S. C., Mitzuguchi, T., and Kummerow, F. A. (1974): Effect of dietary fat on the release of cholesterol from swine erythrocytes. Proc. Soc. Exp. Biol. Med., 146:236–240.

Phospholipids and Atherosclerosis, edited by
P. Avogaro, M. Mancini, G. Ricci, and
R. Paoletti. Raven Press, New York © 1983.

Phospholipids in Serum Lipoproteins

Angelo M. Scanu

*Departments of Medicine and Biochemistry, The University of Chicago
Pritzker School of Medicine, Chicago, Illinois 60637*

Phosphoglycerides, commonly referred to as phospholipids, are major components of cell membranes and circulating lipoproteins (13,19,21). Characteristically,
because of their amphiphilic structure, they will organize into various types of
aggregates when exposed to aqueous solutions. A phospholipid molecule has an
amphiphilic nature because it contains a strong hydrophilic head group and two
long apolar hydrocarbon chains; lyso derivatives have only one hydrocarbon chain.
Phosphatidylcholine (PC) and sphingomyelin (SP) are usually major components
of biological structures, such as lipoproteins; minor constituents comprise phosphatidylserine (PS), phosphatidylinositol (PI), phosphatidylethanolamine (PE), and
glycosphingolipids (GSL). Both PC and PE at neutral pH have a zwitterionic head
group; whereas, PS and PI bear a net negative charge. In the case of GSL, the
polar properties depend on the nature of the carbohydrate moiety. The fatty acid
chains are usually 16 carbon atoms long although species up to 24 carbon atoms
are also present. With the diacylphospholipids it is common to see an almost equal
distribution between saturated and unsaturated fatty acids occupying the R_1 and R_2
positions, respectively. Like any other amphiphilic molecule, the solubility of phospholipids in water depends on the balance between hydrophilic and hydrophobic
groups. In general, phospholipids form micellar structures, where the hydrophobic
portion segregates into an inner core permitting the polar head group to be in contact
with the outside solvent. According to the thermodynamic treatment of the process
of micelle formation proposed by Tanford (27), the structure of an amphiphile in
water can be predicted from its chemical composition. Although micelles can be
of different shapes—spheres; discoidal, oblate, or prolate ellipsoids; long cylin-
ders—for the purpose of this discussion analyses will be limited to two types of
structures: phospholipids arranged in a planar, single bilayer sheet or as a unilamellar
sealed vesicle. In the planar bilayer arrangement, the amphiphilic head groups of
the phospholipids are tightly packed, as in biological membranes; in turn, the curved
surface of the vesicles permits a greater separation between the phospholipid head
groups. It should also be evident that the number of phospholipid molecules in the
outward half of the bilayer of a unilamellar vesicle is significantly larger than that

in the inner monolayer. Phospholipids can form mixed vesicles with unesterified cholesterol. The surface of these vesicles accommodate amphiphilic proteins, such as those from plasma apolipoproteins. To a certain extent cholesterol-containing phospholipid vesicles when associated with apolipoproteins mimic the structure of a serum lipoprotein, and thus these vesicles serve as useful models for the study of lipoprotein structure. When amphiphilic molecules, such as phospholipids, aggregate into a micellar structure and reach critical micellar concentrations, the constituent molecules in the micelle are in equilibrium with the unassociated or monomer form of the amphiphile. For the predominant types of molecules representing the phospholipids of biological structures, namely two long hydrocarbon chains per head group, the concentration of monomers in solution is extremely small, on the order of 7×10^{-6} to 4.7×10^{-10} moles/liter.

To sum up, phospholipids, because of their chemical characteristics and amphiphilic nature, form predictable aggregates in aqueous solutions where the polar head groups are exposed to the external solvent shielding, with the apolar fatty acid chains away from the aqueous environment. Although predicted from the *in vitro* study of model systems, aggregated structures of phospholipids have biological relevance, as shown through animal experimentation and clinical conditions. Thus, an understanding of the behavior of phospholipids in aqueous solution provides an insight into the structure and metabolism of plasma lipoproteins.

PRINCIPLES OF LIPOPROTEIN STRUCTURE

One of the characteristics of circulating lipoproteins, contrary to the structures discussed in the previous section, is that they contain a relatively large amount of nonpolar lipids, either triglycerides or cholesteryl esters (13,19,21). The triglyceride-rich particles, namely chylomicrons and very low-density lipoprotein (VLDL), at the time of their secretion into the circulation, appear to have the overall structural organization of a mature lipoprotein particle (7). On the other hand, as suggested from studies on liver perfusates containing inhibitors of the enzyme lecithin-cholesterol acyltransferase (LCAT) or on patients with the familial congenital deficiency of this enzyme, the newly secreted nascent high-density lipoprotein (HDL) is a discoidal structure characterized by a bilayer of phospholipid and some unesterified cholesterol peripherally bounded by apoproteins, particularly apo A-I and apo E. These bilayer structures are thought to be suitable substrates for LCAT, which by converting unesterified cholesterol into esterified cholesterol will transform the mixed bilayer into the structure characteristic of all mature plasma lipoproteins. Despite the great diversity in size, density, and chemical composition, all lipoproteins recognize a common underlying structure, which can be inferred from compositional analyses (5,24). All lipoproteins can be considered to conform with a spherical model with a liquid core of cholesteryl esters and triglycerides having a radius of 20.2 Å. This is surrounded by a monolayer of phospholipids and unesterified cholesterol; the former have their hydrophobic ends closely packed on the surface of the core. According to this model, protein and head groups of phospholipids are at the outer surface of the particle and occupy an area of 62.7 and 15.6Å^2/molecule, respectively. Phospholipids play an important structural role by ensuring the interaction of the particle with the aqueous environment via their head groups and by contributing to the particle internal stability through the hydrophobic boundary between the tails of the hydrocarbon chains and the hydrophobic core. Moreover, phospholipids are expected to solubilize the cholesterol molecules located within the surface polar monolayer of the particle and interact with the apoproteins. A model of this kind must have a great deal of fluidity in order to permit each lipoprotein component to exchange with other lipoproteins or membranes. It also predicts that any increase in HDL size must be attended by a proportional increment of the nonpolar and polar components if the same overall geometry is to be maintained. A similar consideration applies for the lipoproteins of the VLDL and the low-density lipoprotein (LDL) classes.

INTERACTION BETWEEN PLASMA APOPROTEINS, VESICLES, AND LIPOPROTEINS

Since phospholipid vesicles can be defined in terms of their physical and chemical properties, they have become a useful model for the study of the interaction of phospholipids with plasma apolipoproteins. These studies have been facilitated by the knowledge of the primary structure of these apolipoproteins and of their behavior in aqueous solutions (13,14,16,20). Apoproteins appear to have structural features in common, namely various lengths of amphiphilic helices having a polar and an apolar surface which permit these apoproteins to interact with amphiphiles, such as phospholipids. The binding of apoproteins with phospholipids has been amply documented, particularly using phospholipid vesicles in the absence and presence of cholesterol. These studies have shown that apoprotein-phospholipid interactions depend on several factors: (a) nature and concentration of the reactants, (b) stoichiometry, (c) temperature, (d) pH and ionic strength, and (e) length of incubation time. The resulting recombinants can be isolated by ultracentrifugation or chromatographic procedures, or by both and shown to represent either vesicular or planar bilayer discoidal structures soluble in water. The properties of these complexes principally depend on the initial stoichiometry of the reactants. For instance, it can be shown that by using mixed PC/cholesterol vesicles of a molar ratio of 4:1, the interaction with human apo A-I is not attended by any disruption of the vesicular structure if the uptake of the apoprotein by the vesicle surface does not surpass seven to eight molecules per vesicle (4,22). This number of molecules is one that allows for maximal occupancy of the area of the vesicle surface in between the polar head groups of phospholipids. If more apoproteins are added to the system, the overall detergency capacity of the apo A-I molecule now disrupts the vesicles. This generates planar discoidal structures corresponding in thickness to the width of a phospholipid bilayer and defined in size by the number of bound apo A-I molecules.

The same principles derived from the study of the interaction between apoproteins, such as apo A-I and apo A-II, and phospholipid vesicles would seem to also apply to the interaction of apoproteins with naturally occurring lipoprotein particles. Recently, Lagocki and Scanu (11) have studied the interaction of human apo A-II with canine HDL, a particle containing essentially only apo A-I (three molecules per particle). When the studies were carried out either at 4° or 27°C, there was a progressive displacement of canine apo A-I by human apo A-II without loss of lipid until the apo A-I was totally displaced. At this point the HDL particles contained essentially only apo A-II (six molecules of apo A-II per particle). However, if human apo A-II was added in excess, canine HDL was disrupted and the new heterogenous structures generated were no longer identifiable with the initial HDL particle. These phenomena can be explained by the greater affinity of apo A-II relative to apo A-I for the HDL surface as indicated from studies using artificial amphiphilic systems (23). Two implications of these studies in regard to HDL are that apoproteins and phospholipids do not interact strongly and that the surface concentration of apoproteins is modulated by the relative affinity of the apoproteins for the lipoprotein surface.

INTERACTION BETWEEN VESICLES AND LIPOPROTEINS WITH PARTICULAR REFERENCE TO HDL

The structural similarities of their surfaces permits an analysis of interactions between phospholipids and lipoproteins, as indicated by the studies which have been recently reviewed (26). Overall, these interactions lead to structural changes of the reactants. For instance, *in vitro* incubation of HDL with synthetic multilamellar liposomes of dipalmitoyl lecithin is attended by the clearing of the initially turbid lipid suspension, owing to the breakdown of the liposomes into bilayer structures containing the apo A-I molecules released from HDL; the resulting HDL has now more apo A-II and phospholipids, the latter being transferred from the liposomes into the HDL surface. Transfer of phospholipids into HDL has also been shown to occur when unilamellar vesicles of egg yolk or rat liver lecithin are incubated with plasma. Transfer is influenced by reactant stoichiometry, time of incubation, and temperature. Depending upon the amount of phospholipids reaching the HDL surface, this lipoprotein can either remain relatively unaltered (HDL can be envisioned as accepting only a small amount of phospholipid without significant alterations in its geometry except, perhaps, for some changes in apoprotein conformation) or can be disrupted as a consequence of the progressive loss of its major amphiphile apo A-I.

A similar transfer process has been shown to occur between the phospholipids of the artificial fat emulsion Intralipid and HDL (R. Weinberg and A. M. Scanu, *unpublished*) leading to changes in lipoprotein density. Thus, regardless of the source of phospholipids, either from a naturally occurring source or from artificial particles, HDL can act as an acceptor of the released phospholipids up to a saturation point, above which the excess phospholipid organizes into vesicular structures. A phospholipid transfer process of this kind can be clearly shown by subjecting triglyceride-rich particles to the hydrolysis by lipoprotein lipase. The reduction in core volume owing to triglyceride cleavage results in the formation of phospholipid bilayer buds which then dislodge and reach the HDL surface. This process has been postulated to occur *in vivo* as a part of the degradation of chylomicrons and VLDL particles.

PHOSPHOLIPIDS, LIPOPROTEINS, AND LIPID MODIFYING ENZYMES

In vitro studies have shown that the phospholipids present at the surface of serum lipoproteins are readily accessible to the action of phospholipases. Particularly well studied has been the action of venom phospholipase A_2 against human LDL (1) and HDL_3 (15) indicating that all of the phospholipids except for sphingomyelin (nonhydrolyzed by phospholipase A_2) are cleaved into their lyso derivatives and fatty acids in the presence of albumin, which acts as a product acceptor. The presence of a phospholipase A_2 enzyme has not been documented in human plasma although the heparin-releasable lipoprotein lipase has a phospholipase A-I action of a yet undetermined physiological importance (12). The first step in the activity of the enzyme LCAT is a phospholipase-A_2-type reaction except that the unsaturated fatty acid, which is released from the C-2 position of the phospholipid, is transferred to the hydroxyl function of cholesterol rather than into the aqueous environment. The actual mechanism for this fatty acid transferase reaction is not known except that it requires apo A-I as a cofactor (phospholipase A_2 has no apoprotein cofactor requirement) and a substrate molar ratio of lecithin/cholesterol of 3:1 to 4:1 (6). The specific requirement of apo A-I for the LCAT action is supported by the recent observation that the inhibition by apo A-II of the LCAT reaction is related to the capacity of this apoprotein to displace apo A-I from the HDL surface (22). The importance of the LCAT reaction in transferring nascent HDL into mature particles is well recognized. The recent development of methods for the immunoquantification of LCAT is expected to shed greater light on the mechanisms of this enzyme's action and its regulation (2,3).

PHOSPHOLIPIDS AND INTERACTIONS WITH CELL SURFACE

Phospholipids and, in particular, lipoprotein phospholipids are also involved in interactions with cell membranes although these interactions have not been clearly defined. Exchange and transfer processes would ensure equilibration of phospholipids between lipoprotein and cell membranes and facilitate the movement of cholesterol from cellular membranes to plasma. All of these processes may be accounted for by the physiochemical makeup of the reactants; however, they may also recognize the participation of specific phospholipid exchange proteins, which have been elegantly shown to play a fundamental role in the intracellular transport of phospholipids (29,30). Also, recent data on the *in vitro* interaction between HDL_3 and polymorphonuclear cells (17) suggest that phospholipids may have an additional specific role in lipoprotein-cell interactions via their transformation into lysophosphatides, probably through the action of a membrane-bound phospholipase. The generation of these lysophosphatides may initiate all biochemical events related to the lipoprotein-dependent regulation of cell metabolism (18). If so, this reaction may be tightly coupled with the process of lysophosphatide reacylation occurring at the cellular level.

CONCLUSIONS

Phospholipids play a major role in the structure of plasma lipoproteins and their metabolism. However, there are still many unknowns which should attract the attention for future research. For instance, there is no knowledge about the function of the minor phospholipid components in lipoproteins and, in particular, sphingomyelin, phosphatidylethanolamine, and phosphatidylinositol. Neither is there a clear insight into their metabolic regulation. Of the phospholipid-modifying enzymes acting in plasma much of our understanding is, at present, confined to LCAT; yet recent studies have provided evidence for a phospholipase action of lipoprotein lipase (12) and hepatic lipase (8,9,28). A reverse LCAT reaction requiring LDL as a cofactor has recently been reported (25), and this observation should bring new leads for understanding the role played by lysophosphatides in lipoprotein metabolism. Phospholipids are at the center of the interactions between lipoproteins and lipid-modifying enzymes, and probably between lipoproteins and cells as well. Important in the latter regard is the very recent observation that HDL_3 can modulate the synthesis and secretion of glycosphingolipids in cultured skin fibroblasts (10). More information is needed on how phospholipids may modulate the interplay between lipoproteins and metabolic events within the cell. The possibility that membrane-bound phospholipases participate in these events also needs exploration.

ACKNOWLEDGMENT

This work was supported by United States Public Health Grant HL-18577.

REFERENCES

1. Aggerbeck, L., Kézdy, F. J., and Scanu, A. M. (1976): Enzymatic probes of lipoprotein structure: Hydrolysis of human serum low-density lipoprotein-2 by phospholipase A_2. *J. Biol. Chem.*, 251:3823–3830.
2. Albers, J., Adolphson, J. L., and Chen, C. H. (1981): Radioimmunoassay of human plasma lecithin-cholesterol acyl transferase. *J. Clin. Invest.*, 67:141–148.
3. Chung, J., Abano, D., and Scanu, A. M. (1981): Mass-activity distribution of lecithin:cholesterol acyl transferase in plasma lipoproteins of human plasma. *Fed. Proc. (in press)*.
4. Chung, J., Abano, D. A., Fless, G. M., and Scanu, A. M. (1979): Isolation, properties and mechanism of in vitro action of lecithin-cholesterol acyl transferase. *J. Biol. Chem.*, 254:7456–7464.
5. Edelstein, C., Kézdy, F. J., Scanu, A. M., and Shen, B. W. (1979): Apolipoproteins and the structural organization of plasma lipoproteins—human plasma lipoprotein-3. *J. Lipid Res.*, 20:143–153.
6. Glomset, J. A. (1979): Lecithin-cholesterol acyl transferase. In: *The Biochemistry of Atherosclerosis*, edited by A. M. Scanu, R. W. Wissler, and G. S. Getz, pp. 247–273. Marcel Dekker, New York.
7. Havel, R. J. (1980): Lipoprotein biosynthesis and metabolism. *Ann. NY Acad. Sci.*, 348:16–27.
8. Jansen, H., and Hulsmann, W. C. (1980): Heparin-releasable (liver) lipase(s) may play a role in the uptake of cholesterol by steroid-secreting tissues. *Trends Biochem. Sci.*, 5:265–268.

9. Kussi, T., Saarinen, L., and Nikkila, E. A. (1980): Evidence for the role of hepatic endothelial lipase in the metabolism of plasma high density lipoprotein in humans. *Atherosclerosis*, 36:589–593.

10. Kwok, B. C. R., Dawson, G., and Ritter, M. C. (1981): Stimulation of glycolipid synthesis and exchange by human serum high density lipoprotein-3 in human fibroblasts and leukocytes. *J. Biol. Chem.*, 256:92–98.

11. Lagocki, P., and Scanu, A. M. (1980): In vitro modulation of the apolipoprotein composition of high density lipoprotein-displacement of apolipoprotein A-I from HDL by apolipoprotein A-II. *J. Biol. Chem.*, 255:3701–3706.

12. Nilsson Ehle, P., Garfinkel, A. S., and Schotz, M. C. (1980): Lipolytic enzymes and plasma lipoprotein metabolism. *Annu. Rev. Biochem.*, 49:667–693.

13. Osborne, J. C., Jr., and Brewer, H. B., Jr. (1977): The plasma lipoproteins. *Adv. Protein Chem.*, 31:253–337.

14. Osborne, J. C., and Brewer, B. H. (1980): Solution properties of the plasma lipoproteins. *Ann. NY Acad. Sci.*, 348:104–120.

15. Pattnaik, N. M., Kézdy, F. J., and Scanu, A. M. (1976): Kinetic study of the action of snake venom phospholipase A₂ on human serum high density lipoprotein-3. *J. Biol. Chem.*, 251:1984–1990.

16. Pownall, H. J., Jackson, R. L., Morrisett, J. D., and Gotto, A. M., Jr. (1979): Structure and dynamics of re-assembled plasma lipoproteins. In: *The Biochemistry of Atherosclerosis*, edited by A. M. Scanu, R. W. Wissler, and G. S. Getz, pp. 123–143. Marcel Dekker, New York.

17. Ritter, M. C., and Scanu, A. M. (1980): Structural changes in human serum high density lipoprotein-3 attending incubation with blood leukocytes. *J. Biol. Chem.*, 255:3763–3769.

18. Scanu, A. M. (1976): Phospholipases as structural and functional probes for circulating lipoproteins. In: *Structure of Biological Membranes*, edited by S. Abrahamson and I. Pascher, pp. 427–441. Plenum Press, New York.

19. Scanu, A. M. (1979): Plasma lipoproteins: An introduction. In: *The Biochemistry of Atherosclerosis*, edited by A. M. Scanu, R. W. Wissler, and G. S. Getz, pp. 3–8. Marcel Dekker, New York.

20. Scanu, A. M., and Teng, T. L. (1979): Apolipoproteins of plasma lipoproteins: behavior in solution. In: *The Biochemistry of Atherosclerosis*, edited by A. M. Scanu, R. W. Wissler, and G. S. Getz, pp. 107–121. Marcel Dekker, New York.

21. Scanu, A. M., and Landsberger, F., eds. (1980): Lipoprotein structure. *Ann. NY Acad. Sci.*, 348:1–436.

22. Scanu, A. M., Lagocki, P., and Chung, J. (1980): Effect of apolipoprotein A-II on the structure of high density lipoproteins: relationship to the activity of lecithin: cholesterol acyl transferase in vitro. *Ann. NY Acad. Sci.*, 348:160–171.

23. Shen, B. W.: Solid water interface as model for apolipoprotein: lipid interactions: absorption of human apo high density lipoprotein to amphiphilic interfaces *(submitted for publication)*.

24. Shen, B. W., Scanu, A. M., and Kézdy, F. J. (1977): The structure of serum lipoprotein inferred from compositional analysis. *Proc. Natl. Acad. Sci. USA*, 76:837–841.

25. Subbaiah, P. V., Albers, J. J., Chen, H. C., and Bagdade, J. D. (1980): Low density lipoprotein-activated lysolecithin acylation by human plasma lecithin-cholesterol acyltransferase. Identify of lysolecithin acyltransferase and lecithin-cholesterol acyltransferase. *J. Biol. Chem.*, 255:9275–9280.

26. Tall, A. R., and Small, D. M. (1980): Body cholesterol removal: Role of plasma high-density lipoproteins. *Adv. Lipid. Res.*, 17:1–51.

27. Tanford, C. (1980): *The Hydrophobic Effect*, pp. 1–233. John Wiley, New York.

28. Van Tol, A., Van Gent, T., and Jansen, H. (1980): Degradation of high density lipoprotein by heparin-releasable liver lipase. *Biochem. Biophys. Res. Commun.*, 94:101–108.

29. Wirtz, K. W. A. (1976): Transfer of phospholipids between membranes. *Biochim. Biophys. Acta*, 346:95–117.

30. Wirtz, K. W. A., Moonen, P., Van Deenen, L. L. M., Radhakrishnan, R., and Khorana, H. G. (1981): Identification of the lipid binding site of the phosphatidyl exchange protein with a photosensitive nitrene and carbene precursor of phosphatidylcholine. *Ann. NY Acad. Sci.*, 348:244–255.

Phospholipids and Atherosclerosis, edited by
P. Avogaro, M. Mancini, G. Ricci, and
R. Paoletti. Raven Press, New York © 1983.

Structure and Function of Plasma Lipoproteins

Henry J. Pownall and Antonio M. Gotto, Jr.

Department of Medicine, Baylor College of Medicine, and The Methodist Hospital,
Houston, Texas 77030

The plasma lipoproteins are a group of macromolecules in the blood that perform numerous tasks related to lipid metabolism (16,25). They are defined according to the density at which they are isolated as high-, low-, and very low-density lipoproteins (HDL, LDL, and VLDL, respectively). A fourth class comprises the chylomicrons, a lipoprotein secreted by the intestine following a dietary fat load. The lipoproteins are not discrete particles but rather form a continuum of densities, sizes, and compositions extending from chylomicrons to HDL (Table 1). In particular, the HDL distribution is bimodal and two quasi-discrete subclasses, HDL_2 and HDL_3, have been isolated. The protein composition also differs with respect to the identity of the lipoprotein class although a given protein, an apolipoprotein as they are usually designated, may appear in more than one class. The distribution and the molecular weights of each of the apoproteins are given in Table 2.

There is no definitive evidence, such as X-ray diffraction, to provide unequivocal support for the structure of the plasma lipoproteins. However, collective consid-

TABLE 1. *Protein and lipid composition of the major lipoprotein classes*[a]

	HDL_3	HDL_2	LDL	IDL	VLDL	Chylomicrons
Protein	55	40	22	19	8	2
Phospholipids	25	33	22	19	18	7
Cholesterol	4	5	8	9	7	2
Cholesteryl esters	13	17	42	29	12	3
Triglycerides	3	5	6	23	55	86
Density (g/cc)	1.15	1.09	1.035	1.012	0.97	0.93
Radius (nm)	3.9	5.1	9.6	15	20	60

[a]HDL, high-density lipoprotein; LDL, low-density lipoprotein; IDL, intermediate density lipoprotein; VLDL, very low-density lipoprotein.
From Shen et al. (41), with permission.

TABLE 2. *Apoprotein content of major lipoprotein classes[a]*

Apoprotein[b]	HDL	LDL	VLDL	Chylomicrons
A-I (28,400)	64	nil	nil	7
A-II (17,400)	20	nil	nil	5
B (255,000)		95	63	19
C-I (6,600)	6	nil	1	11
C-II (8,700)	1	nil	4	15
C-III (8,700)	4	nil	25	41
E (35,000)	2	<5	14	?
D (22,000)	3	nil	nil	nil

[a]HDL, high-density lipoprotein; LDL, low-density lipoprotein; VLDL, very low-density lipoprotein.
[b]Molecular weights given in parentheses do not include the carbohydrate.
From Havel et al. (16), with permission.

eration of a large body of physical data has led to a general model of all lipoproteins, in which the polar components (phospholipids, cholesterol, and protein) form a monolayer around a spherical core of the neutral lipids (triglyceride and cholesteryl esters) (10,38,41,52). This arrangement is depicted in Fig. 1 for HDL_2 and HDL_3, neither of which has enough neutral lipids to form a separate "core" phase. In contrast VLDL and LDL have triglyceride-rich and cholesteryl ester-rich cores, respectively. Calorimetric and X-ray studies have provided evidence that the neutral lipids of intact LDL, exclusive of the polar components, are confined to a separate (core) region of the particle (8,9,42).

Although solubilization of lipid is an important function of all of the apolipoproteins, many of them have other roles related to lipid metabolism (Table 3) (16,25). This includes the activation of two key enzymes of lipid metabolism. One of these is lecithin-cholesterol acyltransferase (LCAT). This enzyme catalyzes the formation of nearly all plasma cholesteryl esters and is activated by apo A-I and apo C-I. Lipoprotein lipase, which hydrolyzes the triglyceride of VLDL and chylomicrons, is activated by apo C-II. Not surprisingly, all of these activators appear in those lipoproteins that are the putative substrates for the enzymes that they activate; HDL is a substrate for LCAT, and VLDL and chylomicrons are substrates for lipoprotein lipase. These enzymes form the cornerstone of any rational consideration of the distribution of apoproteins and lipids among lipoprotein classes since they catalyze the irreversible breaking and forming of covalent bonds. As a consequence, major changes in lipoprotein stability leading to further changes in structure via lipid or protein transfer are observed. Some of these are spontaneous, whereas specific plasma factors for cholesteryl ester, triglyceride, and phospholipid transfer have been identified (5,6,12).

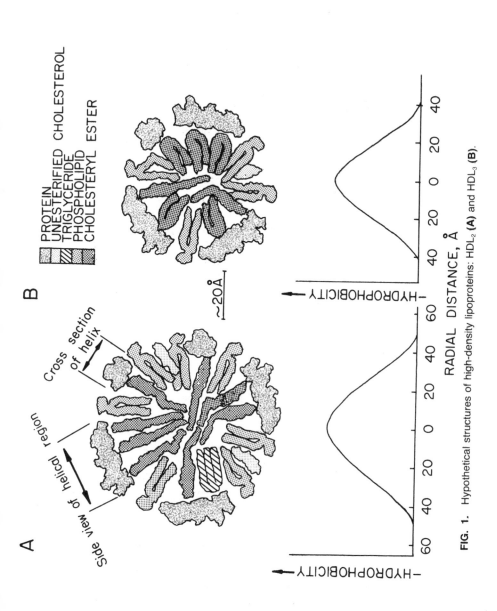

FIG. 1. Hypothetical structures of high-density lipoproteins: HDL$_2$ **(A)** and HDL$_3$ **(B)**.

TABLE 3. *Proposed physiological roles of*
plasma apolipoproteins

Apolipoprotein	Function[a]
apo A-I	LCAT Activator
apo A-II	Hepatic lipase activator
apo C-I	LCAT Activator
apo C-II	Lipoprotein lipase activator
apo E	Focus of receptor-mediated uptake
apo B	Focus of receptor-mediated uptake
apo D	Cholesteryl ester transfer protein

[a]LCAT, lecithin:cholesterol acyltransferase.
From Havel et al. (16), with permission.

APOLIPOPROTEIN STRUCTURE AND PROPERTIES

A large number of studies on the structure and behavior of the human plasma apolipoproteins has led to refinement of the molecular theory first proposed by Segrest et al. (39). All of the water-soluble apoproteins sequenced and studied to date appear to fit the model of a polypeptide chain that can form alpha helixes in which polar and nonpolar faces are formed. In dilute solutions or in presence of denaturants, such as guanidine hydrochloride, the apoproteins are monomeric. In the absence of denaturants and at sufficiently high concentrations, the apoproteins self-associate. Concomitant with this self-association, the polypeptide chain converts from a random chain to one with increased α-helical content. This process is driven by hydrophobic effects; presumably the nonpolar sides of the helical segments are in contact with each other.

Since the appearance of the original paper describing what is now referred to as "the amphipathic helical theory" of apolipoprotein structure, several other apolipoproteins have been sequenced and their solution properties documented (39); these include apo A-I, apo A-II, apo C-I, apo C-II, and a reduced carboxymethylated apo A-II (4,11,23,27,34,40,49,51). All of these apoproteins self-associate and possess multiple amphipathic helical regions.

REASSEMBLY OF LIPOPROTEINS

A number of techniques have been used to achieve the partial and total reassembly of plasma lipoproteins. This includes simple mixing or co-sonication of lipids and proteins. More recently, detergent removal techniques have emerged as a successful method where simple mixing fails and sonication must be avoided.

Ritter and Scanu studied the reassembly of apo A-I (36) and apo A-II (37) with total HDL lipids using sonication. Simple incubation will lead to some lipid-protein association, but sonication is required for maximal incorporation. Both apo A-I and apo A-II gave a heterogeneous mixture of lipid-protein complexes; the reaction is most efficient when the apoproteins are monomeric. The circular dichroic spectra of lipid complexes of apo A-I and apo A-II were consistent with a higher helical content relative to that of the apoproteins in aqueous solutions. Similar results were obtained by Assmann and Brewer who, in addition, suggested that apo A-I and apo A-II associate differently with sphingomyelin and lecithin (1). In their studies, no co-sonication lipid and protein was employed, but the yield of complexes was poor and in some cases was less than 20%.

Subsequent reassembly studies have focused on the thermodynamics and mechanism of lipid-protein association, and for many of these a simpler system, typically a single protein and lipid, was used. Many of these studies utilized apo A-I because of its abundance and dimyristoyl phosphatidylcholine (DMPC), a synthetic lecithin, which has a gel → liquid crystalline phase transition (T_c) at 23.9°C. The spontaneous association of apo A-I with DMPC has been reported in a number of laboratories (18,20,30,47,50). The molecular weight of the complex is between 200,000 and 400,000 with the lipid to protein ratio increasing as the initial ratio of lipid to protein is raised. By electron microscopy the complexes have the appearance of a bilayer disc; the structure proposed is that of a helical apoprotein lying along the circumference of the disc as shown in Fig. 2A (50). In fluorescence depolarization studies (20) and differential scanning calorimetry (13,50), the usually sharp thermal phase transition (T_c) of DMPC is slightly elevated and significantly broadened in the complex. That the transition is retained means that the complex must retain its essential bilayer arrangement. Neutron scattering (53) and X-ray (2) studies are

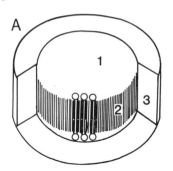

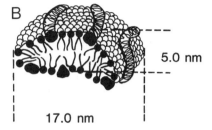

FIG. 2. **A:** Model of reassembled apo A-I/lecithin complex according to Tall et al. (49). **B:** Model of an apo C-I/DMPC complex according to Laggner et al. (21).

consistent with this assignment. Raman spectroscopy (13) has shown that the physical state of DMPC within the complex differs from that of pure lipid. Relative to pure lipid, there is less lateral order among the acyl chains in the complexes below T_c, but above T_c the interactions in the complexes and the pure lipid are indistinguishable. Compared to pure liposomes, DMPC in apo A-I/DMPC complexes has more acyl chain trans isomers between 24° and 30°C; above 30°C the trans isomer content of complexes and liposomes is approximately equal. Within the complex the protein structure is also modified when compared to the apoproteins in solution. Raman data indicate the immobilization of the hydrocarbon side chains. Potentiometric data indicate that within the complex, the charged residues are accessible to the aqueous phase and titrate abnormally, suggesting that they are partially masked.

Of the apo C proteins only the lipid binding of apo C-III has been studied in detail. Apo C-III associates with DMPC at or above T_c (53). As a consequence the helical content of the apoprotein is increased from ~25% to greater than 80%; the thermal behavior of the complexes, as assessed by electron spin resonance (ESR) and fluorescence, indicates that the hydrocarbon region undergoes a phase transition that is elevated and broadened relative to that of pure DMPC (26). The ESR data suggest that within the complex the acyl chain motion is greatly restricted by the presence of protein. Thus, in many ways, the structure is not very different from that of DMPC/apo A-I complexes. However, the X-ray data of Laggner et al. (21) and others (3) have led to a proposed structure that is different in one respect: rather than having all of the protein on the edge of a bilayer disk, the complex is represented as an oblate ellipsoid in which the apoprotein is randomly associated with the particle surface. The appearance is similar to that of a flattened micelle (Fig. 2B).

Apo C-III also forms a vesicular complex with some lecithins (3,24). Aune et al. reported that at low apo C-III to egg lecithin ratios, the complex had the architecture of a single-bilayer vesicle with the apoprotein presumably associated with the surface. At high protein/lipid ratios the chemical and physical properties of the complex are similar to those of the apo C-III/DMPC complex having the same stoichiometry. Recently Jonas et al. observed similar kinds of vesicular complexes of DMPC and apo A-I (17).

The addition of cholesterol to the lipid mixtures that are to be assembled with apolipoproteins is a logical extension of the early reassembly efforts. The association of apo A-I with DMPC/cholesterol mixtures has been described by a number of investigators whose results may be summarized as follows (19,30,47). First, the ratio of cholesterol to phospholipid in the lipid/protein complex is equal to or less than that in the starting incubation mixture. Second, the fraction of cholesterol incorporated into the complex decreases as the ratio of cholesterol to phospholipid in the initial incubation mixture is increased. Third, the fraction of protein incorporated into the complex decreases with the amount of cholesterol that is in the starting mixture. Finally, the size and heterogeneity of the complex increases with increasing cholesterol composition. The latter observation is consistent with the observation that even in the absence of protein, cholesterol/phospholipid vesicles are always larger than those composed of lecithin alone. The lower content of cholesterol in complexes relative to the starting liposomes suggests that apo A-I preferentially associates with pure DMPC and that cholesterol may exclude the apoprotein from the bilayer. Simply speaking, this may be viewed as a competition between apo A-I and cholesterol for the same sites on the DMPC surface.

Some studies of the association of apolipoproteins with single-chained amphiphiles have been conducted, but these are more important as guides for mechanistic or thermodynamic studies than they are for model lipoproteins. The association of apolipoproteins with lysolecithin (15,28,51) and sodium dodecyl sulfate (35) produces changes in the fluorescence and circular dichroic spectra that are similar to those observed when assembly is performed with lecithins. In both instances the spectral properties are similar to those of the intact lipoprotein, suggesting that in all three the apoproteins are α-helical (circular dichroic studies) and the tryptophan residues of the protein reside in a hydrophobic environment (fluorescence shift).

In some cases, there may be a kinetic barrier to the association of lipids to an apolipoprotein so that an indirect method of assembly must be used (43,44,46,47). The mildest and simplest procedure is that of detergent removal, a technique that is widely used in membrane reassembly. One simply combines the lipid and protein in the presence of a detergent, which is then removed by either dialysis or gel filtration. When applied to total HDL lipids and proteins or apo A-I and various lecithins, a homogeneous complex with the molecular weight, density, and composition of HDL can be formed. Moreover, LCAT substrates composed of complexes containing apo A-I, lecithin, and cholesterol are more than 20 times more reactive than HDL, suggesting that these may be used as models for "nascent" HDL. A typical electron micrograph of apo A-I/1-palmitoyl-2-oleoyl phosphatidylcholine complexes is shown in Fig. 3. Based upon analytical ultracentrifugation, gradient gel electrophoresis and analytical gel filtration, this complex has a molecular weight of about 200,000. Because of the simplicity and efficiency of this method it is likely that detergent removal methods will be used in many of the common *in vitro* systems that have been used to study lipid metabolism, such as cell culture and perfusion studies.

KINETICS AND MECHANISM OF *IN VITRO* LIPOPROTEIN ASSEMBLY

One of the important but poorly understood areas of lipid metabolism is that of lipoprotein synthesis and secretion. Several studies have focused on one mechanistic aspect of this process: the mechanism of *in vitro* lipid-protein association. The primary goal of these studies has been the identification of those determinants of the lipid and protein that regulate their rate of association.

There are a number of variables to be considered, including the physical state of the phospholipid, the structure of the protein, the cholesterol content of the lipid, and the size of the apolipoprotein. A number of studies have shown that the rate of association of an apolipoprotein with phospholipids is a direct function of the

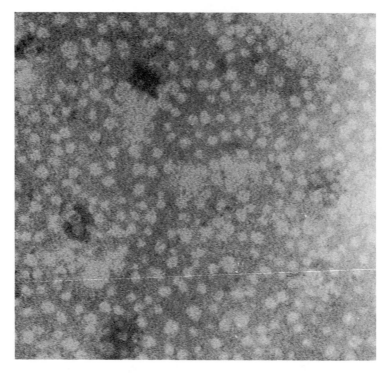

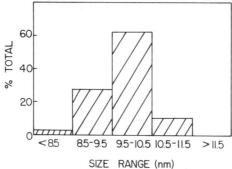

SIZE RANGE (nm)

FIG. 3. A: Electron micrograph of model for nascent high-density lipoprotein composed of 100:1 molar ratio of 1-palmitoyl-2-oleoyl phosphatidylcholine and apo A-I. **B:** Histogram of the size distribution.

permeability of the lipid matrix (29,30,33,45). For the synthetic lipid, DMPC, the maximum permeability of the lipid is at T_c; this high permeability has been assigned to "hole" defects in the lipid matrix that occur at the interface of coexisting gel and liquid crystalline phases. Presumably, the apoprotein can only bind via insertion into one of the preformed holes. In crystal theory, addition of an impurity to a pure substance can increase the number of defects. If the lipid bilayer is considered as a two-dimensional crystalline array, the addition of an impurity would be expected to increase the permeability and thereby provide additional sites for association for the apoprotein. This has been observed for a physiologically important "impurity"—cholesterol (30). When mixed with up to 12 mole % cholesterol, the rate of association with apo A-I is dramatically increased. One model of this process is shown in Fig. 4 in which the calorimetric results of others have been incorporated. Proposed here is that between 0 and 25 mole % cholesterol there exist two phases. One of these is solid and contains 25 mole % cholesterol; the other is a relatively pure phase of DMPC. At the interface between these two phases there are "channel" or "hole" defects that are the sites of selective associations with apolipoproteins. As predicted by the model and observed in our experiments, the rate of association is slowest at 0 and at 25 mole %, and greatest intermediate between these two points. It is important to point out that this is purely a kinetic effect because complexes formed at T_c (24°C), where the rate is fast, are stable at 20° and 30°C, where the rate is very slow; moreover, the product formed at each temperature is the same irrespective of the rate.

The rate of association is also a function of size and structure of the apoprotein. Pownall et al. (33) observed that there is a strong dependence of the rate of association on the molecular weight of the protein. Large proteins associate with DMPC only at or near T_c, and the rates are on the time scale of minutes. Smaller proteins and peptides associate at a rate that is much faster and that has a decreased dependence on the molecular weight. Apo A-I (MW = 28,400) and the synthetic lipid-associating peptide of 20 residues (LAP-20, MW = 2,280) represent extremes in behavior. The association of apo A-I with DMPC is slow and occurs only at T_c but that of LAP-20 is fast and almost independent of temperature. These results suggest that the apolipoproteins bind to preformed holes in the lipid matrix. According to the cluster theory of lipid melting there are a greater number of large holes in DMPC at T_c so that apo A-I associates with this lipid only near T_c. LAP-20 requires smaller preformed holes so that the effects of temperature and size on the number and size of the holes becomes less important.

Finally, there is some evidence that the exposure of hydrophobic residues to the aqueous phase can increase the rate of association of an apolipoprotein with lipid.

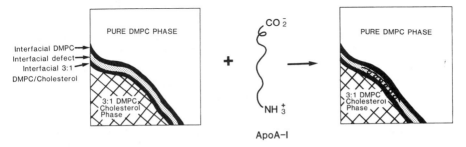

FIG. 4. A hypothetical model for the mechanism by which apo A-I associates with the surface of a liposome in which a dimyristoyl phosphatidylcholine (DMPC) and a 1:3 cholesterol/DMPC phase coexist. Apo A-I may insert into this hole or channel defect to give the initial lipid-protein intermediate on the right.

Apo A-I, apo A-II, apo C-III, and reduced carboxymethylated A-II (RCM-A-II) each undergo significant structural changes as a function of the concentration of a denaturing salt, such as guanidinium chloride (Gdm·Cl). With apo A-I and apo A-II two discrete transitions are observed according to

$$
\begin{array}{ccccc}
\text{folded} & \xrightarrow[\text{0.3 M Gdm·Cl}]{\text{dissociation}} & \text{folded} & \xrightarrow[\text{~1.0 M Gdm·Cl}]{\text{unfolding}} & \begin{array}{c}\text{monomeric} \\ \text{random} \\ \text{coil}\end{array} \\
\text{oligomer} & & \text{monomer} & &
\end{array}
$$

In apo C-III and RCM-A-II, these two transitions are concerted; that is

$$
\begin{array}{ccc}
\text{folded} & \xrightarrow[\text{Gdm·Cl}]{\text{~1.0 M}} & \begin{array}{c}\text{monomeric} \\ \text{random} \\ \text{coil}\end{array} \\
\text{oligomer} & &
\end{array}
$$

The two transitions produced by Gdm·Cl have two common characteristics. First, there is substantial spectroscopic, hydrodynamic, and theoretical evidence that Gdm·Cl promotes and induces the exposure of hydrophobic amino acid residues via both dissociation and unfolding. Second, in recent studies of the kinetics of lipid-apolipoprotein association, it was observed that the rate of association increased dramatically at the Gdm·Cl concentrations at which these transitions occurred (33). Therefore, it was concluded that lipid-protein association can be promoted by exposure of hydrophobic residues although the details of the mechanism require additional investigation. A schematic representation of the mechanism of lipid-apolipoprotein association is given in Fig. 5.

THERMODYNAMICS OF LIPID PROTEIN ASSOCIATION

One of the goals of research on the thermodynamics of lipoproteins has been to identify those structural determinants that regulate lipoprotein stability. It is generally believed that relatively nonspecific hydrophobic forces are involved; however little more than that has been posited. One of the problems is that in native lipoproteins one must deal with too many compositional and structural variables. For this reason, a two-component model system composed of a single lipid and protein offer the best opportunity for measuring the equilibrium constant for lipid-protein association. Two different experimental models have been developed for this kind of study. In one, the apolipoprotein is viewed as the host for a variety of ligands in much the same way that the association of fatty acids with albumin has been studied. This has seen the greatest application with sodium dodecyl sulfate and lysolecithin, which are single-chained amphiphiles that have relatively high critical micelle concentrations. In the other, which will be presented here, the apolipoprotein is regarded as associating with a preformed surface of double-chained amphiphiles that have a relatively low (10^{-12} M) critical micelle concentration. Simply speaking then, this is an attempt to determine the partition coefficient for the distribution of an apolipoprotein between the aqueous phase and the lipid surface.

In aqueous solutions, the unitary free energy of association, ΔG_a, of an amphiphile with a lipoprotein may be calculated from

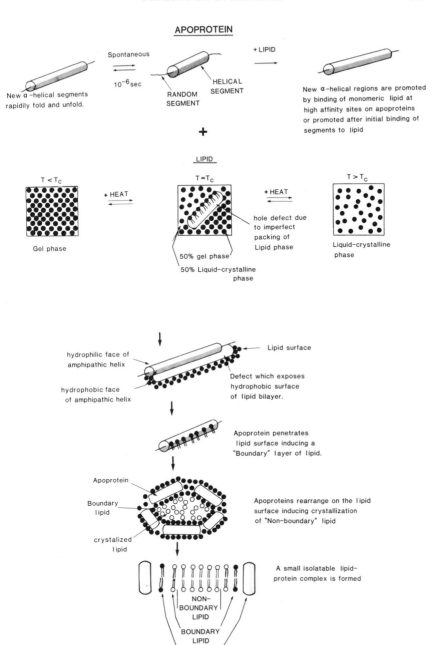

FIG. 5. A schematic representation of the mechanism of lipid-apolipoprotein association.

$$\Delta G = -RT \ln K \qquad [1]$$

$$K = X_L/X_W \qquad [2]$$

where X_L and X_W are the respective mole fractions of the amphiphile in the lipoprotein and aqueous phases.

Using equilibrium methods we have measured ΔG_a for the polypeptides given in Fig. 6 (32). RCM-A-II is the monomeric species produced by reduction and carboxymethylation of human apo A-II; apo C-III is a major apolipoprotein of the high- and very low-density lipoproteins, and the LAP series is a group of model apolipopeptides whose design was based, in part, on the theory proposed by Segrest et al. (39). The free energies of association of these peptides with DMPC are given in Table 4 (32). In addition, the calculated ΔG_a has been tabulated based upon the sum of the free energies of transfer (δG_i) (hydrophobicities) of the individual amino acids according to

$$\Delta G_a = \sum_1 \delta G_i \qquad [3]$$

The values of δG_i were taken from the studies of Bull and Breese (7) and Levitt (22).

<u>A-II</u>

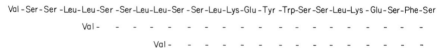

<u>C-III</u>

<u>MODEL PEPTIDES</u>

FIG. 6. The primary structure of apo A-II, apo C-III and model peptides. Apo A-II is shown as the monomer of what exists in plasma as a disulfide-linked dimer. The model peptides are designated from top to bottom as LAP-24, LAP-20, and LAP-16, respectively. (LAP-lipid-associating peptide).

TABLE 4. *Free energy of association (ΔG_a) of lipid-associating peptides (LAP) with dimyristoyl phosphatidylcholine*

Peptide[a]	ΔG_a(kcal)		
	Measured[b]	B&B Calculated[c]	L Calculated[d]
apo C-III	−10	−61	(−53)[e] (+12.1)
+0.3 M Gdm·Cl	−9.3		
RCM A-II	−8.0, −7.2	−66.6	(−53.8) (−1.6)
+0.3 M Gdm·Cl	−6.2		
LAP-16	−6.5[f]	−16.7	(−14.2) (−1.4)
LAP-20	−8.9	−22.4	(−17.8) (−4.4)
LAP-24	−9.5	−28.1	(−21.4) (−7.4)

[a]Gdm·Cl, guanidinium chloride; RCM A-II, reduced carboxymethylated A-II.
[b]First value is for association with single bilayer vesicles; the second was obtained with multilayers.
[c]Based on Bull-Breese parameters (7).
[d]Based on Levitt parameters (22).
[e]Values in parentheses obtained neglecting contribution of hydrophilic side chains.
[f]Measured in 1.0 M NaCl.

The effect of Gdm·Cl on the ΔG_a suggests that the association is hydrophobic. The trend in the ΔG_a of the homologous series of peptides comprising LAP-16, LAP-20, and LAP-24 is in the direction expected for hydrophobic bonding, since LAP-20 and LAP-24 have two and four more leucine residues, respectively, than LAP-16. One of the main differences between Levitt and the Bull-Breese free-energy scales is that the former gives positive values for the polar amino acid residues and in this way reflects the unfavorable transfer of those residues from an aqueous to a hydrocarbon phase. However, according to Segrest et al. (39) the polar amino acid residues of apoproteins in a lipoprotein remain at the surface where they are in contact with water. Thus, according to this model, the δG_a of the polar amino acid residues should not be included in the calculation of ΔG_a. Using the Levitt scale and neglecting the contribution of polar residues, the ΔG_a is calculated, given in the last column of Table 4. Although consistently smaller by 15 to 20%, this gives, as expected, values similar to those based upon the Bull and Breese parameters. These values are still much more exergonic than those observed.

The polarity change at the lipid-water interface is gradual, as is best illustrated in the ESR studies of Griffith et al. (14). With this view, the thermodynamic rol of both polar and nonpolar amino acid residues becomes more apparent. In a real or reassembled lipoprotein the apoprotein is in an α-helical conformation with its polar residues facing the aqueous phase and the nonpolar residues penetrating part way into the hydrocarbon region of the lipid. The charged residues have an unfavorable ($\Delta G_a > 0$) free energy of transfer from water to the hydrophobic region and remain in contact with water. This term is responsible for holding the protein at or near the surface of the lipoprotein. The polar residues have a relatively high affinity for water, whereas the hydrophobic amino acids partition into any less polar phase. These amino acid residues are typically distributed throughout an apolipoprotein such that when placed in an α-helix, a polar and a hydrophobic face are formed. The collective effect of the preferential association of the polar residues with water and nonpolar residues with environments less polar than water is that a driving force for helix formation is provided if there is an interface with which the apoprotein can associate. Because the hydrophobic residues are located near the surface, where the environment is not much less polar than water, the ΔG_a is not fully expressed and peptide transfer from water to the phospholipid surface is faster and less exergonic than predicted. This location permits exposure of the sequence determinants required for enzyme activation and for binding to cell surface receptors.

ACKNOWLEDGMENTS

The authors wish to thank Ms. Sarah Myers for editorial assistance and Mrs. Susan Kelly for providing the line drawings. This research was supported by the National Heart and Blood Vessel Research and Demonstration Center, Baylor College of Medicine, a project of the National Heart, Lung and Blood Institute, National Institutes of Health, Grant HL-17269 and HL-26250. We also wish to thank Mrs. Carol A. Coreathers and Mrs. Diane Moran for assistance in the preparation of the manuscript.

REFERENCES

1. Assmann, G., and Brewer, H. B., Jr. (1974): Lipid-protein interactions in high density lipoproteins. *Proc. Natl. Acad. Sci. USA*, 71:989–993.
2. Atkinson, D., Smith, H. M., Dickson, J., and Austin, J. P. (1976): Interaction of apoprotein from porcine high-density lipoprotein with dimyristoyl lecithin. *Eur. J. Biochem.*, 64:541–547.
3. Aune, K. C., Gallagher, J. G., Gotto, A. M., Jr., and Morrisett, J. D. (1977): Physical properties of the dimyristoylphosphatidylcholine vesicle and of complexes formed by its interaction with apolipoprotein C-III. *Biochemistry*, 16:2151–2156.
4. Barbeau, D. L., Jonas, A., Teng, T., and Scanu, A. M. (1979): Asymmetry of apolipoprotein A-I in solution as assessed from ultracentrifugal, viscometric, and fluorescence polarization studies. *Biochemistry*, 18:362–369.
5. Barter, P. J., Gooden, J. M., and Rajaram, O. V. (1979): Species differences in the activity of a serum triglyceride transferring factor. *Atherosclerosis*, 33:165–169.
6. Brewster, M., Ihm, I., Brainard, J., and Harmony, J. A. K. (1978): Transfer of phosphatidylcholine facilitated by a component of human plasma. *Biochim. Biophys. Acta*, 529:147–159.
7. Bull, H. B., and Breese, K. (1974): Surface tension of amino acid solutions. A hydrophobicity scale of the amino acid residues. *Arch. Biochem. Biophys.*, 161:665–670.
8. Deckelbaum, R. J., Shipley, G. G., and Small, D. M. (1977): Thermal transition in human plasma low density lipoproteins. *J. Biol. Chem.*, 252:744–754.
9. Deckelbaum, R. J., Shipley, G. G., Small, D. M., Lees, R. S., and George, P. K. (1975): Structure and function of lipids in human low density lipoproteins. *Science*, 190:392–394.
10. Edelstein, C., Kezdy, F. J., Scanu, A. M., and Shen, B. W. (1979): Apolipoproteins and the structural organization of plasma lipoproteins: Human plasma high density lipoprotein-3. *J. Lipid Res.*, 20:143–153.
11. Edelstein, C., and Scanu, A. M. (1980): Effect of guanidine hydrochloride on the hydrodynamic and thermodynamic properties of human apolipoprotein A-I in solution. *J. Biol. Chem.*, 255:5747–5754.

12. Fielding, P. E., and Fielding, C. J. (1980): A cholesteryl ester transfer complex in human plasma. *Proc. Natl. Acad. Sci. USA*, 77:3327–3330.
13. Gilman, T., Kauffman, J. W., and Pownall, H. J. (1981): Raman spectroscopy of the thermal properties of reassembled high-density lipoprotein:apolipoprotein A-I complexes of dimyristoyl-phosphatidylcholine. *Biochemistry*, 20:656–661.
14. Griffith, O. H., Dehlinger, P. J., and Van, S. P. (1974): Shape of hydrophobic barrier of phospholipid bilayers. Evidence for water penetration in biological membranes. *J. Membr. Biol.*, 15:159–192.
15. Haberland, M. E., and Reynolds, J. A. (1975): Interaction of L-α-palmitoyl lysophosphatidylcholine with the A-I polypetide of high density lipoprotein. *J. Biol. Chem.*, 250:6636–6639.
16. Havel, R. J., Goldstein, J. L., and Brown, M. S. (1980): Lipoproteins and lipid transport. In: *Metabolic Control and Disease*, 8th edn, edited by P. K. Bondy and L. E. Rosenberg, pp. 393–494. W. B. Saunders, Philadelphia.
17. Jonas, A., Drengler, S. M., and Kaplan, J. S. (1981): Interaction of apolipoprotein A-I with dimyristoylphosphatidylcholine particles of various sizes. *J. Biol. Chem.*, 256:2420–2426.
18. Jonas, A., and Krajnovich, D. J. (1977): Interaction of human and bovine A-I apolipoproteins with L-α-dimyristoyl phosphatidylcholine and L-α-myristoyl lysophosphatidylcholine. *J. Biol. Chem.*, 252:2194–2199.
19. Jonas, A., and Krajnovich, D. J. (1978): Effect of cholesterol on the formation of micellar complexes between bovine A-I apolipoprotein and L-α-dimyristoylphosphatidylcholine. *J. Biol. Chem.*, 253:5758–5763.
20. Jonas, A., Krajnovich, D. J., and Patterson, B. W. (1977): Physical properties of isolated complexes of human and bovine A-I apolipoproteins with L-α-dimyristoyl phosphatidylcholine. *J. Biol. Chem.*, 252:2200–2205.
21. Laggner, P., Gotto, A. M., Jr., and Morrisett, J. D. (1979): Structure of dimyristoylphosphatidylcholine vesicle and the complex formed by its interaction with apolipoprotein C-III: X-ray small-angle scattering studies. *Biochemistry*, 18:164–171.
22. Levitt, M. (1976): A simplified representation of protein conformations for rapid simulation of protein folding. *J. Mol. Biol.*, 104:59–107.
23. Mantulin, W. W., Rohde, M. F., Gotto, A. M., Jr., and Pownall, H. J. (1980): The conformational properties of human plasma apolipoprotein C-II. *J. Biol. Chem.*, 255:8185–8191.
24. Morrisett, J. D., Gallagher, J. G., Aune, K. C., and Gotto, A. M., Jr. (1974): Structure of the major complex formed by interaction of phosphatidylcholine bilamellar vesicles and apolipoprotein-alanine (APO-C-III). *Biochemistry*, 13:4765–4771.
25. Morrisett, J. D., Jackson, R. L., and Gotto, A. M., Jr. (1975): Lipoproteins: Structure and function. *Annu. Rev. Biochem.*, 44:183–207.
26. Novosad, Z., Knapp, R. D., Gotto, A. M., Pownall, H. J., and Morrisett, J. D. (1976): Structure of apolipoprotein-phospholipid complex: ApoC-III induced changes in the physical properties of dimyristoylphosphatidylcholine. *Biochemistry*, 15:3176–3183.
27. Osborne, J. C., Jr., and Brewer, H. B., Jr. (1977): The plasma lipoproteins. *Adv. Protein Chem.*, 31:253–327.
28. Palumbo, G., and Edelhoch, H. (1977): Interaction of ApoA-II from human high density lipoprotein with lysolecithin. *J. Biol. Chem.*, 252:3684–3688.
29. Pownall, H. J., Massey, J. B., Kusserow, S. K., and Gotto, A. M., Jr. (1978): Kinetics of lipid-protein interactions: Interaction of apolipoprotein A-I from human plasma high density lipoproteins with phosphatidylcholines. *Biochemistry*, 17:1183–1188.
30. Pownall, H. J., Massey, J. B., Kusserow, S. K., and Gotto, A. M., Jr. (1979): Kinetics of lipid-protein interactions: Effect of cholesterol on the association of human plasma high-density apolipoprotein A-I with L-α-dimyristoylphosphatidylcholine. *Biochemistry*, 18:574–579.
31. Pownall, H. J., Morrisett, J. D., and Gotto, A. M., Jr. (1977): Composition-structure-function correlations in the binding of an apolipoprotein to phosphatidylcholine bilayer mixtures. *J. Lipid Res.*, 18:14–24.
32. Pownall, H. J., Pao, Q., Hickson, D., Sparrow, J. T., and Gotto, A. M., Jr. (1982): Thermodynamics of lipid-protein association in human plasma lipoproteins. *Biophys. J.*, 37:175–177.
33. Pownall, H. J., Pao, Q., Hickson, D., Sparrow, J. T., Kusserow, S. K., and Massey, J. B. (1981): Kinetics and mechanism of association of human plasma apolipoproteins with dimyristoylphosphatidylcholine: Effect of protein structure and lipid clusters on reaction rates. *Biochemistry*, 20:6630–6635.

34. Reynolds, J. A. (1976): Conformational stability of the polypeptide components of human high density serum lipoprotein. *J. Biol. Chem.*, 251:6013–6015.
35. Reynolds, J. A., and Simon, R. H. (1974): The interaction of polypeptide components of human high density lipoprotein with sodium dodecyl sulfate. *J. Biol. Chem.*, 249:3937–3940.
36. Ritter, M. C., and Scanu, A. M. (1977): Role of apolipoprotein A-I in the structure of human serum high density lipoproteins. *J. Biol. Chem.*, 252:1208–1216.
37. Ritter, M. C., and Scanu, A. M. (1979): Apolipoprotein A-II and structure of human serum high density lipoproteins: *J. Biol. Chem.*, 254:2517–2525.
38. Segrest, J. P. (1976): Molecular packing of high density lipoproteins: A postulated functional role. *FEBS Lett.*, 69:111–115.
39. Segrest, J. P., Jackson, R. L., Morrisett, J. D., and Gotto, A. M., Jr. (1974): A molecular theory of lipid-protein interactions in the plasma lipoproteins. *FEBS Lett.*, 38:247–253.
40. Shen, B. W. (1980): Properties of human apolipoprotein A-I at the air-water interface. *Biochemistry*, 19:3643–3650.
41. Shen, B. W., Scanu, A. M., and Kezdy, F. J. (1977): Structure of human serum lipoproteins inferred from compositional analysis. *Proc. Natl. Acad. Sci. USA*, 74:837–841.
42. Sklar, L. A., Doody, M. C., Gotto, A. M., Jr., and Pownall, H. J. (1980): Serum lipoprotein structure: Resonance energy transfer localization of fluorescent lipid probes. *Biochemistry*, 19:1294–1301.
43. Stoffel, W., and Darr, W. (1976): Human high density apolipoprotein A-I-lysolecithin-lecithin and sphingomyelin complexes. *Hoppe Seylers Z. Physiol. Chem.*, 357:127–137.
44. Stoffel, W., Salm, K., and Langer, M. (1978): A new method for the exchange of lipid classes of human serum high density lipoprotein. *Hoppe Seylers Z. Physiol. Chem.*, 359:1385–1393.
45. Swaney, J. B. (1980): Mechanisms of protein lipid interaction. *Biol. Chem.*, 255:8791–8797.
46. Swaney, J. B. (1980): Properties of lipid-apolipoprotein association products. *J. Biol. Chem.*, 255:8798–8803.
47. Tall, A. R., and Lange, Y. (1978): Incorporation of cholesterol into high density lipoprotein recombinants. *Biochem. Biophys. Res. Commun.*, 80:206.
48. Tall, A. R., Shipley, G. G., and Small, D. M. (1976): Conformational and thermodynamic properties of apoA-I of human plasma high density lipoproteins. *J. Biol. Chem.*, 251:3749–3755.
49. Tall, A. R., Small, D. M., Deckelbaum, R. J., and Shipley, G. G. (1977): Structure and thermodynamic properties of high density lipoprotein recombinants. *J. Biol. Chem.*, 252:4701–4711.
50. Teng, T., Barbeau, D. L., and Scanu, A. M. (1978): Sedimentation behavior of native and reduced apolipoprotein A-II from human high density lipoproteins. *Biochemistry*, 17:17–21.
51. Verdery, R. B., III, and Nichols, A. V. (1974): Interaction of lysolecithin micelles and lecithin vesicles with apolipoprotein Gln-I from serum high density lipoproteins. *Biochem. Biophys. Res. Commun.*, 57:1271–1278.
52. Verdery, R. B., III, and Nichols. A. V. (1975): Arrangement of lipid and protein in human serum high density lipoproteins: A proposed model. *Chem. Phys. Lipids*, 14:123–134.
53. Wlodawer, A., Segrest, J. P., Chung, B. H., Chiovetti, R., Jr., and Weinstein, J. N. (1979): High-density lipoprotein recombinants: Evidence for a bicycle tire micelle structure obtained by neutron scattering and electron microscopy. *FEBS Lett.*, 104:231–235.

Phospholipids and Atherosclerosis, edited by
P. Avogaro, M. Mancini, G. Ricci, and
R. Paoletti. Raven Press, New York © 1983.

Photochemical and Bifunctional Crosslinker Studies on the Structure of Human Serum High-Density Lipoprotein

Wilhelm Stoffel

Institut für Physiologische Chemie der Universität zu Köln, West Germany

Considerable information has been accumulated in recent years about the structure of particles belonging to the serum high-density lipoprotein (HDL) class with alpha-electrophoretic mobility. The functional aspects of HDL and its metabolic role require a thorough knowledge of the structural basis of these spherical particles, which show dispersion ranging from 80 to 120 Å in diameter. This led to the classification of subgroups, such as HDL_2, HDL_3, and so on, by density ranging from 1.063 to 1.21 g/ml (1,3,6). The lipid apoprotein ratio is the basis of these different densities although the relative ratios among the lipid classes are very constant. About 40% (wt) (50 moles) of phosphatidyl choline (PC), mostly substituted with polyunsaturated fatty acids ($C_{18:2}$ and $C_{20:4}$), 6% sphingomyelin (SM) and 2% (4 moles) lysolecithin as opposed to approximately 10% cholesterol (25 moles) and the hydrophobic cholesteryl esters with ~25 to 30% (45 moles) and ~5 to 6% triglycerides (7 moles). These water insoluble lipid classes are transported

TABLE 1. *Spin lattice relaxation time of ^{13}C-labeled lysolecithin recombined apolipoprotein A-I (after agarose chromatography)*

Lysolecithin species	Apo A-I/Lyso-PC molar ratio	T_1-time (msec)	
		Micelle	Recombinant
16-^{13}C-16:0	1:55	1940 ± 15	1540 ± 135
11-^{13}C-18:0	1:56	221 ± 5	180 ± 135
14-^{13}C-18:0	1:56	290 ± 10	215 ± 15
11-^{13}C-18:1	1:50	344 ± 10	203 ± 18
14-^{13}C-18:2	1:57	728 ± 40	360 ± 25
N-^{13}CH$_3$	1:51	633 ± 30	632 ± 20

TABLE 2a. *Spin lattice relaxation times* (T_1 *in sec) of ^{13}C-labeled phosphatidylcholines in vesicles and in apo A-I/lyso-PC/PC complexes*[a]

Phosphatidylcholine species	Vesicles	T_1-time (msec) Lipoprotein complex	Stoichiometry apo A-I/lyso-PC/ PC
18:0/[14^{13}C]18:0	629 ± 16	424 ± 28	1:35:69
	652 ± 16	430 ± 3	
[14-^{13}C]18:2/14-^{13}C]18:2	636 ± 32	384 ± 31	1:22:29
	631 ± 13		
[14-^{13}C]18:2/14-^{13}C]18:2	790 ± 14	559 ± 9	1:16:68
16:0(18:2)/[14-^{13}C]18:2	632 ± 24	437 ± 14	1:24:29

[a]Lyso-PC was prepared from soya-lecithin by phospholipase A_2 hydrolysis and recylated with 18:2. It contained 25% 16:0, 8% 18:0, 11% 18:1, 52% 18:2, and 5% 18:3 in the 1-position.

TABLE 2b. *Spin lattice relaxation times* (T_1) *of ^{13}C-labeled sphingomyelin and the respective sphingomyelin/lyso-PC/apo A-I complexes*

^{13}C labeled SM	T_1(msec) of nuclei in		Molar ratio of apo A-I/SM/lyso-PC
	Liposomes	Lipoprotein	
^{13}C-stearoyl-sphingosyl-phosphorylcholine			
N-^{13}CH$_3$	274 ± 8[a]	389 ± 31	1:75:27
^{13}C-11	<50	183 ± 28	
^{13}C-14	<50	234 ± 11	1:121:16
^{13}C-oleoyl-sphingosyl-phosphorylcholine			
N-^{13}CH$_3$	341 ± 6	435 ± 7	1:84:44
^{13}C-11	227 ± 12	206 ± 12	
^{13}C-linoloyl-sphingosyl-phosphorylcholine			
N-^{13}CH$_3$	360 ± 12	414 ± 13	1:72:24
^{13}C-14	594 ± 13	468 ± 17	

[a]Indicate the maximal error possible.

in the water phase of the blood plasma by the main two polypeptide species: apo A-I, with its corrected structure of 243 amino acids, and apo A-II, a dimer with 77 amino acids each, linked by a disulfide bond. The two apoproteins are characterized by a high alpha-helical content in delipidated form and much more so in lipid complexes. These helical sequences, when translated into creatine phosphokinase (CPK) molecular models, exhibit an amphipathic structure (4) with a hydrophilic and a hydrophobic side.

The calculated hydrophobicity indices ($H\phi$) of the residues facing the apolar side far exceeded the averaged hydrophobicity index; for example, those of the ten α-helical regions of apo A-I and three of A-II have an $H\phi$ of 1,750 cal/residue as

TABLE 2c. *Spin lattice relaxation time (T₁) of specifically ¹³C-labeled phosphatidylcholines and cholesterol integrated into human high-density lipoprotein (HDL) by the cholate-exchange method, native HDL, liposomes, and cholate-lipid micelles*

Lipid species	Chemical shift (ppm)	T_1-time (msec)				
		Vesicles	Lipid apo-HDL	Cholate lipid micelles	Exchanged lipid in HDL	Native HDL
[N-¹³CH₃]PC	54.0	430	462	453	451	450
18:0/14-¹³C-18:2-PC	27.0	700	438	632	268	218
18:0/11-¹³C-18-1PC	27.0	210	147	303	182	218
26-¹³C-Cholesterol	23.0	760	—	766	560	—
14-¹³C-18:2-CE					209	
18:2-26¹³C-CE					485	
11-¹³C-18:1-SPM	27.0	238	199			
14-¹³C-18:2-SPM	27.0					

compared to 1,100 cal/residue of the total sequences. It is tempting to assume that these sequences are prone to hydrophobic binding of lipids. Among the possible lipid and protein interactions relevant experiments must prove whether the protein (a) is interdigitated in a lipid bilayer, (b) interacts as a monolayer by ionic interactions with the lipid polar head group, (c) forms autonomous domains in a phospholipid matrix, or (d) interacts by a combination of the three. In an attempt to localize the apo A-I and A-II present in ratios of two or three depending on the density range, limited proteolytic degradation studies have been carried out by Camejo (2). Schonfield and Pfleger (8) approached the problem with immunological methods and demonstrated the different accessibility of the antigenic sites of apo A-I and A-II in native HDL. By the nature of this method, detailed instructions of the molecular arrangement cannot be expected.

Physical techniques so far have given valuable information on binding forces and the modes of interactions of the hydrophilic and hydrophobic segments of amphiphilic lipids and apoproteins (9,13,14). Simple lipoprotein complexes consisting of isolated HDL apolipoproteins A-I and A-II and single lipid species, such as phospholipids labeled with ¹³C in the hydrophilic polar head or in specific positions of their acyl chains, have led via spin lattice relaxation time measurements to the conclusion that only hydrophobic interactions (i.e., interactions of the acyl chains with the hydrophobic regions of apoproteins) stabilize these complexes; polar and ionic interactions do not. This insight derived from model complexes ranging from micelles of ¹³C-lysolecithin apo A-I to ¹³C-phosphatidycholine and SM-apo A-I and apo-HDL complexes was confirmed finally, and objections against model recombinants were circumvented by the lipid exchange method described recently (12). This procedure allows the unperturbed exchange of the lipid species of the native HDL particle against labeled species. The following five tables summarize *selected* data in support of the aforementioned statement that the integrity of the HDL particle, of spherical appearance in electron microscopy, is maintained by hydrophobic interactions.

STRUCTURE OF HDL

TABLE 3. *Stoichiometry of azido-labeled lipid classes and apoproteins in HDL after lipid exchange, photoactivation and delipidation*

Azido lipid	Lipid/apo HDL after exchange	Lipid/apo HDL after delipidation	Crosslinks (%)	Lipid/apo A-I	Lipid/apo A-II	Lipid/A-I: Lipid/A-II ratio
A. PC						
12-N_3-18:1	30.0:1	5.7:1	19	1.34:1	1.43:1	0.94
	10.0:1	2.4:1	24	0.54:1	0.54:1	1.00
	7.4:1	1.4:1	19	0.38:1	0.40:1	0.95
	3.8:1	0.8:1	21	0.24:1	0.25:1	0.96
18-N_3-18:2	8.0:1	1.6:1	20	0.34:1	0.24:1	1.42
	8.3:1	1.6:1	19	0.36:1	0.26:1	1.39
5-N_3-16:0	12.8:1	1.1:1	9	0.26:1	0.24:1	1.08
	10.8:1	0.8:1	7	0.23:1	0.20:1	1.15
16-N_3-16:0	6.7:1	1.2:1	18	0.37:1	0.24:1	1.54
	7.4:1	1.2:1	16	0.33:1	0.23:1	1.43
B. SM						
12-N_3-18:1	7.9:1	1.3:1	16	0.28:1	0.30:1	0.93
	6.0:1	0.7:1	12	0.17:1	0.19:1	0.89
18-N_3-18:2	7.5:1	0.8:1	11	0.21:1	0.24:1	0.88
	7.3:1	0.6:1	8	0.15:1	0.16:1	0.94
16-N_3-16:0	12.0:1	1.4:1	12	0.35:1	0.38:1	0.92
	12.0:1	1.3:1	11	0.35:1	0.36:1	0.97
C.						
25-N_3-Nor-	14.2:1	1.4:1	10	0.41:1	0.27:1	1.52
cholesterol	14.1:1	1.2:1	9	0.33:1	0.25:1	1.32
D. CE						
12-N_3-18:1	3.2:1	0.3:1	9	0.12:1	0.06:1	2.00
	5.1:1	0.5:1	9	0.15:1	0.07:1	2.14
18-N_3-18.2	15.4:1	1.3:1	8	0.35:1	0.18:1	1.94
	25.1:1	2.4:1	10	0.67:1	0.40:1	1.68
16-N_3-16:0	21.3:1	2.3:1	11	0.65:1	0.35:1	1.86
	19.7:1	2.4:1	12	0.69:1	0.35:1	1.97
25-N_3-Norcho-	18.2:1	1.5:1	8	0.50:1	0.26:1	1.92
lesteryloleate	1.37:1	1.4:1	10	0.48:1	0.22:1	2.18

The first table documents the strong immobilization of the monoacyl residue of different ^{13}C-enriched lysolecithins with free, uninhibited motion of the choline methyl groups (Table 1). Lysolecithin can be discharged from the apoproteins by diacylphospholipids, the basis of a recombination method which yields spherical particles. The transition from the lysolecithin apo A-I micelle to spherical particles is accompanied by dramatic changes in secondary structure, induced by the lipid binding which can be followed by circular dichroism measurement. A molar elipticity at 222 nm indicative of α-helix content (f_H) is reached comparing with that of the native HDL $(f_H \sim 70\%)$. It is suggestive that the same sites of the apoproteins are involved in recombinants and in native particles. This is also supported by the T_1-times of lecithin (PC) (Table 2a) and sphingomyelin (Fig. 2b) molecules associated with the apoproteins in recombinants and lipid-exchanged HDL particles

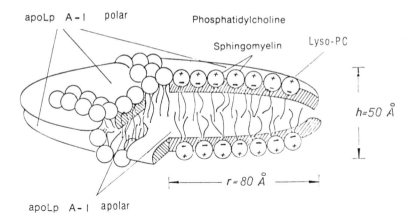

apoLp A - I polar
Phosphatidylcholine
Sphingomyelin Lyso-PC
$h=50\ \overset{\circ}{A}$
$r = 80\ \overset{\circ}{A}$
apoLp A- I apolar

FIG. 1. Proposed model of the lipid-protein arrangement in the apoLp A-I-sphingomyelin-lysolecithin particles.

(Table 2c). Schematically shown in Fig. 1 is a proposed model of an apo A-I-PC-lipoprotein complex.

The phospholipid polar head groups are oriented only to the outer surface of the particle. Chemical shift reagents interact with all phosphate groups, as documented by the ^{31}P-NMR (nuclear magnetic resonance) lines of PC and SM, which collapse and shift as a whole downfield (Fig. 2). All these data are in support of a model of HDL given previously (14) (Fig. 3). An X-ray crystallographic analysis has not been possible, so far, to be applied. Attempts to elucidate the topological molecular arrangement of the HDL apoprotein and lipid components have failed because of the lack of obtaining crystals. Thus, neither this physical technique nor NMR can give an answer about the molecular arrangement of the HDL particle. Two new chemical strategies have, therefore, been developed to overcome this problem.

In order to identify the nearest neighbor or whether there are specific peptide sequences in the apoproteins for binding phospholipids, cholesterol, and cholesteryl esters, a precursor group was located, such as an azido functional group, in different positions of the fatty acyl chains of PC and cholesteryl ester and in the side chain of cholesterol (Fig. 4). On far ultraviolet (UV) irradiation, it forms nitrene which is highly reactive and in a fast reaction crosslink to its nearest neighbor by insertion into C-H bonds or addition to double bonds (Fig. 5). Since these azido lipids carry a high specific radioactivity, the radioactive lipid-lipid and lipid-protein crosslinks can be traced.

The second method, which is exemplified with an apo A-II-PC recombinant, approaches the *topography* of the polypeptide chains in a lipoprotein complex. A scheme is given in Fig. 6. Bifunctional crosslinkers, such as radioactive tartryl-diazide, dimethylsuberimidate (DMS), and preferably dithiobisbutyrimidate (DTBB), were reacted with ε-aminogroups of surface-located lysines, which are 6, 12, and 13Å apart, respectively. Because of the known amino-acid sequence, radioactive

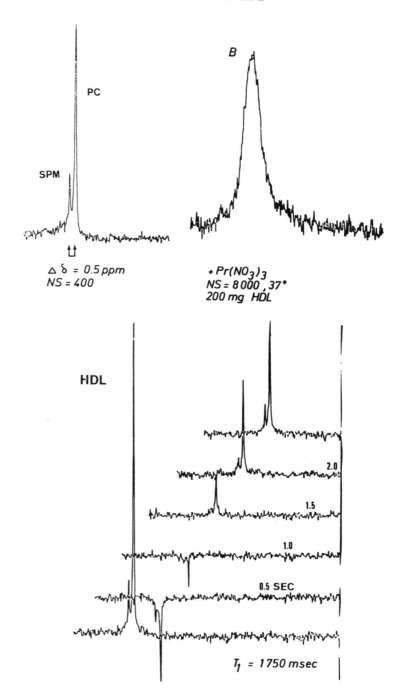

FIG. 2. Top: ^{31}P-NMR spectra of high-density lipoprotein A without B with chemical shift reagent [Pr (NO$_3$)$_3$]. **Bottom:** Spin lattice relaxation time measurement of HDL enriched with (N-^{13}CH$_3$) choline labeled lecithin.

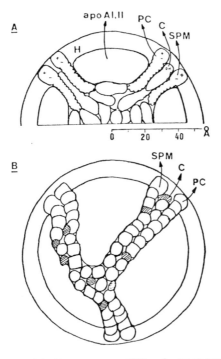

FIG. 3. Schematic model of human serum HDL. **A:** cross-section; **B:** top view.

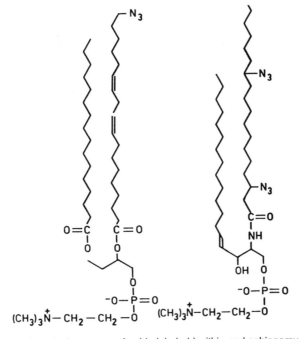

FIG. 4. Chemical structure of azido-labeled lecithin and sphingomyelin.

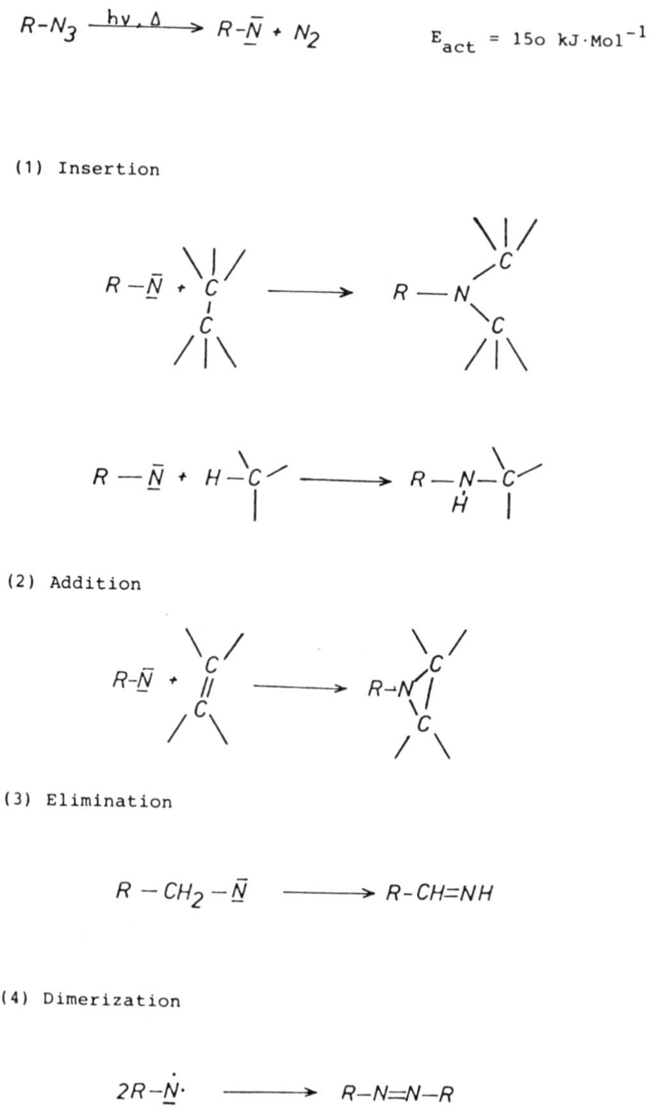

$$R\text{-}N_3 \xrightarrow{\text{h}\nu,\Delta} R\text{-}\underline{\bar{N}} + N_2 \qquad\qquad E_{act} = 150\ kJ\cdot Mol^{-1}$$

(1) Insertion

$$R-\underline{\bar{N}} + \underset{/|\backslash}{\overset{\backslash|/}{C}} \longrightarrow R-N$$

$$R-\underline{\bar{N}} + H-\overset{\backslash}{\underset{|}{C}}\diagdown \longrightarrow R-\underset{\dot{H}}{N}-\overset{\backslash}{\underset{|}{C}}\diagdown$$

(2) Addition

$$R\text{-}\underline{\bar{N}} + \overset{\backslash/}{\underset{/\backslash}{\overset{C}{\underset{C}{\parallel}}}} \longrightarrow R\text{-}N$$

(3) Elimination

$$R - CH_2 - \underline{\bar{N}} \longrightarrow R\text{-}CH{=}NH$$

(4) Dimerization

$$2R-\underline{\dot{N}}\cdot \longrightarrow R-N{=}N-R$$

FIG. 5. Reactions of nitrenes liberated by photolysis from azido-precursors.

proteolytic (thermolysin) fragments separated by two-dimensional thin-layer chromatography will carry one or, in most cases, two peptides at the foot points of the bifunctional crosslinker. Cleavage of the disulfide bond caused the amidine groups to release the two peptides. The peptides were again separated by two-dimensional thin-layer chromatography and acid hydrolyzed; and then the amino-acid composition of the peptides was determined and assigned to the lysine-containing sequence.

By this approach, as will be demonstrated later, it is possible to draw far reaching conclusions about the arrangement and folding of the apoprotein in the particle. On

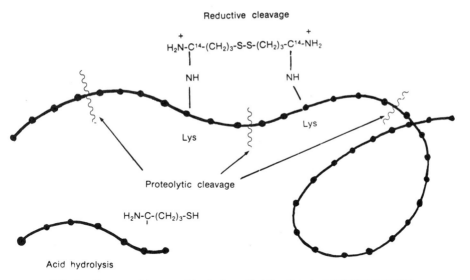

Reductive cleavage

$$H_2N-\overset{+}{C}{}^{14}\text{-}(CH_2)_3\text{-}S\text{-}S\text{-}(CH_2)_3\text{-}\overset{+}{C}{}^{14}\text{-}NH_2$$

NH   NH

Lys

Lys

Proteolytic cleavage

$$H_2N-\underset{|}{C}-(CH_2)_3\text{-}SH$$

Acid hydrolysis

FIG. 6. Strategy of topographic studies with bifunctional crosslinking reagents.

the following discussion of the results of the first approach, namely, the crosslinking of azido-labeled PC, cholesterol, and cholesteryl esters (CE) after photolysis, interlipid-crosslinking will be disregarded and only one set of examples will be discussed.

Lecithin, cholesterol, and CE of native HDL were exchanged against the three PC species: di-12-N_3-oleoyl-2-18-N_3-18:2-PC, and 2-16- and 5-N_3-16:0-PC, 25-N_3-norcholesterol, 25-norcholesteryl linolate and cholesteryl-18-N_3-linoleate by the procedure reported in Stoffel et al. (14). When amounts and molar ratios of the labeled photosensitive PCs, cholesterol (C), and CE as liposomes identical with the lipids of HDL are equilibrated with native HDL (PC/SM/C/CE 80/16/53/24) 44–50% PC, 58% C, and 15% CE are exchanged. After photolysis (>300 nm) of the purified HDL under the necessary precautions (oxygen free at 4°C, cut-off filter 300 nm), the apoproteins were delipidated either by the standard chloroform-methanol-ether (2:1:1.5) extraction procedure (7) or via Sephadex LH-20 chromatography (5), the radioactive crosslinked apoproteins were separated by Sephadex G-150 with detergent (0.5% sodium duodecyl sulfate in Tris pH 8.4, 8 M urea) containing buffer and the purified apolipoprotein, A-I and A-II, obtained in purified form. From the specific radioactivities the stoichiometry of crosslinking could be quantified. The results are summarized in Table 3.

What are the conclusions which can be drawn from this new chemical approach? In the first series increasing concentrations of 2-(12-N_3-18:1)-PC were exchanged via mixed cholate micelles against HDL-PC and accumulated up to 40%. On the average, 20% of the photosensitive PC were covalently linked to the apoproteins after photolysis, linearly increasing with the amount of exchanged azido-PC. If the distribution of the crosslinked PC with the reactive nitrene in the 5- and 16-positions of palmitate linked to apo A-I and A-II are compared, the 16-N_3-16:0-PC binding

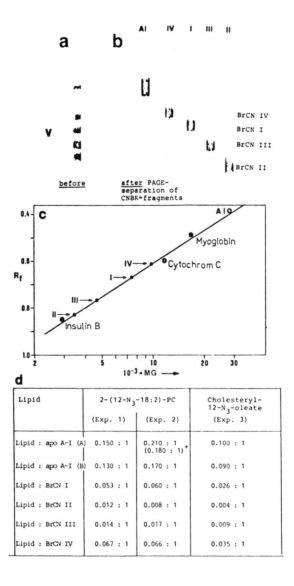

a b AI IV I III II

V

BrCN IV
BrCN I
BrCN III
BrCN II

before after PAGE-separation of CNBR-fragments

c

0.4 — A I

Myoglobin

0.6 — IV → Cytochrom C

R_f I →

III →

0.8 — II →

Insulin B

1.0 —

2 5 10 20 30

$10^{-3} \times MG \longrightarrow$

d

Lipid	2-(12-N_3-18:2)-PC		Cholesteryl-12-N_3-oleate
	(Exp. 1)	(Exp. 2)	(Exp. 3)
Lipid : apo A-I (A)	0.150 : 1	0.210 : 1 (0.180 : 1)[+]	0.100 : 1
Lipid : apo A-I (B)	0.130 : 1	0.170 : 1	0.090 : 1
Lipid : BrCN I	0.053 : 1	0.060 : 1	0.026 : 1
Lipid : BrCN II	0.012 : 1	0.008 : 1	0.004 : 1
Lipid : BrCN III	0.014 : 1	0.017 : 1	0.009 : 1
Lipid : BrCN IV	0.067 : 1	0.066 : 1	0.035 : 1

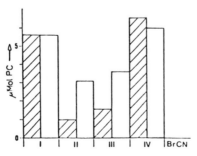

μMol PC

5

0

I II III IV BrCN

A

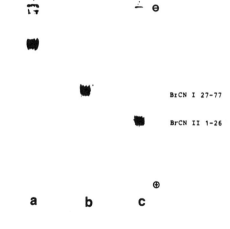

BrCN I 27-77

BrCN II 1-26

⊕

a   b   c

Lipid	2-(12-N_3-18:2)-PC		Cholesteryl-12-N_3-oleate
	(Exp. 1)	(Exp. 2)	(Exp. 3)
Lipid : apo A-II-77	0.130 : 1	0.060 : 1	0.090 : 1
Lipid : BrCN-I	0.120 : 1	0.057 : 1	0.075 : 1
Lipid : BrCN-II	0.009 : 1	0.005 : 1	0.015 : 1

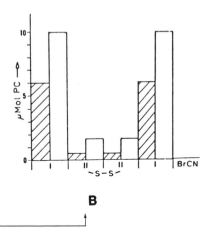

B

FIG. 7. A: Distribution of radioactive phosphatidylcholines photocrosslinked to CNBr-fragments of apo A-I. Dodecyl sulfate polyacrylamide (17%) gel electrophoresis of CNBr-cleavage fragments of apolipopolypeptide A-I **(a)** and of the four fragments separated by preparative dodecyl sulfate polyacrylamide gel electrophoresis **(b)**. I: sequence 1–86; II: 87–112; III: 113–148; IV: 149–243. **(c)** Determination of molecular mass of fragments. **(d)** Stoichiometry of covalently linked phospholipid and cyanogen fragments. *Hatched columns:* nmol PC/µmol CNBr fragment; *open columns:* nmol PC/amino acid residue. **B:** Distribution of radioactive phosphatidylcholines photocrosslinked to CNBr-fragments of apo A-II. Dodecylsulfate polyacrylamide (17%) gel electrophoresis of CNBr-cleavage fragments of **(a)** apolipoprotein A-II/2, **(b)** CNBr I 27-77, **(c)** CNBr II 1–26. Stoichiometry of covalently linked phospholipid linked to CNBr-fragments. *Hatched columns:* nmol PC/µmol CNBr-fragment; *open columns:* nmolPC/amino acid residue.

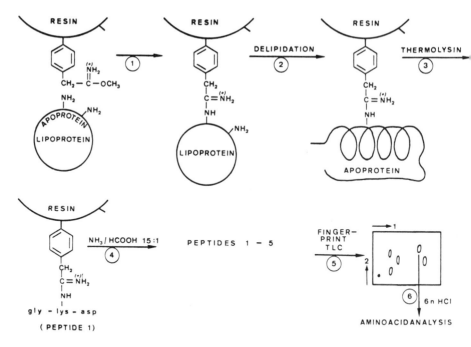

FIG. 8. Schematic presentation of analytical steps. (1) Coupling of lipoprotein complex to imidoester resin. (2) Delipidation. (3) Thermolysin hydrolysis. (4) Cleavage of peptides from resin (exemplified for peptide 1). (5) Thin-layer chromatographic separation of peptides. (6) Amino acid analysis of single peptides.

to apo A-I exceeds that of apo A-II by 40%. The same is observed with the 18-N_3-18:2-PC. If the reactive group is shifted from the terminal methylene group to the 12-position of oleic acid in PC a similar stoichiometry as for the 5-position is obtained. The 5-N_3-16:0-PC crosslinks only to about 8% as compared to the 12-nitrene with 20%. The accessibility of the water phase to the reactive nitrene may lead to intramolecular reactions rather than to intermolecular crosslinks. The binding of the PCs with the photogenerated nitrene closer toward the omega-position (16-N_3-16:0, 18-N_3-18:2), preferably to apo A-I, indicates that regions of apo A-I are embedded deeper into the monomolecular phospholipid layer (see CNBr fragments below). Since apo A-I and A-II bind similarly to the 5- and 12-N_3-oleoyl-PC, but since the distance between the azido group in 12 N_3- and 16-N_3-palmitoyl-PC is about 5Å, these compounds can act as "rulers" to estimate the depth of protein integration into the lipid phase. The azido function of 25-N_3-norcholesterol is about 17Å away from the 3-hydroxy group. The distribution of this cholesterol analog over apo A-I and A-II after photochemical crosslinking is comparable with that of 18-N_3-18:2-PC and therefore supports the idea that cholesterol is arranged, along with the fatty acyl chains of PC, with its 3-OH group at the surface of the HDL particle. The fatty acyl chain as well as the side chain of exchanged 25-N_3 nor-cholesterol-18-N_3-linoleate were azido substituted. In both cases twice the molar amount of this cholesteryl ester was linked to apo A-I compared to apo A-II. The

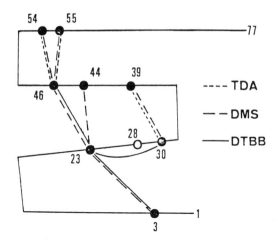

FIG. 9. Schematic presentation of crosslinks between ^{14}C-DMS and ^{14}C-4,4'-DTBB and lysine residues in apo A-II. TDA = Tartryldiazide; DMS = dimethylsuberimidate; DTBB = 4,4'-dithiobisbutyrimidate.

total crosslinking yield was one-half that of the corresponding PC, indicating that, on the average, fewer cholesteryl ester molecules than lecithins interact with the hydrophobic sites of the apoproteins (Table 3). Independent of the method, e.g., whether single apoproteins or HDL apoproteins are recombined with 12-N_3-oleoyl-lyso-PC or PC, the molar ratios of the crosslinking to apo A-I and A-II are identical. This supports the idea that these lipids bind to the apoproteins in the same way in the recombinants, micelles, and native HDL.

The next step then consisted in the cyanogenbromide (CNBr) cleavage of the purified apo A-I and A-II and in the separation of the fragments for further analysis. Whereas lipoapopeptide A-II fragments could be separated on Biogel P-30 with 25% formic acid, the CNBr fragments of apo A-I were separated by preparative SDS-gel electrophoresis (17% SDS) (Fig. 7a,b). The graphic representation of the analyses of the four cyanogenbromide fragments of apo A-I clearly demonstrate that sequences from 1 to 86 and from 149 to 243 carry most of the crosslinked radioactive phospholipids. In the case of apo A-II less than 10% of the radioactivity is associated with sequence 1 to 26 but more than 90% with the sequence 27 to 77. The observation made in binding studies with the fragments of apo A-II are thus confirmed chemically. If it is considered that apo A-II consists of two identical peptides linked by a disulfide bridge, then the center of the apoprotein BrCN-II-S-S-BrCN-II is hardly accessible for the acyl residues of lecithins. This is similar to the low binding capacity of the central two cyanogenbromide fragments of apo A-I. Present work now aims at further confirming the peptide domains responsible for the lipid binding.

Results were obtained with radiolabeled *bifunctional crosslinkers* regarding the folding of apo A-II on the surface of an apo A-II-PC spherical particle. These studies were initiated by first demonstrating chemically that apo A-II is distributed in the surface shell of the complex (10). Benzimidoester-substituted polystyrene

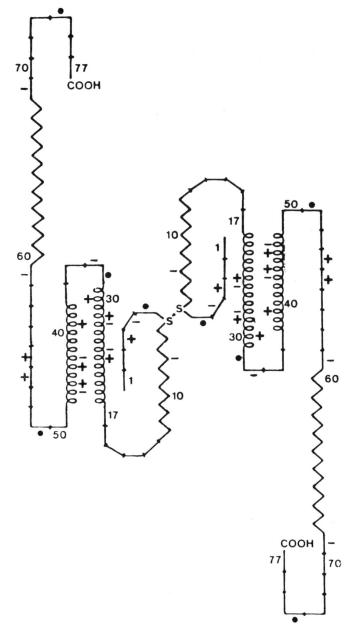

FIG. 10. Suggested conformation and alignment of apo A-II on the apo A-II-polyenephos-phatidylcholine-lysophosphatidylcholine-particle surface.

beads of the Merrifield resin type were continuously percolated with the lipoprotein solution. The particles were bound to the resin via an amidine linkage with the ε-amino groups of all those lysines exposed at the surface. Thermolysin hydrolysis of the polypeptide after delipidation left only these peptides behind. They were cleaved with triethylamine/formic acid, separated by two-dimensional thin-layer chromatography, hydrolyzed, and assigned to the sequence (Fig. 8).

The result was that five lysines (positions 23, 39, 46, 54, 55) containing peptides were linked to the resin. They must have had to protrude far enough to be accessible for the imidoester groups at the resin surface. In order to determine the lysines 10 to 15Å apart, the bifunctional crosslinker DTBB with the aforementioned reconstituted apo A-II-PC particle were reacted, and the folding of the polypeptide chains on the surface was determined. Naturally, this method is limited to only those sequences that contain lysine residues. After taking into account the numerous two-dimensional peptide separations with the intact DTBB-bridge, reduction of oxidation with subsequent amino-acid analysis, and assignment to the sequence, the following topographical allocation of the apo A-II polypeptide chain in the surface of the particle can be developed (Fig. 9).

DTBB, like DMS and tartryldiazide, bridges lysines of three regions. Only lys-28 is not accessible for the crosslinkers. The accumulation of helical regions joined by being bent in the center become obvious from the chemical studies. Tetradecenyl acetate (TDA) (6–7Å) crosslinks three out of nine and DMS and DTBB crosslinks eight out of nine lysines per half molecule apo A-II. No cross-bridges between the two apo A-II halves were formed. In summary, these experiments show that the lipoproteins surface has protein domains of plain, and not globular, arrangement. Not all of the lysine residues of apo A-II are oriented toward the water interphase. Proline residues of the chain bring together three peptide regions of apo A-II, two of which are helical and the carboxy terminus oriented very likely parallel to these in a planar beta-sheet structure. The two halves of apo A-II are not associated as mirror images but diagonally oriented (Fig. 10). Further sophistication of the two apoprotein components of HDL and other lipoprotein complexes will advance the detailed knowledge about this important class of macromolecular arrangements in high-density lipoproteins.

REFERENCES

1. Anderson, D. W., Nichols, A. V., Forte, T. M., and Lindgren, F. R. (1977): Particle distribution of human serum high-density lipoproteins. *Biochim. Biophys. Acta*, 493:55–68.
2. Camejo, G. (1969): The structure of human density lipoprotein: a study of the effect of phospholipase A and trypsin on its components and of the behavior of the lipid and protein moieties at the air–water interphase. *Biochim. Biophys. Acta*, 175:290–300.
3. Eisenberg, S., and Levi, R. I. (1975): Lipoprotein metabolism. *Adv. Lipid Res.*, 13:1–89.
4. Jackson, R. L., Morrisett, J. D., Gotto, A. M., and Segrest, J. P. (1975): The mechanism of lipid-binding by plasma lipoproteins. *Mol. Cell Biochem.*, 6:43–50.
5. Rudman, D., Garcia, L. A., and Howard, C. W. (1970): A new method for isolating the nonidentical protein subunits of human plasma α-lipoprotein. *J. Clin. Invest.*, 49:365–372.
6. Scanu, A. M. (1966): Forms of human serum high-density lipoprotein. *J. Lipid Res.*, 7:295–306.
7. Scanu, A. M., and Edelstein, C. (1971): Solubility in aqueous solutions of ethanol of the small molecular weight peptides of the serum very low density and high density lipoproteins: relevance to the recovery problem during delipidation of serum lipoproteins. *Anal. Biochem.*, 44:576–588.
8. Schonfield, G., and Pfleger, G. (1974): The structure of human high density lipoprotein and the levels of apolipoprotein A-I in plasma as determined by radioimmunassay. *J. Clin. Invest.*, 54:236–246.
9. Stoffel, W., Därr, W., and Salm, K. (1977): Lipid-protein interactions between human apolipoprotein A-I and defined sphingomyelin species. *Z. Physiol. Chem.*, 358:1–11.

10. Stoffel, W., and Preissner, K. (1979): Surface localization of apolipoprotein AII in lipoprotein-complexes. *Z. Physiol. Chem.*, 360:685–690.
11. Stoffel, W., and Preissner, K. (1979): Conformational analysis of serum apolipoprotein AII in lipoprotein complexes with bifunctional crosslinking reagents. *Z. Physiol. Chem.*, 360:691–706.
12. Stoffel, W., Salm, K., and Langer, M. (1978): A new method for the exchange of lipid classes of human serum high-density lipoprotein. *Z. Physiol. Chem.*, 359:1385–1393.
13. Stoffel, W., Salm, K., and Tunggal, B. D. (1979): Chemical proof of lipid protein interaction by crosslinking photosensitive lipids to apoproteins. *Z. Physiol. Chem.*, 360:523–428.
14. Stoffel, W., Zierenberg, O., Tunggal, B. D., and Schreiber, E. (1974): ^{13}C-nuclear magnetic resonance spectroscopic evidence for hydrophobic lipid-protein interactions in human high-density lipoproteins. *Proc. Natl. Acad. Sci. USA*, 71:3696–3700.

Phospholipids and Atherosclerosis, edited by
P. Avogaro, M. Mancini, G. Ricci, and
R. Paoletti. Raven Press, New York © 1983.

Properties of Nascent Lipoproteins Secreted by Rat Liver

Sebastiano Calandra, Ermanno Gherardi, and Patrizia Tarugi

*Instituto di Patologia Generale, Università degli Studi di Modena,
41100 Modena, Italy*

In this chapter some of the recent advances on the hepatic synthesis of plasma lipoproteins are reviewed. Attention is focused on the lipid and apoprotein composition of nascent lipoproteins. In addition, the experimental models that are currently used for the study of lipoprotein secretion by rat liver are examined.

LIVER AS A SITE OF SYNTHESIS OF PLASMA LIPOPROTEINS

The liver is a major site of production of plasma lipoproteins in the rat. Studies conducted *in vivo* demonstrated that after partial hepatectomy there is a marked although transient decrease of plasma very low-density lipoprotein (VLDL) and high-density lipoprotein (HDL) (34). Also, there is severe hypolipoproteinemia following the administration of orotic acid (52) and 4-aminopyrazolopyrimidine (44)—compounds that induce a marked increase in the neutral lipid content in the liver. Furthermore, the concentration of plasma lipoproteins usually decreases following toxic damage to the liver, such as with galactosamine-induced liver injury (43). More direct evidence of the role of the liver in the synthesis and secretion of plasma lipoproteins has emerged from studies conducted *in vitro* by using a variety of experimental models, such as liver slices (14,31,39), liver microsomes (1,26), isolated and perfused rat liver (3,10,17,20,21,25,29,30,32,33,36,37,41,42,53), and isolated rat hepatocytes (4,22,24,46). Attempts have also been made to isolate nascent plasma lipoproteins from the Golgi apparatus (5,13,27,28,35,47) and the endoplasmic reticulum (15) of rat liver. Although these studies have unequivocally demonstrated the ability of rat liver to synthesize and secrete lipoproteins under a variety of physiological and pathological conditions, only a few have allowed for a correct assessment of the mass of lipoproteins secreted by the liver *in vitro* and an accurate characterization of the physicochemical properties of the newly secreted lipoproteins.

131

EXPERIMENTAL MODELS FOR THE STUDY OF
LIPOPROTEINS SECRETION

In most of the early *in vitro* studies conducted with liver slices, liver microsomes, isolated hepatocytes, and perfused liver, hepatic tissue was incubated or perfused with medium containing a radioactive precursor of the lipid or, more often, the protein moiety of plasma lipoproteins. The rate of lipoprotein secretion was measured by the radioactivity incorporated into the lipoproteins released into the medium, to which plasma carrier had been added prior to the isolation of the lipoproteins. However, this experimental approach could not give an exact quantification of the secreted lipoproteins for two reasons: (a) the intracellular pool of the precursor (usually [14]C- or ^{3}H-labeled amino acid) was unknown, and (b) the intracellular pool of preformed lipoproteins or apolipoproteins, or both, had never been estimated. A further limitation of those studies was that carrier plasma was added to the incubation, or perfusion medium, to ensure an adequate recovery of labeled lipoproteins after their isolation by preparative ultracentrifugation. Thus, since the labeled lipids or apolipoproteins, or both, present in the newly secreted lipoproteins may exchange with those present in the lipoproteins of the carrier plasma, it is difficult to establish whether the radioactivity found in one lipoprotein class truly reflects that originally incorporated into the same lipoprotein during its assembly in the liver.

In order to overcome some of these drawbacks two experimental models have been adopted in the last decade: (a) isolated rat hepatocytes (4,22,24,46), and (b) isolated rat liver perfused with a lipoprotein-free medium (3,10,17,20,25,29, 30,33,36,37). Although the use of rat hepatocytes has provided useful information about the net output and chemical composition of newly secreted VLDL (49), it does not seem to be suitable for the study of newly secreted HDL. In addition to lipoproteins, rat hepatocytes secrete biliary lipids (cholesterol and lecithin) which may interact with lipoproteins or peptides, or both, present in the medium, thus producing lipoprotein-like particles floating in the HDL range (24). Because of these technical problems, the isolated and perfused liver appears to be, at present, the most reliable method for the study of the net output and the physicochemical properties of newly secreted lipoproteins.

As mentioned above some plasma lipoprotein classes can be isolated from the Golgi apparatus of rat liver (5,13,27,28,35,47). Usually this experimental model involves the isolation of a Golgi-rich subcellular fraction, the rupture of the vesicles by some drastic treatment (6), and the isolation of lipoproteins by preparative ultracentrifugation. Although VLDL and LDL can be isolated from the Golgi vesicles in adequate amounts, the attempts to isolate lipoproteins of higher density have been, so far, unsuccessful (18).

LIVER PERFUSION STUDIES

In 1974, Marsh (29) studied the hepatic secretion of lipoproteins by perfusing rat liver with a nonrecirculating medium (single-pass perfusion) devoid of plasma lipoproteins. Despite the short duration of the perfusion (40 min), the material recovered in the perfusate allowed the separation of lipoproteins at 1.006, 1.040, 1.060, and 1.210 g/ml, and an analysis of their lipid and protein composition. The main advantages of this experimental model are its simplicity, the preservation of liver viability during the short-term perfusion, and the prevention (or high reduction) of the catabolism of newly secreted lipoproteins in the liver. On the other hand, the main disadvantages are the large volumes of perfusate which require concentration and the minute amounts of lipoproteins available for study. In order to overcome these problems Hamilton et al. (19) proposed a liver perfusion model in which the perfusate, containing glucose and erythrocytes but no plasma proteins, was recirculated for several hours. By using appropriate oxygenators (Silastic lungs) (19) that could prevent the structural damage of secreted lipoproteins, this prolonged perfusion (up to 6 hr) yielded sufficient material for a complete characterization of both VLDL and HDL (20). In a recent study a recirculating system similar to that proposed by Hamilton et al. was used, with the exception that bovine serum albumin was added to the medium (3). The addition of albumin [with a low content of contaminating apolipoproteins apo A-I and E (8)] prevents the hemolysis of the erythrocytes and greatly delays the deterioration of liver viability (2). Under these experimental conditions the recovery of perfusate lipoproteins is satisfactory (3).

Needless to say that in both the noncirculating and recirculating liver perfusion systems, the experimental conditions are far from physiological with regard to pressure, flow rate, and, above all, medium composition. It is conceivable that the net output, as well as the composition, of lipoproteins secreted by a liver perfused with portal blood (as occurs *in vivo*) is remarkably different from that observed *in vitro* under the experimental conditions described above.

The main disadvantage of prolonged liver perfusion with a recirculating medium is the catabolism of newly secreted lipoproteins which may be taken up and degraded by the liver cells (38,45,50,51). Furthermore, the composition of newly secreted lipoproteins may be modified during the perfusion by the action of lipoprotein lipases (23) and lecithin-cholesterol acyltransferase (LCAT) released by the liver (17).

ISOLATION OF LIPOPROTEINS FROM THE LIVER PERFUSATE

Lipoproteins secreted by perfused liver are usually separated by sequential preparative ultracentrifugation (3,10,17,20,25,29,30,33,36,37) within density intervals fairly similar to those adopted for separation of plasma lipoproteins. The choice of the density cut-off points for the perfusate lipoproteins is, however, rather arbitrary since there are no systematic studies on the flotation properties, density, and size distribution of perfusate lipoproteins. Attempts to investigate these problems were made in the past by Heimberg and Wilcox (21), and more recently by Marsh and Sparks (33) and by Gherardi and Calandra (unpublished observations), but the results are still inconclusive. Heimberg and Wilcox (21) isolated the perfusate lipoproteins by ultracentrifugation in a zonal rotor and identified various fractions: chylomicron-like particles, VLDL ($d < 1.020$ g/ml), LDL, and a residual fraction which included HDL and heavier plasma proteins. No attempts were made in that study to define precise density cut-off points for LDL or HDL. Marsh and Sparks (33) correlated the size distribution of perfusate lipoproteins with their flotation properties. They showed that when perfusate lipoproteins ($d < 1.210$ g/ml) were applied to an agarose column, three fractions could be eluted. The first, corresponding to the void volume of the column, floated at 1.006 g/ml and chemically resembled VLDL; the second contained heterogeneous material with regard to density which could be isolated at the densities of 1.006, 1.020, and 1.060 g/ml; the third contained lipoproteins floating at a density higher than 1.060 g/ml. In a recent study (Gherardi and Calandra, *unpublished observations*) separation of perfusate lipoproteins by ultracentrifugation was tried using a continuous salt density gradient (40) in order to compare the separation profile of perfusate lipoproteins with that of rat plasma lipoproteins. As a result, the major lipoprotein fraction of perfusate lipoproteins could be isolated at $d < 1.020$ g/ml, but lipoprotein material was present above that density up to 1.210 g/ml. In the density interval from 1.070 to 1.210 g/ml two overlapping classes of HDLs could be identified, which were characterized by a different apo E to apo A-I ratio. In view of these considerations the data concerning the properties of perfusate lipoproteins, especially those isolated at $d > 1.020$ g/ml by preparative ultracentrifugation, should be taken with caution. This should be kept in mind when investigating the effects of those factors that are potentially capable of altering the net output or the chemical composition, or both, of the lipoproteins secreted by the liver (e.g., dietary manipulations and the administration of drugs, hormones, and so on).

CONCENTRATION OF LIPOPROTEINS IN THE LIVER PERFUSATE

The mass of the lipoproteins in the various density classes released by the perfused liver varies in relation to the viability of the liver, the conditions of the perfusion (short- versus long-term perfusion), and the method of separation and quantification of perfusate lipoproteins. The output of lipoproteins secreted by the perfused liver under various experimental perfusion systems is shown in Table 1. Despite the difference in the absolute values reported by various authors (3,20,29,33,37), the data summarized in Table 1 clearly indicate that VLDL and HDL represent the major lipoprotein density classes secreted by rat liver perfused *in vitro* with a lipoprotein-free medium. Whether isolated and perfused rat liver secretes an LDL fraction similar to plasma LDL, is still a matter of controversy. Several investigators (3,10,29,33,37) have isolated a lipoprotein fraction in the density range 1.006 to 1.075 g/ml with a somewhat different lipid composition from that of perfusate VLDL. This may be taken as an indication that rat liver secretes an LDL species or that the LDL is formed from the catabolism of perfusate VLDL, which may occur in the hepatic vascular bed by the action of a lipoprotein lipase. Further studies are needed to clarify these points. It is interesting to compare the net secretion rate of lipoproteins obtained in the liver perfusion studies with those reported in

TABLE 1. Secretion of lipoproteins by rat liver perfused with a lipoprotein-free medium[a]

Density class (g/ml)	Ref. 29	Ref. 20[b]	Ref. 33	Ref. 37[c]	Ref. 3
Very low-density lipoprotein					
1.006	39 ± 1.9	44	55 ± 5.4	23.9	17.5 ± 3.4
Low-density lipoprotein					
1.006–1.050					7.2 ± 0.6
1.006–1.060	15 ± 1.8		33.9 ± 4.9		
1.006–1.087				0.5	
High-density lipoprotein					
1.050–1.090					6.3 ± 0.5
1.060–1.210	20.0 ± 1.5		21.0 ± 3.4		
1.075–1.210		12.5			
1.087–1.210				2.9	
1.090–1.210					9.0 ± 1.0

[a]Data in micrograms of apolipoprotein per gram of liver per hour.
[b]Recalculated by assuming a mean liver weight of 9 g in a 350 g rat.
[c]Recalculated from the value given in micrograms of apolipoprotein per gram of liver per 4 hr.

studies with isolated hepatocytes (4,22,24,46). By using hepatocytes in suspension, Jeejeebhoy et al. (22) found that the secretion of VLDL protein was about 35 μg/ g of hepatocytes per hour, in good agreement with the results of Marsh (29). However, the rate of secretion of VLDL protein by rat hepatocytes in culture (4) was found to be much lower (30–50%) than that reported in liver perfusion studies (Table 1). No comparison is possible with regard to HDL since there are no conclusive data on the net output of HDL by isolated hepatocytes. In a recent study Kempen (24) isolated lipoprotein particles containing phospholipid and cholesterol from a medium of freshly isolated hepatocytes, at densities from 1.030 to 1.080 g/ml and from 1.100 to 1.240 g/ml. These particles however did not correspond to the HDLs secreted by the perfused rat liver with regard to the content of both cholesteryl esters and apoproteins.

ELECTROPHORETIC MOBILITY OF PERFUSATE LIPOPROTEINS

Heimberg and Wilcox (21) reported that perfusate lipoproteins of $d < 1.006$ g/ ml behave as plasma VLDL in paper electrophoresis. They also noticed that the perfusate lipoproteins ($d < 1.006$) contained a minor component which did not move in paper electrophoresis (chylomicron-like particles). Other authors reported that both VLDL (20,37) and HDL (20) from liver perfusate moved slower than plasma VLDL and HDL in both paper and agarose electrophoresis. In addition, perfusate VLDL and HDL are heterogeneous, since they have been reported to exhibit trailing and diffusion in paper electrophoresis. A similar trailing was observed for VLDL isolated from the Golgi apparatus of rat liver (27).

LIPID COMPOSITION OF PERFUSATE LIPOPROTEINS

The lipid composition of the various lipoprotein classes isolated from liver perfusate differs from that of the corresponding plasma fractions. Marsh and Sparks (33) reported that perfusate VLDL and LDL contained less cholesteryl esters but more cholesterol and phospholipids than plasma VLDL, whereas the lipid to protein ratio was the same. In the study by Hamilton et al. (20) the difference between perfusate and plasma VLDL was also documented although it was less striking than that found by others (33). They reported that the lipid composition of perfusate HDL differed substantially from that of plasma HDL (20); perfusate HDL contained more triacylglycerols, free cholesterol, and phospholipids but much less cholesteryl esters than plasma HDL. Hamilton et al. (10,20) demonstrated that this peculiar lipid composition of perfusate HDL was related to the fact that during liver perfusion, the secreted lipoproteins had little chance to be exposed to the enzyme LCAT. When LCAT present in the perfusate was blocked by the addition of an inhibitor [5-5'-dithionitrobenzoic acid (DTNB)] to the perfusate, the relative content of phospholids, triacylglycerols, and free cholesterol in HDL increased, whereas that of cholesteryl esters decreased (17,20). It is not clearly understood whether the low cholesteryl ester concentration of perfusate VLDL is related to a reduced exposure of these particles to LCAT. Hamilton et al. reported that perfusate VLDLs secreted in the presence of DTNB were fairly similar to those secreted in the absence of the inhibitor (20).

The perfusate HDLs, secreted in the presence of DTNB, and predominantly made of phospholipids and cholesterol, are structurally similar to lipid bilayers. In negative-staining electron microscopy they appear as disk-shaped particles, which in appropriate conditions, assume a "rouleaux" configuration (17,20). Perfusate HDLs secreted in the absence of DTNB consist of small HDLs (about 75%) and some discoidal particles similar to those observed in the presence of DTNB. These discoidal HDL particles bear strong similarities in size and shape to those found in the HDL of patients suffering from LCAT deficiency (48). Further evidence of the role of LCAT in determining the lipid composition of newly secreted HDL is that perfusate HDL secreted both in the absence and in the presence of DTNB is a more suitable substrate for LCAT than the HDL isolated from rat plasma (17,20).

As mentioned above perfusate HDLs contained an unexpected high proportion of triacylglycerols (20). This is probably due to the presence of a contaminating lipoprotein, rich in triacylglycerols, which is isolated in the density interval 1.075 to 1.175 (9). This lipoprotein, which contains mainly apo B, could be successfully separated from HDL by concanavallin A/Sepharose affinity chromatography (9). It is not known whether these "HDL" particles containing apo B are (a) directly secreted by the liver, (b) artifacts formed during the ultracentrifugation of the perfusate, or (c) products of the catabolism of lipoproteins of lower density. Although it is unclear if these particles are present in normal rat plasma, it is worth mentioning that a lipoprotein fraction, rich in triacylglycerols and containing predominantly apo B, has been recently isolated from rat plasma HDL_1 (1.050–1.090 g/ml) (12).

It is interesting to compare the lipid composition of perfusate lipoproteins to that of lipoproteins secreted by rat hepatocytes or isolated in the Golgi apparatus of rat liver. For the technical reasons specified above (see section on experimental models), this comparison is confined to VLDL and LDL. VLDLs secreted from cultured rat hepatocytes (49) resemble those isolated from both recirculating (10,20) and non-recirculating liver perfusate (29,33). VLDLs isolated from tubules and vesicles of the Golgi apparatus were fairly similar to plasma VLDL, with two exceptions: a low relative content of cholesteryl esters and a high content of fatty acids (27). The reduced content of cholesteryl esters in Golgi VLDL, similar to that found in perfusate VLDL, has been repeatedly confirmed in other recent studies (13,47).

APOPROTEIN COMPOSITION OF PERFUSATE LIPOPROTEINS

In 1973 Windmueller et al. (53) demonstrated the ability of perfused rat liver to synthesize the various apoproteins of VLDL and HDL. They also reported that the rate of ^{3}H-lysine incorporation was greater in large molecular weight apoproteins of VLDL (predominantly Apo B) than in proteins of intermediate (presumably apo E) or low molecular weight (apo C). The ^{3}H content was greater in the intermediate molecular weight apoproteins (Apo E and apo A-I) of perfusate HDL than in the other peptides of this fraction. No conclusive data emerged from that study with regard to the apoprotein composition of perfusate VLDL and HDL because the liver had been perfused with a medium that contained plasma lipoproteins. In a nonre-circulating liver perfusion system, Marsh (30) found that perfusate VLDL resembled serum VLDL in apoprotein composition, at least qualitatively, and the proportion of the apoproteins soluble in tetramethylurea (TMU) in perfusate and plasma VLDL was the same. Furthermore, no evidence was found that perfusate LDL (d 1.006–1.040 g/ml) resembled serum LDL in apoprotein composition. In striking contrast, perfusate HDL contained much less apo A-IV and apo A-I and twice as much apo E as did its plasma counterpart.

In the recirculating liver perfusion system Hamilton et al. (20) observed that the apoprotein composition of perfusate VLDL was fairly similar to that of plasma VLDL with the exception of the "C" apoproteins, which in 8 M urea polyacrylamide gels were less intensely stained than the major apoprotein (apo E). In perfusate HDL most of the stainable material detected in urea gels migrated in the apo E region rather than in the apo A-I region, as found in plasma HDL. This important observation was fully confirmed by Felker et al. (10) who reported that the apo E/apo A-I ratio in perfusate HDL_2 (1.075–1.175 g/ml) and HDL_3 (1.075–1.210 g/ml) was 1.8 and 1.3, respectively; whereas, in plasma HDL_2 and HDL_3 this ratio was much lower (0.14 and 0.045, respectively). The apo E/apo A-I ratio increased considerably in HDL secreted in the presence of the LCAT inhibitor DTNB (10,17). Recently Marsh and Sparks (33) attempted to quantify the apoprotein composition of perfusate lipoproteins by measuring the staining intensity of the various peptides separated in sodium dodecyl sulfate (SDS)-polyacrylamide gel electrophoresis. In contrast to other studies (10) they found that the apo B/apo E ratio in perfusate

VLDL was lower than that observed in plasma VLDL, and the "C" peptides accounted for about 50% of the total apoprotein complement of perfusate VLDL. They also reported a high apo E/apo A-I ratio in perfusate HDL, as previously documented (10,30). Some recent studies (3,37) confirmed the observation of Hamilton et al. (10,20) that perfusate VLDL contained apo B and apo E but only minute amounts of "C" peptides. Some controversy exists about the peptide composition of perfusate LDL (d 1.006–1.050 g/ml). Noel et al. (37) found only apo B in perfusate LDL, whereas other authors claimed that perfusate LDL is almost undistinguishable from perfusate or plasma VLDL (3,30).

Few data are available about the concentration of the various apoproteins in the whole liver perfusate. By using a sensitive radioimmunoassay technique Felker et al. (10) found that the apo E/apo A-I ratio in the whole liver perfusate was about 13. A similar value was observed in rat liver perfused with a lipoprotein-free medium for 3 hr (3). Of course, it would be most desirable to repeat these studies by measuring also the other major apoproteins by immunological techniques.

It is interesting to compare the apoprotein composition of perfusate VLDL to that of VLDL or LDL, or both, isolated from the Golgi vesicles of rat liver. In 1970 Mahley et al. (28) reported that the apoproteins of Golgi VLDL resembled those found in VLDL isolated from both plasma and liver perfusate, at least qualitatively. However, other studies (5,35) demonstrated that Golgi VLDL were either devoid of "C" peptides (apo C-II and apo C-III) or contained them in a reduced proportion as compared to plasma VLDL. This observation was recently confirmed by Swift et al. (47) and Gherardi et al. (13). It should be emphasized that VLDL deficient in apo C-II and apo C-III are secreted by rat hepatocytes either in suspension (24) or in culture (4).

NASCENT LIPOPROTEINS

On the basis of the above-mentioned studies, there is good evidence that the lipoproteins secreted by rat liver, perfused with a lipoprotein-deficient medium, differ considerably from the corresponding plasma fractions for one or more of the following properties: lipid and apoprotein composition, ultrastructure, and ability to act as substrate for LCAT. It seems therefore appropriate to designate these lipoproteins "nascent lipoproteins" (20,29), as opposed to circulating lipoproteins, which are those isolated from plasma. Now, the question can be raised as to whether or not nascent lipoproteins demonstrated in liver perfusion studies are secreted as such in the *in vivo* situation. It is likely that *in vivo* the newly secreted VLDL resemble nascent VLDL because the latter are almost undistinguishable from those VLDL directly isolated by the liver cells before their release from the Golgi apparatus. The same conclusion cannot be applied to HDL since there is no evidence, as yet, that perfusate HDL (nascent HDL) is similar to the HDL present intracellularly in the cisternae and vacuoles of the Golgi apparatus. The above question cannot be answered until a more reliable method has been found to isolate HDL from the liver cell before they are discharged into the extracellular environment.

UNSOLVED PROBLEMS

If the study of the physicochemical properties of nascent lipoproteins is well in progress in several laboratories, the characterization of the process of assembly and secretion of nascent lipoproteins, as well as that of their biological properties, is still in its infancy. Among the numerous unanswered questions, the ones presented below were chosen for their paramount importance for the understanding of the metabolism of plasma lipoproteins.

First, what are the mechanisms whereby nascent lipoproteins exchange lipids and peptides with circulating lipoproteins on their entry into the circulation, and what are the roles played by LCAT, lipoprotein lipase, and the cholesteryl ester transfer factor? Is the secretion of lipoproteins and that of LCAT and cholesteryl ester transfer factor by the liver coordinate or independent events (11)? (That is, do factors capable of stimulating the secretion of one lipoprotein class induce also a parallel overproduction of LCAT or cholesteryl ester transfer factor, or both?)

Second, are the VLDL produced by the liver different from those released by the intestine? It has been recently shown (7) that apo B of rat plasma VLDL consists of three peptides (PI, PII, PIII), whereas apo B present in chylomicrons consists predominantly of the PIII peptide. Therefore, it would be interesting to know if rat liver secretes VLDL having predominantly PI and PII peptides.

Third, are nascent HDL secreted as a single lipoprotein class, containing particles having both apo E and apo A-I as constituent peptides, or as two classes of particles each having one single constituent peptide?

Last, what are the biological properties of nascent lipoproteins? Do nascent lipoproteins interact with cells and influence cellular lipid homeostasis? Does the peculiar lipid and apoprotein composition of nascent lipoproteins render them more susceptible to the uptake and degradation by tissues? The recent studies of Windler et al. (50,51), who found that the hepatic uptake of nascent VLDL with low apo C content is different from that of circulating VLDL, have given a preliminary answer to these questions.

REFERENCES

1. Bungenberg de Jong, J., and Marsh, J. B. (1968): Biosynthesis of plasma lipoproteins by rat liver ribosomes. *J. Biol. Chem.*, 243:192–199.
2. Calandra, S., Gherardi, E., Bartošek, I., and Guaitani, A. (1981): Impiego del fegato isolato e perfuso nello studio della secrezione delle lipoproteine del plasma. *Atti del 1° convegno per lo studio degli organi isolati* (Capizzi, F. D. ed.), pp. 131–138. Patron, Bologna.
3. Calandra, S., Gherardi, E., Fainaru, M., Guaitani, A., and Bartošek, I. (1982): Secretion of lipoproteins, apolipoprotein A-I and apolipoprotein E by isolated and perfused liver of rat with experimental nephrotic syndrome. *Biochim. Biophys. Acta*, 665:331–338.
4. Davis, R. A., Engelhorn, S. C., Pangburn, S. H., Weistein, D. B., and Steinberg, D. (1979): Very low density lipoprotein synthesis and secretion by cultured rat hepatocytes. *J. Biol. Chem.*, 254:2010–2016.
5. Dolphin, P. J., and Rubinstein, D. (1977): Glycosylation of apoproteins of rat very low density lipoproteins during transit through the hepatic Golgi apparatus. *Can. J. Biochem.*, 55:83–90.
6. Enrenheich, J. H., Bergeron, J. J. M., Siekevitz, P., and Palade, G. E. (1973): Golgi Fractions prepared from rat liver homogenate. *J. Cell Biol.*, 59:46–72.

7. Elovson, J., Huang, Y. O., Baker, N., and Kannan, R. (1981): Apolipoprotein B is structurally and metabolically heterogenous in the rat. *Proc. Natl. Acad. Sci. USA*, 78:157–161.
8. Fainaru, M., and Deckelbaum, R. (1979): Lipid binding protein (apolipoprotein A-I) contamination of high grade commercial albumins. *FEBS Lett.*, 97:171–174.
9. Fainaru, M., Felker, T. E., Hamilton, R. L., and Havel, R. J. (1977): Evidence that a separate particle containing B-apoproteins is present in high density lipoproteins from perfused rat liver. *Metabolism*, 26:999–1004.
10. Felker, T. E., Fainaru, M., Hamilton, R. L., and Havel, R. J. (1977): Secretion of the arginin rich and A-I apolipoproteins by the isolated perfused rat liver. *J. Lipid Res.*, 18:465–473.
11. Fielding, P. E., and Fielding, C. J. (1980): A cholesteryl ester transfer complex in human plasma. *Proc. Natl. Acad. Sci. USA*, 77:3327–3330.
12. Gherardi, E. (1980): Isolation of a lipoprotein containing the arginin rich peptide from rat HDL₁ (1.050–1.090 g/ml). Abstract of the VII International Symposium on Drugs Affecting Lipid Metabolism, p. 38. Milano, 28–31 May.
13. Gherardi, E., Calandra, S., Bartošek, I., and Guaitani, A. (1980): Isolation of nascent low density lipoproteins from Golgi vescicles and perfusate of isolated and perfused rat liver. Abstracts of the 15th EASL Meeting, Beograd, 4–6 September, p. 6.
14. Gherardi, E., Messori, M., Rozzi, R., and Calandra, S. (1980): Experimental nephrotic syndrome in the rat induced by puromycin aminonucleoside: Hepatic synthesis of lipoproteins and apolipoproteins. *Lipids*, 15:858–863.
15. Glaumann, H., Bergstrand, A., and Ericsson, L. E. (1975): Studies on the synthesis and intracellular transport of lipoprotein particles in rat liver. *J. Cell Biol.*, 64:356–377.
16. Haft, D. E., Roheim, P. S., White, A., and Eder, H. A. (1962): Plasma lipoprotein metabolism in perfused rat livers. I. Protein synthesis and entry into the plasma. *J. Clin. Invest.*, 41:842–849.
17. Hamilton, R. L. (1978): Hepatic secretion and metabolism of high density lipoproteins. In: *Disturbance in Lipid and Lipoprotein Metabolism*, edited by J. M. Dietschy, A. M. Gotto, and J. A. Ontko, pp. 155–171. American Physiological Society, Bethesda, Maryland.
18. Hamilton, R. L. (1980): Nascent VLDL and nascent HDL from liver. In: *Atherosclerosis, Vol. 5: Proceedings of the 5th International Symposium on Atherosclerosis*, edited by A. M. Gotto, L. C. Smith, and B. Allen, pp. 164–167. Springer-Verlag, New York.
19. Hamilton, R. L., Berry, M. N., Williams, M. C., and Severinghous, E. M. (1974): A simple and inexpensive membrane "lung" for small organ perfusion. *J. Lipid Res.*, 15:182–186.
20. Hamilton, R. I., Williams, M. C., Fielding, C. J., and Havel, R. J. (1976): Discoidal bilayer structure of nascent high density lipoproteins from perfused rat liver. *J. Clin. Invest.*, 58:667–680.
21. Heimberg, M., and Wilcox, H. G. (1972): The effect of palmitic and oleic acids on the properties and composition of the very low density lipoprotein secreted by the liver. *J. Biol. Chem.*, 247:875–880.
22. Jeejeebhoy, K. N., Ho, J., Breckenridge, C., Bruce-Robertson, A., Steiner, G., and Jeejeebhoy, J. (1975): Synthesis of VLDL by isolated rat hepatocytes in suspension. *Biochim. Biophys. Res. Commun.*, 66:1147–1153.
23. Jensen, G. L., Baly, L. D., Brannon, P. M., and Bensadoun, A. (1980): Synthesis and secretion of lipolytic enzymes by cultured chicken hepatocytes. *J. Biol. Chem.*, 255:11141–11148.
24. Kempen, H. J. M. (1980): Lipoprotein secretion by isolated rat hepatocytes: Characterization of the lipid carrying particles and modulation of their release. *J. Lipid Res.*, 21:671–680.
25. Kook, A. I., and Rubinstein, D. (1973): A comparison of the secretion of two components of very low density lipoproteins by perfused rat liver. *Can. J. Biochem.*, 51:490–494.
26. Lo, C. H., and Marsh, J. B. (1970): Biosynthesis of plasma lipoproteins. *J. Biol. Chem.*, 245:5001–5006.
27. Mahley, R. W., Hamilton, R. L., and LeQuire, V. S. (1969): Characterization of lipoprotein particles isolated from the Golgi apparatus of rat liver. *J. Lipid Res.*, 10:433–439.
28. Mahley, R. W., Bersot, T. P., LeQuire, V. S., Levy, R. I., Windmueller, H. G., and Brown, W. V. (1970): Identity of very low density lipoprotein apoproteins of plasma and liver Golgi apparatus. *Science*, 168:380–382.
29. Marsh, J. B. (1974): Lipoproteins in a nonrecirculating perfusate of rat liver. *J. Lipid Res.*, 15:544–550.
30. Marsh, J. B. (1976): Apoproteins of the lipoproteins in a nonrecirculating perfusate of rat liver. *J. Lipid Res.*, 17:85–90.

31. Marsh, J. B., and Drabkin, D. L. (1958): Metabolic channeling in experimental nephrosis. *J. Biol. Chem.*, 230:1073–1081.

32. Marsh, J. B., and Whereat, A. F. (1959): The synthesis of plasma lipoproteins by rat liver. *J. Biol. Chem.*, 234:3196–3200.

33. Marsh, J. B., and Sparks, C. E. (1979): Hepatic secretion of lipoproteins in the rat and the effect of experimental nephrosis. *J. Clin. Invest.*, 64:1229–1237.

34. Narayan, K. A., Mary, G. E. S., and Kummerow, F. A. (1968): Rat serum lipoproteins after partial hepatectomy. *Proc. Soc. Exp. Biol. Med.*, 129:2–10.

35. Nestruck, A. C., and Rubinstein, D. (1976): The synthesis of apoproteins of very low density lipoproteins isolated from the Golgi apparatus of rat liver. *Can. J. Biochem.*, 54:617–628.

36. Noel, S. P., and Rubinstein, D. (1974): Secretion of apolipoproteins in very low density and high density lipoproteins by perfused rat liver. *J. Lipid Res.*, 15:301–308.

37. Noel, S. P., Wong, L., Dolphin, P. J., Dory, L., and Rubinstein, D. (1979): Secretion of cholesterol-rich lipoproteins by perfused livers of hypercholesterolemic rats. *J. Clin. Invest.*, 64:674–683.

38. Quarfordt, S., Hanks, J., Scott Jones, R., and Shelbourne, F. (1980): The uptake of high density lipoprotein cholesteryl ester in the perfused rat liver. *J. Biol. Chem.*, 255:2934–2937.

39. Radding, C. M., and Steinberg, D. (1960): Studies on the synthesis and secretion of serum lipoproteins by rat liver slices. *J. Clin. Invest.*, 39:1560–1569.

40. Redgrave, T. G., Roberts, A. C. K., and West, C. E. (1975): Separation of plasma lipoproteins by density gradient ultracentrifugation. *Anal. Biochem.*, 65:42–49.

41. Roheim, P. S., Miller, L., and Eder, H. A. (1965): The formation of plasma lipoproteins from apoprotein in plasma. *J. Biol. Chem.*, 240:2994–3001.

42. Ruderman, N. B., Richards, K. C., Valles de Bourges, V., and Jones, A. L. (1968): Regulation of production and release of lipoprotein by the perfused rat liver. *J. Lipid Res.*, 9:613–619.

43. Sabesin, S. M., Kuiken, L. B., and Ragland, J. B. (1975): Lipoprotein and lecithin:cholesterol acyltransferase changes in galactosamine induced rat liver injury. *Science*, 190:1302–1304.

44. Shiff, T. S., Roheim, P. S., and Eder, H. A. (1971): Effects of high sucrose diets and 4-aminopyrazolopyrimidine on serum lipids and lipoproteins in the rat. *J. Lipid Res.*, 12:596–603.

45. Sigurdsson, G., Noel, S. P., and Havel, R. (1978): Catabolism of the apoprotein of low density lipoproteins by the isolated and perfused rat liver. *J. Lipid Res.*, 19:628–634.

46. Sundler, R., Akesson, B., and Nilsson, A. (1973): Triacylglycerol secretion in very low density lipoproteins by isolated rat liver parenchymal cells. *Biochim. Biophys Res. Commun.*, 55:961–968.

47. Swift, L. L., Manowitz, N. R., Dunn, G. D., and LeQuire, V. S. (1980): Isolation and characterization of hepatic Golgi lipoproteins from hypercholesterolemic rats. *J. Clin. Invest.*, 66:415–425.

48. Torsvik, H., Solaas, M. H., and Gjone, E. (1970): Serum lipoproteins in plasma lecithin:cholesterol acyltransferase deficiency, studied by electron microscopy. *Clin. Genet.*, 1:139–150.

49. Weistein, D. B., Davis, R. A., Engelhorn, S. C., and Steinberg, D. (1980): Synthesis and secretion of very low density lipoprotein by cultured rat hepatocytes. In: *Atherosclerosis, Vol. 5: Proceedings of the 5th International Symposium on Atherosclerosis*, edited by A. M. Gotto, L. C. Smith, and B. Allen, pp. 168–172. Springer-Verlag, New York.

50. Windler, E., Chao, Y., and Havel, R. J. (1980): Determinants of hepatic uptake of triglyceride-rich lipoproteins and their remnants in the rat. *J. Biol. Chem.*, 255:5475–5480.

51. Windler, E., Chao, Y., and Havel, R. J. (1980): Regulation of the hepatic uptake of triglyceride-rich lipoproteins in the rat. *J. Biol. Chem.*, 255:8303–8307.

52. Windmueller, H. G. (1964): An orotic acid-induced, adenine-reversed inhibition of hepatic lipoprotein secretion in the rat. *J. Biol. Chem.*, 239:530–537.

53. Windmueller, H. G., Herbert, P. N., and Levy, R. I. (1973): Biosynthesis of lymph and plasma lipoprotein apoproteins by isolated perfused rat liver and intestine. *J. Lipid Res.*, 14:215–223.

Phospholipids and Atherosclerosis, edited by
P. Avogaro, M. Mancini, G. Ricci, and
R. Paoletti. Raven Press, New York © 1983.

Interrelationship Between Plasma Phospholipids and Low-Density Lipoprotein Turnover

Gilbert R. Thompson

*Medical Research Council Lipid Metabolism Unit, Hammersmith Hospital,
London, W12 OHS, England*

This chapter discusses two aspects of the relationship between plasma phospho-lipids and low-density lipoprotein (LDL) turnover. One is the manner in which exogenous phospholipids affect the fatty acid composition of LDL lipids, and thus the turnover of the entire LDL particle, when introduced directly into the circulation. The other aspect discussed is how those diseases or drugs that directly affect LDL turnover can alter the pattern of endogenous phospholipids, which comprise about 25% of the LDL particle. A brief description of the structure and function of phospholipids in plasma, and the factors which influence their metabolism in both health and disease, is presented first.

STRUCTURE AND FUNCTION OF PLASMA PHOSPHOLIPIDS

The two main classes of phospholipid found in human plasma are glycerophos-pholipids, notably phosphatidylcholine or lecithin, and sphingophospholipids, such as sphingomyelin (see Fig. 1). Glycerophospholipids contain glycerol esterified with phosphoric acid at the 3-position and with fatty acids at the 1- and 2-positions. The fatty acid at the 1-position is usually saturated, whereas that at the 2-position is usually unsaturated. In lecithin the phosphoric acid is further esterified with choline. Sphingophospholipids contain sphingosine, instead of glycerol, similarly esterified with phosphoric acid and linked to a single, usually saturated fatty acid by an amino group; the phosphoric acid in sphingomyelin is secondarily esterified with choline, as in lecithin. Under normal circumstances roughly two-thirds of the total phospholipid in plasma is lecithin; approximately 20%, sphingomyelin, and the remainder, mainly lysolecithin and phosphatidylethanolamine. However, there is considerable variation between different lipoprotein classes in this respect. Both very low-density lipoprotein (VLDL) and LDL are richer in sphingomyelin than is high-density lipoprotein (HDL), which contains relatively more lecithin (43).

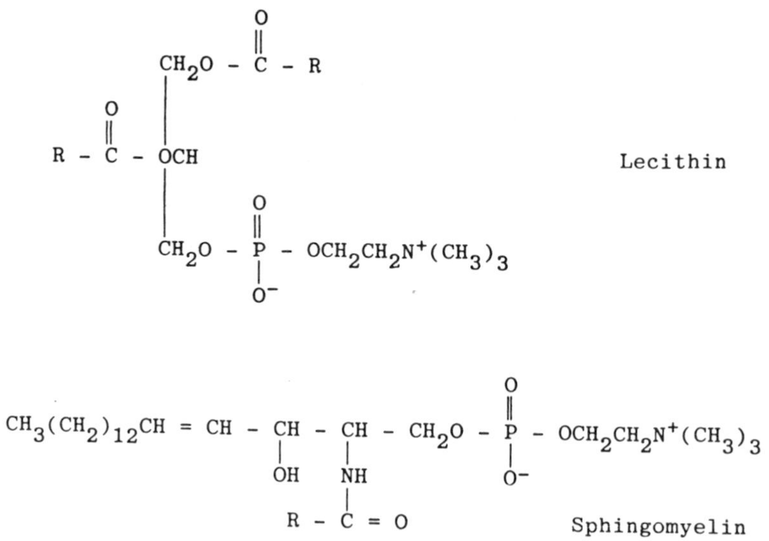

$$CH_2O - \overset{\overset{\displaystyle O}{\|}}{C} - R$$

$$R - \overset{\overset{\displaystyle O}{\|}}{C} - OCH$$

Lecithin

$$CH_2O - \overset{\overset{\displaystyle O}{\|}}{\underset{\underset{\displaystyle O^-}{|}}{P}} - OCH_2CH_2N^+(CH_3)_3$$

$$CH_3(CH_2)_{12}CH = CH - \underset{\underset{\displaystyle OH}{|}}{CH} - \underset{\underset{\displaystyle NH}{|}}{CH} - CH_2O - \overset{\overset{\displaystyle O}{\|}}{\underset{\underset{\displaystyle O^-}{|}}{P}} - OCH_2CH_2N^+(CH_3)_3$$

$$R - C = O$$

Sphingomyelin

FIG. 1. Formulas of the two principal phospholipids of human plasma.

Phospholipid synthesis takes place in most tissues, but plasma phospholipids are derived mainly from the liver and small intestine. The hepatic contribution consists of those phospholipids contained in newly synthesized VLDL and HDL, and significant quantities of lecithin are contributed by the small intestine in the form of chylomicrons; the actual amount entering the circulation is dependent on dietary fat intake. The nature of the fat in the diet markedly influences the fatty acid composition of plasma phospholipids, as exemplified by the studies of Spritz and Mishkel (45). Those authors showed that the percentage of lecithin molecules in plasma with linoleic acid in the 2-position increased from 40% during a saturated fat-rich diet to 64% when the diet was enriched in polyunsaturated fat.

Phospholipids are important constituents of all cell membranes, not the least being red cell membranes. Exchange of lecithin, and to a lesser extent sphingomyelin, between plasma and red cells plays an important role in maintaining the functional integrity of mature erythrocytes, which cannot synthesize their own phospholipids (38). As mentioned above, phospholipids are present in plasma as constituents of lipoproteins, where they interact with apoproteins to play a key role in solubilizing nonpolar lipids, such as triglycerides and cholesteryl esters. This property reflects the amphipathic nature of phospholipids. Their nonpolar fatty acyl chains interact with a lipid environment; their polar head groups, with an aqueous environment (20).

PLASMA PHOSPHOLIPID METABOLISM

There are three main pathways involved in the overall turnover of phospholipids in plasma: (a) exchange between cell membranes and lipoproteins, and between different lipoproteins, (b) hydrolysis by phospholipases, and (c) applicable only to lecithin, conversion into lysolecithin by the action of the enzyme lecithin-cholesterol acyltransferase (LCAT).

The triglyceride component of injected chylomicrons or an artificial fat emulsion is cleared from the plasma far more rapidly than the phospholipid component; the half-life of disappearance of triglyceride is from 1 to 15 min compared with 3 to 6 hr for phospholipid (28). Part of the reason for the longer half-life of the latter is that net transfer and exchange of phospholipids occur between chylomicrons and other lipoproteins, notably HDL, which have a much slower turnover rate than chylomicrons (30). Phospholipid exchange between LDL and HDL has also been demonstrated *in vivo* and is more rapid with lecithin than sphingomyelin (19). This process can be minimized *in vitro*, as during preparative ultracentrifugation, by maintaining plasma at 5°C. Exchange of phospholipids between subcellular fractions of liver and artificially prepared phospholipid dispersions or lipoproteins *in vitro* has also been shown and can be accelerated by addition of a so-called phospholipid exchange protein derived from the liver (21,51). In a similar manner this exchange protein enhances phospholipid exchange between LDL and HDL *in vitro* (18). The relevance of these observations to phospholipid exchange *in vivo*, however, remains to be determined.

Eisenberg and Schurr (9) studied the removal of phospholipid from VLDL during its catabolism to LDL. They showed that considerable hydrolysis of lecithin resulted from the action of both extrahepatic and hepatic lipases with the formation of lysolecithin, which was then rapidly removed. In addition, they observed some transfer of intact lecithin to HDL. As a result of these processes the VLDL remnant became relatively enriched in sphingomyelin; in this respect, it resembled the final product of VLDL catabolism, namely LDL. The above results, which were obtained *in vitro*, did not indicate any dependence upon LCAT of the processes involved. However, *in vivo*, this enzyme exerts an important influence on plasma phospholipid metabolism, as exemplified by the increased levels of lecithin and decreased levels of lysolecithin found in familial LCAT deficiency (34). Under normal circumstances this enzyme transesterifies the free cholesterol of HDL, and probably LDL, with a poly- or monounsaturated fatty acid derived from the 2-position of lecithin, thus generating cholesteryl ester and lysolecithin (13). Subsequently, much of the cholesteryl ester gets transferred to other lipoproteins, initially to VLDL and eventually to LDL; whereas, the lysolecithin gets taken up mainly by albumin.

One result of LCAT deficiency is the accumulation in plasma of an abnormal LDL, rich in free cholesterol and lecithin, known as Lp-X. This lipoprotein also occurs in patients with biliary obstruction, largely as a result of the reflux into plasma of large amounts of biliary lecithin and free cholesterol, although deficiency of LCAT consequent upon hepatic dysfunction is undoubtedly a contributing factor in some instances. In an analogous manner, infusion of Intralipid, a fat emulsion which contains egg lecithin, can result in the appearance of Lp-X in the plasma of neonates. This is caused by an overloading of their clearance mechanisms (16). In both these situations the deficiency of LCAT can be regarded as relative rather than absolute. This is in contrast with what occurs in familial LCAT deficiency. Interestingly, the amount of Lp-X in the plasma of patients with the latter disorder can be reduced by restricting their intake of dietary fat, and thus the input of chylomicron lecithin and free cholesterol (12).

INFLUENCE OF EXOGENOUS PHOSPHOLIPIDS ON SERUM LIPIDS

There is little evidence that orally administered phospholipids have any effect on serum lipids other than that attributable to the amount and composition of their constituent fatty acids. Thus Greten et al. (15) failed to demonstrate any difference between the effects of equivalent masses of polyunsaturated fatty acids, whether administered as lecithin or triglyceride. This is not surprising in view of (a) the inability of Scow et al. (40) to increase the lecithin content of chylomicrons by feeding oral lecithin and (b) evidence that the latter undergoes extensive hydrolysis during absorption (39).

In contrast, intravenously administered phospholipids can influence serum lipids to a profound extent. Friedman and Byers (10) gave intravenously an emulsion of soybean phospholipids to rats and demonstrated well-correlated increases in both serum cholesterol and phospholipid, but not triglyceride. These effects were exaggerated by partial or total hepatectomy, suggesting that the liver normally plays a role in phospholipid catabolism (5). Those authors also showed that the hypercholesterolemia was dependent upon the maintenance of excess phospholipid in plasma (6). In subsequent studies they showed that the rise in serum cholesterol preceded any increase in hepatic cholesterol synthesis (7) and concluded that the bulk of the increase in cholesterol in plasma was derived from mobilization of tissue cholesterol by circulating phospholipid (8). There is little doubt, however, that hepatic cholesterol synthesis does increase, presumably because of a phospholipid-induced decrease in hepatocyte cholesterol content, as has been shown in rats given intravenous egg lecithin (23). The ability of both lecithin and sphingomyelin to promote efflux of free cholesterol from cells is well documented (4), especially when combined with apo A, as in HDL (46). That this property may well have therapeutic potential is suggested by the demonstration that intravenous lecithin of animal origin caused regression of experimentally induced aortic atheroma in rabbits (11). Subsequent studies showed that this property was also exhibited by Lipostabil, a preparation in which the lecithin fatty acids are mainly polyunsaturated and are derived from soybeans; however, it was not exhibited by egg lecithin, which contains chiefly saturated and monounsaturated fatty acids (1). Interestingly the rise in serum phospholipids was less after Lipostabil than egg lecithin, suggesting that the polyunsaturated phospholipid was cleared faster from plasma.

EFFECTS OF INTRAVENOUS PHOSPHOLIPIDS
ON LDL METABOLISM

Intralipid is a fat emulsion of 10 or 20% soybean triglyceride in 1.2% egg lecithin, which is used extensively in the realm of parenteral nutrition. In 1975, Thompson et al. (48) investigated the contrasting effects, on the plasma lipoproteins of control subjects, of Intralipid administered via oral and intravenous routes. All subjects were on a low-fat diet and each received 500 ml of 10% Intralipid daily for 5 days, via intragastric tube during one study period and intravenously during the other. Blood samples were taken daily and LDL (*d* 1.006–1.063), obtained by ultracentrifugation of plasma, was assayed for cholesterol, phospholipid, and protein content. In addition, the fatty acid composition of LDL lecithin and cholesteryl ester was determined. As illustrated in Fig. 2 a zone of opaque lipid was visible in

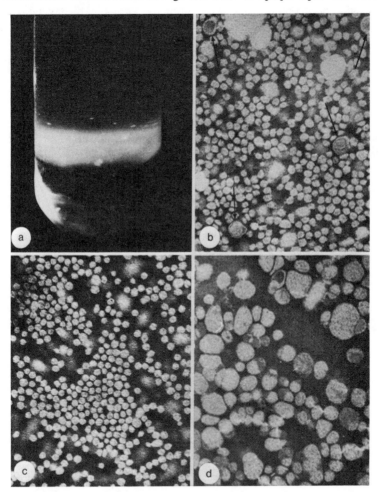

FIG. 2. **a:** Plasma from control subject obtained 12 hr after last of five daily infusions of intravenous Intralipid, showing zone of opaque lipid which has sedimented during ultracentrifugation at *d* 1.006. **b:** Electron micrograph of plasma (*d* 1.006–1.063) from same subject showing low-density lipoprotein particles and phospholipid vesicles *(arrows)*. **c:** Normal low-density lipoprotein. **d:** Phospholipid component of Intralipid × 100,000. (From Thompson et al., ref. 48, with permission.)

ultracentrifuged plasma from at least one subject, obtained the day after the fifth dose of intravenous Intralipid. Electron microscopy confirmed that this consisted of phospholipid vesicles, similar to the egg lecithin vesicles present in Intralipid. This phenomenon was not seen after intragastric Intralipid.

The effects of Intralipid on LDL concentration and composition are illustrated in Fig. 3. As can be seen, there was a fall in LDL protein after intragastric Intralipid but no change in the phospholipid/protein ratio. In contrast, intravenous Intralipid caused a progressive rise in LDL protein and in the phospholipid/protein ratio. Note that the latter decreased to basal levels during the week after the last infusion, but that the elevation of LDL protein persisted. This suggests that the effects of intravenous Intralipid on LDL were apparent even after all the excess phospholipid infused (6 g/day) had disappeared from plasma. Although not shown, changes in LDL cholesterol occurred in parallel with LDL protein.

Analysis of the fatty acid composition of LDL lecithin showed a change similar to that of egg lecithin after intravenous, compared with intragastric, Intralipid— especially in respect to oleic ($C_{18:1}$) and linoleic ($C_{18:2}$) acids (Fig. 4). Comparable changes were observed in LDL cholesteryl esters, presumably because of the interaction between LCAT and the altered pattern of fatty acids in LDL lecithin (Table 1).

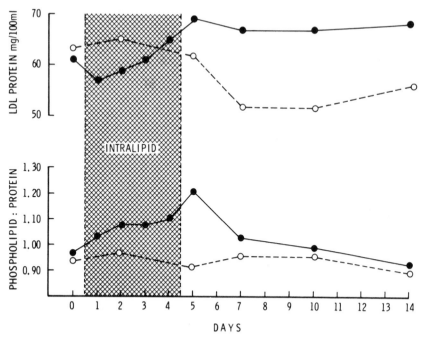

FIG. 3. Concentration of low-density lipoprotein (LDC) protein and protein/phospholipid ratio in a fraction of plasma (d 1.006–1.063) from three subjects receiving intravenous Intralipid (●) and from two subjects receiving intragastric Intralipid (○). (From Thomspon et al., ref. 48, with permission.)

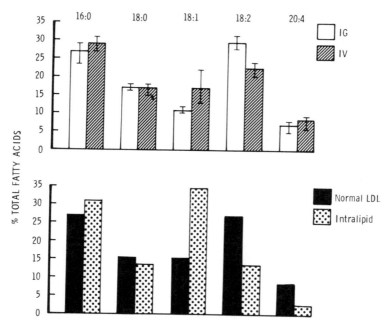

FIG. 4. Fatty acid composition of low-density lipoprotein (LDL) phospholipid from subjects given intragastric (IG) and intravenous (IV) Intralipid, compared with normal LDL and phospholipid component of Intralipid.

TABLE 1. *Fatty acid pattern of cholesteryl esters in the 1.006–1.063 density fraction of plasma after Intralipid*

	Total fatty acids (%)					
	$C_{16:0}$	$C_{18:0}$	$C_{18:1}$	$C_{18:2}$	$C_{20:4}$	$C_{18:1}/C_{18:2}$
Intragastric	11.5	8.4	8.7	46.4	7.3	0.19
Intravenous	11.3	11.0	13.1	41.8	8.7	0.31

In vitro studies confirmed that endogenous LDL lecithin readily exchanges with, and is partly replaced by, egg lecithin—the latter having a higher content of oleic acid and a lower content of linoleic acid than LDL. Similar changes have since been reported in rats infused with Intralipid (25).

The mechanism responsible for the rise in LDL after intravenous Intralipid was further explored by performing non-steady-state LDL turnover studies in control subjects given intragastric and intravenous Intralipid as before, and in some instances intravenous egg lecithin (49). As illustrated in Fig. 5 intravenous administration of either Intralipid or egg lecithin caused a prolongation of the half-life of 125I-labeled LDL in the plasma of the recipient. Quantitative measurements, shown in Fig. 6, confirmed that intragastric Intralipid failed to cause any increase in LDL protein

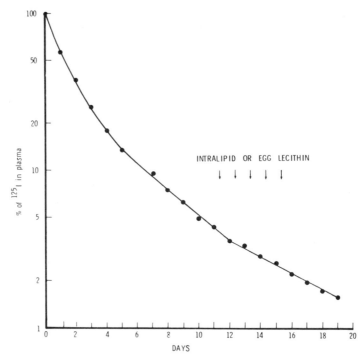

FIG. 5. Effects of five daily infusions of intravenous Intralipid or egg lecithin on plasma half-life of ^{125}I-labeled low-density lipoprotein in control subject. (Adapted from Thompson et al., ref. 49, with permission.)

or cholesterol and did not influence the fractional catabolic rate (FCR) of LDL. In contrast, intravenous Intralipid caused a rise in both LDL cholesterol and protein, and a decrease in FCR. Since there was very little change in the rate of synthesis of LDL, it was assumed that the decrease in FCR was largely responsible for the rise in LDL concentration. Analogous results were obtained when intravenous egg lecithin (1.2%), without any triglyceride, was infused instead of Intralipid (Fig. 7 and Table 2).

In summary, these studies show that intravenous administration of solutions containing egg lecithin (with or without triglyceride) leads to exchange between endogenous and exogenous phospholipids, resulting in modification of the fatty acid composition of both the lecithin and, via the action of LCAT, the cholesteryl ester of the recipients's LDL. The resultant increase in the ratio of oleate/linoleate in these lipids is accompanied by a decrease in the FCR and a rise in the concentration of LDL in plasma. Since opposite changes in respect to the oleate/linoleate ratio, FCR, and concentration of LDL in plasma occur in subjects on highly polyunsaturated fat diets (42), the fatty acid composition of LDL lipids exert an important influence on the rate of catabolism of the entire particle. The well-established link

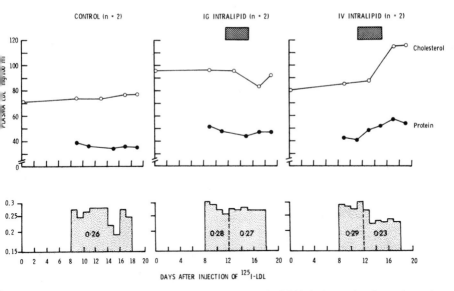

FIG. 6. Concentration in plasma of low-density lipoprotein (LDL) cholesterol and protein, and fractional catabolic rate (urine/plasma ratio) of LDL in pairs of control subjects on low-fat diet alone or receiving intragastric (IG) or intravenous (IV) Intralipid (2,500 ml of 10%), over the periods shown by the hatched rectangles.

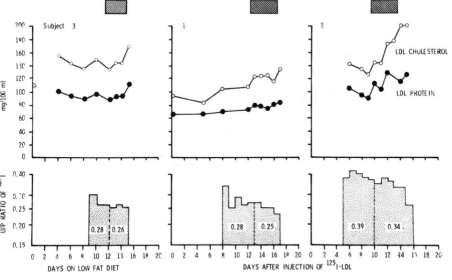

FIG. 7. Concentration in plasma of low-density lipoprotein (LDL) cholesterol and protein, and fractional catabolic rate (urine/plasma ratio) of LDL in three control subjects receiving intravenous egg lecithin (30 g, equivalent to that infused in Fig. 6) over period shown by hatched rectangles.

TABLE 2. Effect of intravenous egg lecithin (6 g/day for 5 days) on fatty acid composition of high-density lipoprotein in a normal subject[a]

	Total fatty acids (%)					
	$C_{16:0}$	$C_{18:0}$	$C_{18:1}$	$C_{18:2}$	$C_{20:4}$	$C_{18:1}/C_{18:2}$
PC						
Pre	31	16	9	30	10	0.30
Post	33	20	15	23	7	0.65
CE						
Pre	12	1	16	61	5	0.26
Post	11	1	22	55	5	0.40

[a]PC, phosphatidylcholine; CE, cholesteryl ester.

between bile acid excretion and LDL catabolism suggests the possibility that changes in the fatty acid composition of LDL cholesteryl esters affect LDL catabolism by influencing the rate of hydrolysis of cholesteryl esters to free cholesterol and thus increasing the availability of the latter for conversion into bile acids. In contrast to egg lecithin, intravenous administration of Lipostabil, largely containing polyunsaturated lecithin, has been shown to decrease the oleate/linoleate ratio of plasma phospholipids and cholesteryl esters, and to decrease LDL levels (3). Whether or not Lipostabil achieves the latter effect by increasing the FCR of LDL remains to be determined however.

Finally, a brief comment on the possible clinical consequences of infusing phospholipids intravenously. Although Lp-X was not found in the plasma of any of the patients studied here who were given intravenous Intralipid or egg lecithin (49), this phenomenon has been well described in both rats (25) and human neonates (16) who were given the fat emulsion at relatively high infusion rates. As mentioned previously, this presumably results from a deficiency of LCAT relative to the amount of substrate entering plasma, namely free cholesterol and phospholipid. The prolonged presence of Lp-X in plasma, as in familial LCAT deficiency and primary biliary cirrhosis, can lead to changes in red cell morphology and a hemolytic tendency. In addition, Intralipid infusion can also cause transient hypertriglyceridemia in healthy adults which in some (14), but not all (35), studies was accompanied by a slight impairment of pulmonary function. However, serious and even fatal pulmonary dysfunction has been described in premature neonates infused with 20% Intralipid (26), which was presumed to be due to inadequate rates of hydrolysis of triglyceride by lipoprotein lipase.

INFLUENCE OF TURNOVER RATE ON PHOSPHOLIPID COMPOSITION OF LDL

Hypocatabolism of LDL is an integral feature of familial hypercholesterolemia (FH or familial type II hyperlipoproteinemia), a disease stemming from a dominantly inherited defect of LDL receptors and characterized by a reduced FCR of LDL. The resultant increase in plasma LDL levels is greater in homozygotes than in heterozygotes, not only because they have a more marked catabolic defect but also because they exhibit a greater increase in LDL synthesis (22). The reduced FCR and accompanying hypercholesterolemia can both be partially reversed by treatment with anion-exchange resins, such as cholestyramine, which impair bile acid reabsorption and thus stimulate hepatic synthesis of bile acids from cholesterol.

In addition to having an increased concentration of LDL in plasma, patients with FH show certain abnormalities of LDL composition, most marked in homozygotes. Slack and Mills (44) described an increase in the cholesteryl ester content and a decrease in the triglyceride content of LDL from FH patients. Mills et al. (29) subsequently noted that the lecithin/sphingomyelin ratio was reduced in two homozygotes. An increase in the cholesterol/phospholipid ratio and a decrease in the lecithin/sphingomyelin ratio of LDL had been decribed previously in several patients who were probably FH heterozygotes (17). Recently, larger-scale studies have confirmed an increase in cholesterol/phospholipid ratios in LDL of both homozygotes and heterozygotes (27,41), although in neither instance were lecithin/sphingomyelin ratios determined. Investigation of patients attending the Hammersmith Hospital Lipid Clinic, London, confirmed the findings of these various groups of workers and demonstrated that (a) the ratios of cholesterol and of sphingomyelin to protein were increased and the lecithin/protein ratio was decreased in the LDL of subjects with FH, and (b) these changes were more marked in homozygotes than in heterozygotes (22), as illustrated in Fig. 8.

In order to investigate whether these abnormalities were primary, for example, because of the synthesis and secretion of an abnormal LDL particle, or were secondary to the catabolic defect, LDL composition was studied in FH patients undergoing plasma exchange for therapeutic reasons (22). As shown in Fig. 9 both the elevated cholesterol/phospholipid ratio and the decreased lecithin/sphingomyelin ratio became less abnormal following plasma exchange. The partial normalization of LDL composition, which was most marked on the day after plasma exchange, was presumably due to the removal of most of the circulating LDL particles and their subsequent replacement with newly synthesized LDL. This observation implies that the composition of LDL changes as it ages and suggests that both the increased cholesterol and sphingomyelin content of LDL and the decreased lecithin and triglyceride content observed in homozygotes were consequences of the reduced FCR. Further evidence in favor of hypocatabolism as an explanation for these abnormalities can be gleaned by considering data obtained in heterozygotes, the composition of whose LDL is intermediate between that of homozygotes and controls, as is its FCR and half-life in plasma. Treatment with an anion-exchange resin has been shown both to increase the FCR and to decrease the cholesterol content of their LDL, relative to either phopholipid (24) or protein (50). Analogous changes have been observed in hypothyroid patients before and after treatment with thyroxine (2).

PLASMA PHOSPHOLIPIDS AND LDL

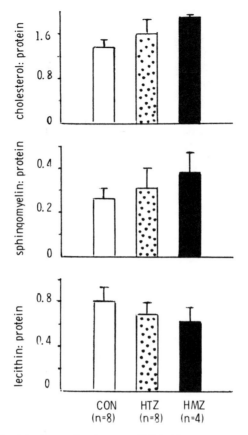

FIG. 8. Lipid/protein mass ratios (mean ± SD) in LDL of control subjects (CON), FH heterozygotes (HTZ), and homozygotes (HMZ).

Decreases in the lecithin/sphingomyelin ratio similar to that seen in FH have been observed in the LDL of monkeys fed a diet rich in cholesterol and saturated fat; whereas, the ratio increased when the animals were switched to a high-sucrose diet (36), as shown in Table 3. Other workers have shown that the FCR of LDL is reduced by saturated fat feeding (37) but increased by sucrose (32). Thus when LDL turnover is slow, LDL particles become enriched in cholesterol and sphingomyelin at the expense of triglyceride and lecithin, whereas the reverse occurs when turnover is rapid.

Any discussion of the mechanism for the changes in lipid composition that occur during LDL ageing must inevitably be speculative. However, exchange of cholesteryl ester takes place between HDL on the one hand, and VLDL and LDL on the other (31,33). Perhaps the longer each LDL particle circulates in plasma, the more cholesteryl ester it accumulates from HDL, with a reciprocal decrease in triglyceride. The changes in phospholipid composition are less easily explained. One possibility is that LDL lecithin is consumed to a greater extent because of the

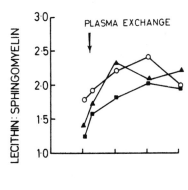

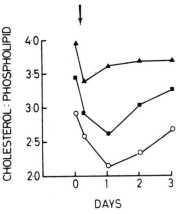

FIG. 9. Sequential measurements of lipid/protein molar ratios in low-density lipoprotein from two familial hypercholesterolemic homozygotes (▲,■) and a heterozygote (○) before and after plasma exchange with plasma protein fraction. (From Jadhav and Thompson, ref. 22, with permission.)

TABLE 3. *Effect of diet on serum lipids and mass ratio of lecithin:sphingomyelin in low-density lipoprotein of chimpanzees*

Diet	N	Total cholesterol (mg/dl)	Triglyceride (mg/dl)	Phospholipid (mg/dl)	Lecithin/ Sphingomyelin ratio
Control	4	259	60	295	3.73
High fat	6	606	65	459	2.93
High sucrose	4	231	122	275	4.14

From Peeters (36), with permission.

prolonged action of LCAT. Alternatively, lecithin may be progressively displaced by sphingomyelin, possibly derived from VLDL hydrolysis, as has been demonstrated *in vitro* with HDL (47). None of these explanations is entirely satisfactory, but they do help illustrate the dynamic state of lipoproteins in the circulation and the close relationship between the turnover rate and lipid composition of LDL.

REFERENCES

1. Adams, C. W. M., Abdulla, Y. H., Bayliss, O. B., and Morgan, R. S. (1967): Modification of aortic atheroma and fatty liver in cholesterol-fed rabbits by intravenous injection of saturated and polyunsaturated lecithins. *J. Pathol. Bacteriol.*, 94:77–87.
2. Ballantyne, F. C., Epenetos, A. A., Caslake, M., Forsythe, S., and Ballantyne, D. (1979): The composition of low density lipoprotein and very low density lipoprotein subfractions in primary hypothyroidism and the effect of hormone replacement therapy. *Clin. Sci.*, 57:83–88.
3. Blaton, V., Soetewey, F., Vandamme, D., Declercq, B., and Peeters, H. (1976): Effect of polyunsaturated phosphatidyl-choline on human types II and IV hyperlipoproteinemias. *Artery*, 2:309–325.
4. Burns, C. H., and Rothblat, G. H. (1969): Cholesterol excretion by tissue culture cells: Effect of serum lipids. *Biochim. Biophys. Acta*, 176:616–625.
5. Byers, S. O., and Friedman, M. (1956): Independence of phosphatide induced hypercholesteremia and hepatic function. *Proc. Soc. Exp. Biol. Med.*, 92:459–462.
6. Byers, S. O., and Friedman, M. (1958): Hypercholesterolemic effect of various phospholipid preparations. *Am. J. Physiol.*, 193:435–438.
7. Byers, S. O., Friedman, M., and Sugiyama, T. (1962): Mechanism underlying phosphatide-induced hypercholesterolemia. *J. Biol. Chem.*, 237:3375–3380.
8. Byers, S. O., and Friedman, M. (1969): Probable sources of plasma cholesterol during phosphatide induced hypercholesterolemia. *Lipids*, 4:123–128.
9. Eisenberg, S., and Schurr, D. (1976): Phospholipid removal during degradation of rat plasma very low density lipoprotein *in vitro. J. Lipid Res.*, 17:578–587.
10. Friedman, M., and Byers, S. O. (1956): Role of hyperphospholipidemia and neutral fat increase in plasma in the pathogensis of hypercholesteremia. *Am. J. Physiol.*, 186:13–18.
11. Friedman, M., Byers, S. O., and Rosenman, R. H. (1957): Resolution of aortic atherosclerotic infiltration in the rabbit by phosphatide infusion. *Proc. Soc. Exp. Biol. Med.*, 95:586–588.
12. Gjone, E. (1974): Familial lecithin:cholesterol acyltransferase deficiency—A clinical survey. *Sand. J. Clin. Lab. Invest.*, 33 (Suppl. 137):73–82.
13. Glomset, J. A., and Norum, K. R. (1973): The metabolic role of lecithin:cholesterol acyltransferase: Perspectives from pathology. *Adv. Lipid Res.*, 11:1–65.
14. Greene, H. L., Hazlett, D., and Demaree, R. (1976): Relationship between Intralipid-induced hyperlipemia and pulmonary function. *Am. J. Clin. Nutr.*, 29:127–135.
15. Greten, H., Raetzer, H., Stiehl, A., and Schettler, G. (1980): The effect of polyunsaturated phosphatidylcholine on plasma lipids and fecal sterol excretion. *Atherosclerosis*, 36:81–88.
16. Griffin, E., Breckenridge, W. C., Kuksis, A., Bryan, M. H., and Angel, A. (1979): Appearance and characterization of lipoprotein during continuous Intralipid infusions in the neonate. *J. Clin. Invest.*, 64:1703–1712.
17. Howard, A. N., Blaton, V., Vandamme, D., Van Landschoot, N., and Peeters, H. (1972): Lipid changes in the plasma lipoproteins of baboons given an atherogenic diet Part 3. A comparison between the lipid changes in the plasma of the baboon and chimpanzee given atherogenic diets and those in human plasma lipoproteins of type II hyperlipoproteinaemia. *Atherosclerosis*, 16:257–272.
18. Illingworth, D. R., and Portman, O. W. (1972): Independence of phospholipid and protein exchange between plasma lipoproteins *in vivo* and *in vitro. Biochim. Biophys. Acta*, 280:281–289.
19. Illingworth, D. R., and Portman, O. W. (1972): Exchange of phospholipids between low and high density lipoproteins of squirrel monkeys. *J. Lipid Res.*, 13:220–227.
20. Jackson, R. L., and Gotto, A. M. (1974): Phospholipids in biology and medicine. *N. Engl. J. Med.*, 290:24–29, 87–93.
21. Jackson, R. L., Westerman, J., and Wirtz, K. W. A. (1978): Complete exchange of phospholipids between microsomes and plasma lipoproteins mediated by liver phospholipid-exchange proteins. *FEBS Lett.*, 94:38–42.
22. Jadhav, A. V., and Thompson, G. R. (1979): Reversible abnormalities of low density lipoprotein composition in familial hypercholesterolaemia. *Europ. J. Clin. Invest.*, 9:63–67.
23. Jakoi, L., and Quarfordt, S. H. (1974): The induction of hepatic cholesterol synthesis in the rat by lecithin mesophase infusions. *J. Biol. Chem.*, 249:5840–5844.
24. Jones, R. J., and Dobrilovic, L. (1970): Lipoprotein lipid alterations with cholestyramine administration. *J. Lab. Clin. Med.*, 75:953–966.

25. Kuksis, A., Breckenridge, W. C., Myher, J. J., and Kakis, G. (1978): Replacement of endogenous phospholipids in rat plasma lipoproteins during intravenous infusion of an artificial lipid emulsion. *Can. J. Biochem.*, 56:630–639.
26. Levene, M. I., Wigglesworth, J. S., and Desai, R. (1980): Pulmonary fat accumulation after Intralipid infusion in the preterm infant. *Lancet*, ii:815–819.
27. Mabuchi, H., Tatami, R., Ueda, K., Ueda, R., Haba, T., Kametani, T., Watanabe, A., Wakasugi, T., Ito, S., Koizumi, J., Ohta, M., Miyamoto, S., and Takeda, R. (1979): Serum lipid and lipoprotein levels in Japanese patients with familial hypercholesterolemia. *Atherosclerosis*, 32:435–444.
28. McCandless, E. L., and Zilversmit, D. B. (1958): Fate of triglycerides and phospholipids of lymph and artificial fat emulsions: Disappearance from the circulation. *Am. J. Physiol.*, 193:294–300.
29. Mills, G. L., Taylaur, C. E., and Chapman, M. J. (1976): Low-density lipoproteins in patients homozygous for familial hyperbetalipoproteinaemia. *Clin. Sci. Mol. Med.*, 51:221–231.
30. Minari, O., and Zilversmit, D. B. (1963): Behavior of dog lymph chylomicron lipid constituents during incubation with serum. *J. Lipid Res.*, 4:424–436.
31. Nestel, P. J., Reardon, M., and Billington, T. (1979): *In vivo* transfer of cholesteryl esters from high density lipoproteins to very low density lipoproteins in man. *Biochim. Biophys. Acta*, 573:403–407.
32. Nestel, P. J., Reardon, M., and Fidge, N. H. (1979): Sucrose-induced changes in VLDL- and LDL-B apoprotein removal rates. *Metabolism*, 28:531–535.
33. Nichols, A. V., and Smith, L. (1965): Effect of very low density lipoproteins on lipid transfer in incubated serum. *J. Lipid Res.*, 6:206–210.
34. Norum, K. R., and Gjone, E. (1967): Familial plasma lecithin:cholesterol acyltransferase deficiency. *Scand. J. Lab. Clin. Invest.*, 20:231–243.
35. Partridge, M. R., Hughes, J. M. B., and Thompson, G. R. (1979): Effect of hyperlipidaemia on pulmonary diffusing capacity for carbon monoxide. *Thorax*, 34:265–268.
36. Peeters, H. (1976): The biological significance of the plasma phospholipids. In: *Phosphatidylcholine: Biochemical and Clinical Aspects of Essential Phospholipids*, edited by H. Peeters, pp. 10–33. Springer-Verlag, Berlin.
37. Portman, O. W., Alexander, M., Tanaka, N., and Soltys, P. (1976): The effects of dietary fat and cholesterol on the metabolism of plasma low density lipoprotein apoproteins in squirrel monkeys. *Biochem. Biophys. Acta*, 450:185–196.
38. Reed, C. F. (1968): Phospholipid exchange between plasma and erythrocytes in man and dog. *J. Clin. Invest.*, 47:749–760.
39. Saunders, D. R. (1970): Insignificance of the enterobiliary circulation of lecithin in man. *Gastroenterology*, 59:848–852.
40. Scow, R., Stein, Y., and Stein, O. (1967): Incorporation of dietary lecithin and lysolecithin into lymph chylomicrons in the rat. *J. Biol. Chem.*, 242:4919–4924.
41. Shattil, S. J., Bennett, J. S., Colman, R. W., and Copper, R. A. (1977): Abnormalities of cholesterol-phospholipid composition in platelets and low-density lipoproteins of human hyperbetalipoproteinemia. *J. Lab. Clin. Med.*, 89:341–353.
42. Shepherd, J., Packard, C. J., Grundy, S. M., Yeshurun, D., Gotto, A. M., and Taunton, O. D. (1980): Effects of saturated and polyunsaturated fat diets on the chemical composition and metabolism of low density lipoproteins in man. *J. Lipid Res.*, 21:91–99.
43. Skipski, V. P. (1972): Lipid composition of lipoproteins in normal and diseased states. In: *Blood Lipids and Lipoproteins: Quantitation, Composition and Metabolism*, edited by G. J. Nelson, pp. 471–583. Wiley-Interscience, New York.
44. Slack, J., and Mills, G. L. (1970): Anomalous low density lipoproteins in familial hyperbetalipoproteinaemia. *Clin. Chim. Acta*, 29:15–25.
45. Spritz, N., and Mishkel, M. A. (1969): Effects of dietary fats on plasma lipids and lipoproteins: An hypothesis for the lipid-lowering effect of unsaturated fatty acids. *J. Clin. Invest.*, 48:78–86.
46. Stein, O., and Stein, Y. (1973): The removal of cholesterol from Landschütz ascites cells by high-density apolipoprotein. *Biochim. Biophys. Acta*, 326:232–244.
47. Stoffel, W., Salm, K-P., and Langer, M. (1978): A new method for the exchange of lipid classes of human serum high density lipoprotein. *Hoppe Seylers Z. Physiol. Chem.*, 359:1385–1393.
48. Thompson, G. R., Segura, R., Hoff, H., and Gotto, A. M. (1975): Contrasting effects on plasma lipoproteins of intravenous versus oral administration of a triglyceride-phospholipid emulsion. *Europ. J. Clin. Invest.*, 5:373–384.

49. Thompson, G. R., Jadhav, A., Nava, M., and Gotto, A. M. (1976): Effects of intravenous phospholipid on low denisty lipoprotein turnover in man. *Eur. J. Clin. Invest.*, 6:241–248.
50. Witztum, J. L., Schonfeld, G., Weidman, S. W., Giese, W. E., and Dillingham, M. A. (1979): Bile sequestrant therapy alters the compositions of low-density and high-density lipoproteins. *Metabolism*, 28:221–229.
51. Zilversmit, D. B. (1971): Stimulation of phospholipid exchange between mitochondria and artificially prepared phospholipid aggregates by a soluble fraction from liver. *J. Biol. Chem.*, 246:2645–2649.

Phospholipids and Atherosclerosis, edited by
P. Avogaro, M. Mancini, G. Ricci, and
R. Paoletti. Raven Press, New York © 1983.

In Vivo and *In Vitro* Uptake of Lecithin by High-Density Lipoproteins

M. Rosseneu

Department of Clinical Biochemistry, Ruddershovelaan 10, B-8000 Brugge, Belgium

A postulated function for the serum high-density lipoproteins (HDL) is the removal of free cholesterol from peripheral tissues, followed by cholesterol esterification by the lecithin-cholesterol acyltransferase (LCAT) enzyme and cholesterol transport to the liver, the organ primarily responsible for the metabolism and excretion of cholesterol (3,8). Recent work has shown that HDL and HDL apoproteins are able to remove lipids from cells in tissue culture. According to Stein et al. (27), HDL can remove cholesterol from smooth muscle cells, and Jackson et al. (10) have shown that apo A-I can remove phospholipids from ascites cells. The exchange process between serum lipoproteins and erythrocyte membranes can also contribute to this mechanism (13). It is, therefore, essential to understand the role played by the HDL phospholipids in this metabolic process. There is a close interaction between apoprotein, phospholipid, and free cholesterol in HDL (6,9). It can, therefore, be expected that the three components will play an active part in the cholesterol transport and incorporation in HDL, as indicated by studies of Jonas (12), Tall (29), and Scherphof et al. (26).

The aim of this paper is to summarize a series of observations obtained both *in vivo* and *in vitro*, which document the active role played by HDL phospholipids and apoproteins in the lipid metabolism. The *in vivo* results were obtained by feeding polyunsaturated and saturated lecithin to chimpanzees and then investigating the compositional and physicochemical modifications occuring within the plasma HDL fraction. The *in vitro* observations relate to the formation of phospholipid-rich HDL obtained by incubation of native human HDL with phospholipids. The relative contribution of the apo A-I and apo A-II proteins to the formation of phospholipid-apoprotein complexes is also analyzed.

IN VIVO INCORPORATION OF PHOSPHOLIPIDS INTO PRIMATE HDL

The compositional changes occurring in the lipids and fatty acids of chimpanzee plasma high-density lipoproteins, after oral treatment with polyunsaturated and saturated lecithin, were followed in the course of this study. These experiments were conducted in chimpanzees since their lipoproteins and apoproteins closely resemble those of humans (4) and since this animal easily responds to dietary treatment (20).

Four 7-year-old male chimpanzees were successively placed on three types of diet for 1 month each: a control diet (I), a diet enriched in polyunsaturated phospholipids (II), and a diet enriched in saturated phospholipids (III). The composition of the three diets was adjusted so that each diet contained the same percentages of protein, carbohydrate, and fat and the same number of calories (Table 1). This was achieved using a basic ape diet providing protein, carbohydrate, and minerals, to which fat was added as soyabean oil and whole milk (diet I), skimmed milk and polyunsaturated lecithin (diet II), or palm oil and saturated lecithin (diet III). The total fat content and number of fatty acids per unit weight were the same in the three diets. The ratio of unsaturated to saturated fat was increased from 0.95 in the control diet to 3.6 in the polyunsaturated diet (II) and decreased to 0.22 in the saturated diet (III). The polyunsaturated lecithin consisted of purified essential phospholipid (EPL) (Natterman, Köln, West Germany) containing 67% linoleic, 11% oleic, 4% stearic, 13% palmitic, and 6% linoleic acid (7). The saturated lecithin was obtained from the above by complete hydrogenation.

After each dietary period (1 month duration), blood was drawn from the animals after overnight fasting and collected into ethylene diamine tetraacetic acid (EDTA). The HDL lipoproteins were isolated by ultracentrifugation according to the standard procedure (20) in the density range of $1.12 < d < 1.21$ g/ml. The fraction was purified by a second centrifugation step. Chemical determination of the protein and lipid composition of the lipoproteins and fatty acid distribution were carried out as previously described (4). The lipoprotein concentration was calculated as the sum of the protein moiety, determined according to the method of Lowry et al. (14), and the various lipid components. Fluorescence depolarization of HDL was measured, after labeling with diphenylhexatriene (DPH), using an Elscint microviscosimeter (18).

TABLE 1. *Composition of control unsaturated and saturated chimpanzee diets*

Composition[a]	Control	Unsaturated	Saturated
Protein (%)	29	29	29
Carbohydrate (%)	63	63	63
Fat (%)	4	4	4
Minerals (%)	4	4	4
Phospholipids (g/day)	3.6	37.6	26.6
Calories/day	2030	2030	2030
P/S ratio[b]	0.95	3.6	0.22

[a]The phospholipids are part of the 4% fat.
[b]Ratio of polyunsaturated (P) to saturated (S) fat.

Lipid and Protein Composition of Chimpanzee HDL

Compared with the control diet, the phospholipid treatment induces drastic changes in the HDL subclass, probably because of the high phospholipid content in this fraction (Table 2). The most striking feature is the increase in cholesteryl esters and lysolecithin under the polyunsaturated diet from, respectively, 15 to 23% and 0.3 to 3.4%. These increases are accompanied by a decrease in the triglyceride content from 6.5 to 3.2%. The percentage of esterified cholesterol increases from 73.6 to 85% as a consequence of the increase in cholesteryl esters and of the slight decrease in free cholesterol. The polyunsaturated lecithin diet has no influence on the lecithin (PC) and sphingomyelin (SM) content so that the SM/PC ration remains constant. These effects are reversed during the saturated diet period, except for the protein content which increases slightly.

The fluidity of the HDL lipid, as measured by fluorescence polarization, is plotted in Fig. 1. The fluorescence polarization ratio of HDL lipids is not significantly affected by the dietary compositions despite the changes observed in the lipid and protein composition. The fluidity measurement provides a mean value for the organization of the lipid phase and for the extent of protein-lipid interaction (16). Treatment with polyunsaturated lecithin makes the HDL surface more fluid and the HDL core more dense, resulting in an unchanged mean value of the fluidity of the HDL particle.

Fatty Acid Composition of Chimpanzee HDL

A comparison of the fatty acid patterns of the HDL triglycerides, cholesteryl esters, and phospholipids is given in Table 3 for the three diets. The major triglyceride fatty acids are oleic and palmitic acid, followed by linoleic acid. The cholesteryl esters are mostly esterified with linoleic, oleic, and palmitic acid. In the phospholipid class, palmitic and linoleic acid are the major constituents; stearic and oleic acid occur as secondary components. The major compositional change induced by the polyunsaturated diet in the triglyceride fraction is an increase by 13% of the linoleic acid content of HDL_3 with a concomitant decrease of palmitic and oleic acid.

The polyunsaturated diet slightly decreases the percentages of the saturated and monounsaturated fatty acids. The most significant changes are, however, induced by the saturated diet, which inuced a drop by 25% from 62 to 37% of the linoleic content of HDL. A concomitant increase of $C_{16:0}$ ($\Delta = 6\%$) and $C_{18:1}$ ($\Delta = 13\%$) is observed during the saturated lecithin diet.

The phospholipid fatty acid pattern is the least sensitive to the degree of saturation of the lecithin diet. The pattern observed after treatment with unsaturated lecithin is close to that observed after the control diet; however, the saturated diet slightly increases the oleic acid content in HDL phospholipids ($\Delta = 6\%$). The percentages of palmitic and stearic acid remain constant.

TABLE 2. Percentage composition of chimpanzee plasma high-density lipoprotein (HDL$_3$) (mean values ± SEM)[a]

	Chemical composition						Phospholipids				
Diet	Protein	FCH	CE	TG	PL	% est. chol.	OH-PC	SM	PC	PE	SM/PC ratio
I	46.4 ±1.1	3.2 ±1.1	15.0 ±0.5	6.5 ±1.0	28.9 ±0.4	73.6 ±0.4	0.3 ±0.1	7.8 ±0.3	83.5 ±0.7	7.4 ±0.7	0.1 ±0.002
II	47.0 ±0.6	2.4 ±0.1	23.4 ±0.6	3.2 ±0.3	24.0 ±0.6	85.0 ±0.7	3.4 ±0.3	7.6 ±0.5	80.9 ±0.5	5.8 ±0.8	0.1 ±0.0006
III	51.8 ±1.5	2.0 ±0.03	16.7 ±1.0	5.0 ±0.4	24.6 ±0.5	83.3 ±1.0	0.7 ±0.1	3.3 ±0.4	84.1 ±0.4	5.2 ±0.3	0.1 ±0.005

[a]FCH = free cholesterol; % est. chol. = % esterified cholesterol; PL = phospholipids; OH-PC = lysolecithin; SM = sphingomyelin; PC = lecithin; PE = phosphatidylethanolamine; CE = cholesteryl esters; TG = triglycerides.

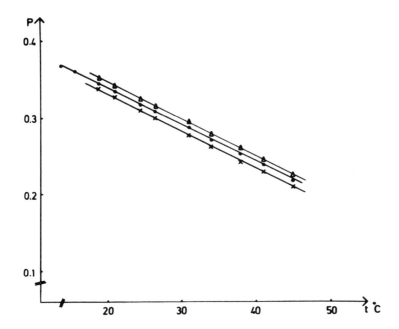

FIG. 1.   Fluorescence polarization ratio (P) of chimpanzee high-density lipoprotein as a function of temperature. (●) control diet, (x) polyunsaturated diet, (Δ) saturated diet.

Mechanism of Actions of the Diets

Treatments with unsaturated phospholipids affects mostly the composition of the HDL_3 fraction. According to the model of Jackson et al. (11) confirmed by X-ray scattering observations, the outer layer of these spherical particles consists of protein and phospholipid with free cholesterol; the core consists of triglycerides and cholesteryl esters. The dietary effect of the polyunsaturated lecithin is an increase in the lysolecithin and cholesteryl esters and a slight decrease in the triglyceride content. The new HDL_3 particles are, therefore, characterized by a more fluid outer surface and a denser core, and these particles might be able to act as better cholesterol carriers from cells and play a protective role in the development of atherosclerosis.

The following mechanism can be postulated: dietary lecithin is converted into lysolecithin and fatty acid is used for cholesterol esterification through the action of LCAT. The observed increase in lysolecithin and cholesteryl esters together with the decrease in free cholesterol support this hypothesis. This mechanism favors the synthesis of the more unsaturated cholesteryl esters. LCAT is activated by the apo A-I protein of the HDL, in agreement with the observation that an increase in lysolecithin and cholesteryl esters is most pronounced in the HDL_3 subclass. This mechanism is enhanced by an increase in the unsaturation of the lipoprotein phospholipids because polyunsaturated lecithins are better substrates for LCAT activity (2).

TABLE 3. *Average fatty acid composition of the lipids from chimpanzee high-density lipoprotein (HDL₃) under control, polyunsaturated, and saturated diets*

Lipids	Fatty acid	Control diet	Unsaturated diet	Saturated diet
Triglycerides	16:0	30.2	26.2	28.9
	16:1	4.3	0.7	5.4
	18:0	3.6	6.1	5.7
	18:1	30.9	24.0	37.5
	18:2	22.7	35.7	16.4
	20:4	1.5	1.3	1.2
	18:1/18:2	1.4	0.7	2.4
Cholesteryl esters	16:0	10.8	13.8	16.2
	16:1	2.8	2.5	6.2
	18:0	0.9	2.0	3.3
	18:1	15.4	13.3	28.2
	18:2	62.1	62.0	37.3
	20:4	5.7	3.9	5.9
	18:1/18:2	0.3	0.2	0.8
Phospholipids	16:0	26.8	27.7	25.7
	16:1	1.5	1.7	2.1
	18:0	16.7	17.9	15.4
	18:1	11.1	10.5	17.7
	18:2	18.7	32.2	21.6
	20:4	10.3	5.2	11.7
	18:1/18:2	0.4	0.3	0.8

The mode of action of the lecithin diets seems to differ from that of the unsaturated and saturated triglyceride diets (16). The data indicate that the fatty acid composition of the triglycerides is most sensitive to the unsaturated lecithin diet; whereas, the unsaturated triglyceride diet selectively influenced the low-density lipoprotein (LDL) triglycerides and the very low-density lipoprotein (VLDL) phospholipids and cholesteryl esters (16). In a study by Rosseneu et al. the cholesteryl esters' fatty acid composition was most modified by the saturated lecithin diet (20). The fluidity of the HDL, measured after labeling with diphenylhexatriene, did not change significantly.

Oral treatment with unsaturated phospholipids has positive effects on the regression of atherosclerosis in chimpanzees; namely, it induces the synthesis of HDL₃ particles with a fluid surface and a denser core, increases the linoleic acid content, and decreases the palmitic and oleic acid content of the lipoprotein lipids. A saturated phospholipid diet favors the formation of cholesteryl esters that might easily deposit on the arterial walls and contribute a supplementary risk factor to the progression of the disease.

IN VITRO INCUBATION OF PHOSPHOLIPIDS WITH HUMAN HDL

These *in vitro* incubation experiments were aimed at the characterizations of the phospholipid and cholesterol uptake by human HDL. The phospholipid-cholesterol vesicles consisted of synthetic dimyristoyl lecithin and cholesterol; this particular phospholipid was selected because Tall et al. (28) had suggested that the incubation of dimyristoyl lecithin with HDL can induce the dissociation of the apo A-I protein from HDL.

Human HDL was isolated by preparative ultracentrifugation from fresh plasma at $1.08 < d < 1.21$ g/ml and by recentrifugation at the same densities. The dimyristoyl lecithin (DMPC)-cholesterol vesicles were prepared by sonication using a Branson sonifier equipped with a microtip (18,19). The unilamellar vesicles were characterized by chromatography on a Sepharose 6B column. The cholesterol/DMPC molar ratio in the mixed vesicles varied between 0 and 50. The HDL fraction was incubated for 3 hr at 25°C with the mixed lipid vesicles at a 2:1 ratio (2 mg DMPC/mg HDL protein) and the mixture was separated by gel chromatography on a Sepharose 6B column, equilibrated in a Tris-HCl buffer pH 8.0,0.01 M Tris, 0.10 M NaCl, to which a 2 to 3 mg sample was added (21).

The fractionation of human HDL and of the HDL after incubation with DMPC vesicles is shown in Fig. 2A, B. The Stokes radius of human HDL is about 50 Å and the phospholipid/protein ratio is 0.7 (wt/wt). After incubation with the DMPC vesicles, the fractionation pattern is identical (Fig. 2B), as the HDL migrates as a single peak and no free lipids are detected. The elution volumes are identical, although the phospholipid/protein ratio increases to 2.1 (wt/wt) in the complex (Table 4).

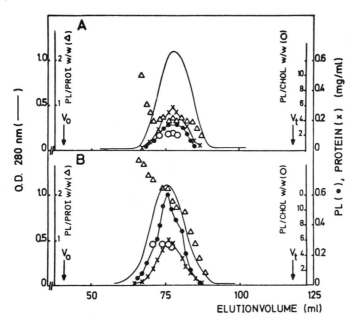

FIG. 2. Isolation of native human HDL **(A)** and HDL incubated with DMPC vesicles **(B)** on a Sepharose 6B column equilibrated in a Tris-HCl Buffer: pH 8.0, 0.01 M Tris, 0.01 N NaCl.

TABLE 4. *Chromatographic separation of high-density lipoprotein (HDL)
after incubation with dimyristoyl lecithin (DMPC)-cholesterol vesicles[a,b]*

Sample	V_e (ml)	K_{av}	PC/Protein (wt/wt)	PC/Chol. (wt/wt)	Protein/Chol. (wt/wt)
Human HDL	76.2	0.392	0.70	2.4	3.0
HDL + DMPC	75.3	0.392	2.1	5.8	2.7
HDL + Chol./DMPC 10 mole % Chol.	75.1	0.41	1.9	6.3	3.4
HDL + Chol./DMPC 50 mole % Chol.	75.5	0.397	0.7	2.3	3.3

[a]Column: Sepharose 6B, buffer: Tris-HCl pH 8.1, 0.01 M Tris, 0.15 N NaCl.
[b]PC = lecithin; Chol. = cholesterol; K_{av} = distribution coefficient = $(V_e\text{-}V_0)/$ $(V_t\text{-}V_0)$ with V_e = elution volume of sample; V_t = total column volume, and V_0 = void volume.

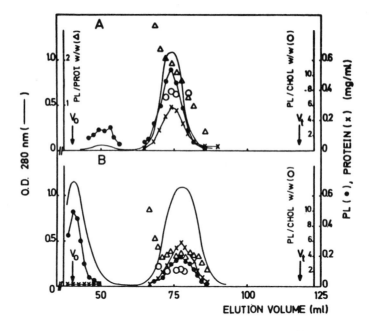

FIG. 3. Isolation of human HDL incubated with DMPC vesicles containing **(A)** 10 mole %; **(B)** 50 mole % cholesterol (for conditions, see Fig. 2 legend).

Similar experiments carried out with DMPC-cholesterol vesicles containing 10 and 50 mole % cholesterol are depicted in Fig. 3A, B. The incubation of HDL with DMPC vesicles containing 10 mole % cholesterol yields results identical to those obtained with pure DMPC vesicles. The phospholipid uptake by HDL amounts to 2 g lecithin/g protein with no significant cholesterol uptake observed. When the incubation is performed with vesicles containing 50 mole % cholesterol, no significant uptake of phospholipids was detected and the free lipids eluted in the void volume (Fig. 3B).

The chromatographic and compositional data summarized in Table 4 indicate that the dimensions of the phospholipid-rich HDL are similar to those of the native particle. The human HDL incorporates twice the quantity of phospholipid present in the native particle, with no significant amount of cholesterol incorporated, as shown by the stability of the protein/cholesterol ratio in the HDL fraction.

In the course of these experiments no free apo A-I was detected and no indication of an apo A-I-phospholipid complex was obtained, for the protein/phospholipid ratio was constant throughout the HDL peak. The vesicles containing 50 mole % cholesterol did not react with HDL, in agreement with the observations of Scherphof et al. (26) and Jonas (12). The presence of a high percentage of cholesterol prevents the transition from gel to liquid-crystalline structure of the DMPC (30), which might be a prerequisite for protein-lipid interaction.

The fluidity of the human HDL, native and enriched with phospholipids, is shown in Fig. 4. No significant change was observed in the fluidity of the HDL fraction despite the incorporation of large amounts of DMPC. This observation suggests that DMPC interacts with the HDL apoprotein, thereby increasing the fluorescence polarization ratio of pure DMPC (0.22) up to that of the DMPC-apoprotein complexes (0.32)—a value close to that of native HDL (30). The disappearance of the DMPC transition around 23°C can also be attributed to protein-DMPC interactions, which decrease the mobility of the lecithin acyl chains (15).

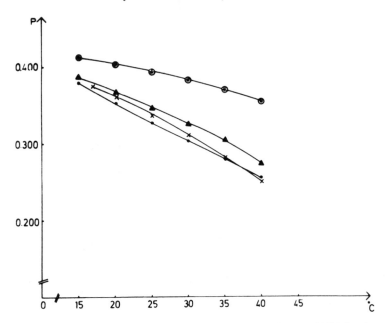

FIG. 4. Fluorescence polarization ratio of native human HDL (⊙) and of HDL incubated with DMPC vesicles containing: (●) 0, (x) 10, (▲) 50 mole % cholesterol.

IN VITRO INTERACTION OF HUMAN HDL APOPROTEINS WITH PHOSPHOLIPIDS

Eachhe two major human HDL apoproteins, apo A-I and apo A-II, have a specific affinity for phospholipids (1). In view of the significant uptake of lecithin by human HDL, as described above, the association of lecithin and lecithin-cholesterol vesicles with these two apoproteins was investigated. The relative contribution of apo A-I and apo A-II to the formation of apo-HDL-lipid complexes was analyzed from the behavior of mixtures of apo A-I with apo A-II in the presence of lipids.

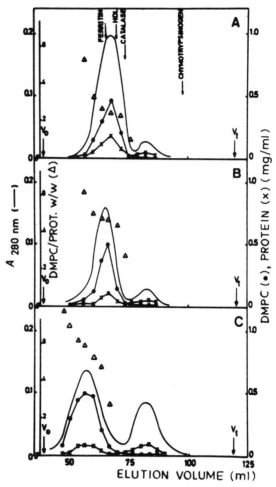

FIG. 5. Isolation of apo A-I-DMPC-cholesterol mixtures by gel chromatography on a Sepharose 6B column. **A:** apo A-I-DMPC; **B:** apo A-I-DMPC-10 mole % cholesterol; **C:** apo A-I-DMPC-50 mole % cholesterol.

The apo A-I and A-II proteins were prepared by delipidation of HDL, and chromatographic separation on a DEAE-cellulose column in 7 M urea (22). The lecithin and lecithin-cholesterol vesicles were prepared as described above, and the apoprotein-lipid reassembly was carried out by incubation, for 3 hr at 25°C, of a lipid-protein mixture at a 2:1 (wt/wt) lipid/protein ratio.

The complexes were isolated by gel filtration on a Sepharose 6B column as described above. The relative affinity of apo A-I and apo A-II for HDL lipids was studied by following the displacement of apo A-I by apo A-II after *in vitro* incubation of HDL with apo A-II. In these experiments 1 to 2 mg HDL was incubated with 2 to 6 mg apo A-II for 12 hr, and the mixture was fractionated by gel chromatography. The apoproteins A-I and A-II were quantitated separately by immunonephelometry (23,24); the phospholipids and cholesterol, by colorimetric assay (31). Complexes were generated between the apo A-I and apo A-II proteins and phos-

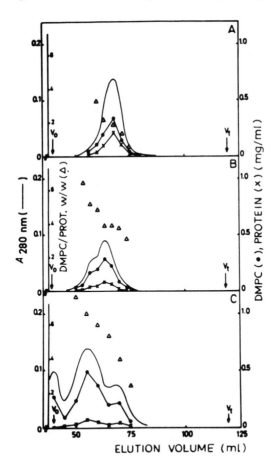

FIG. 6. The same as Fig. 5 but with apo A-II instead of apo A-I.

pholipid-cholesterol vesicles containing 0.5, 10, and 20 mole % cholesterol. These complexes were isolated by gel filtration on a Sepharose 6B column (Figs. 5 and 6) and their composition followed by chemical analysis.

The apoproteins A-I and A-II were incorporated into particles of a size intermediate between that of the original vesicles and of HDL. The size of the complexes did not vary significantly with the cholesterol content of the vesicles between 0 and 20 mole % and is around 59Å. The apo A-I-lipid complexes consist of 100 and 200 moles DMPC/mole apo A-I for DMPC vesicles and for mixed DMPC 10 mole % cholesterol vesicles, respectively. The corresponding molar ratio for the apo A-II-DMPC complexes are 60 and 120, respectively. At higher cholesterol-DMPC ratios (20 mole %), a well-defined complex could not be isolated.

The fluidity of the apoprotein-lipid complexes, isolated as described above, was measured by fluorescence polarization after labeling with diphenylhexatriene. The apo A-I and apo A-II-lipid complexes have identical fluorescence polarization ratios at temperatures between 15° and 40°C (Fig. 7). Compared to the lipid vesicles, the gel to crystalline transition of the lecithin in the complexes has a decreased amplitude and a midpoint temperature which is shifted from 23.5° to 28°C at 0.5 and 10 mole % cholesterol. The DMPC transition disappears in the apoprotein-lipid complexes containing 20 mole % cholesterol; however, it is still observed up to 30 mole % in the pure lipid vesicles. These results indicate that both apo A-I and apo A-II are involved in the phospholipid-apoprotein association in HDL and that apoprotein-lipid interaction decreases the mobility of the lecithin acyl chains in the lipoprotein (15).

The relative contribution of the apo A-I and apo A-II proteins to the ultimate composition of HDL and to the phospholipid/protein ratio in HDL_2 and HDL_3 was

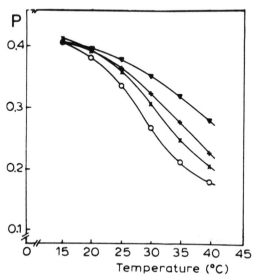

FIG. 7. Fluorescence polarization ratio (P) as a function of temperature for apoprotein A-I and A-II-DMPC-cholesterol complexes with: (○), 0; (x), 5; (+), 10; (▼), 20 mole % cholesterol.

studied by following the competition between apo A-I and apo A-II for HDL lipids. The incubation of human HDL with increasing amounts of human apo A-II induces a progressive release of apo A-I from the HDL particle until 2 moles of apo A-II have substituted for 1 mole of apo A-I in HDL (Fig. 8A–C) (31). The apo A-II-rich HDL has the same elution volume as native HDL, and the substitution of apo A-I by apo A-II is not accompanied by an loss of lipid as the protein/lipid ratio remains constant (Table 5). The apo A-I/A-II molar ratio decreases from 1.3 in native HDL to 0.04 after incubation with apo A-II at a ratio of 4 moles apo A-II/mole apo A-I.

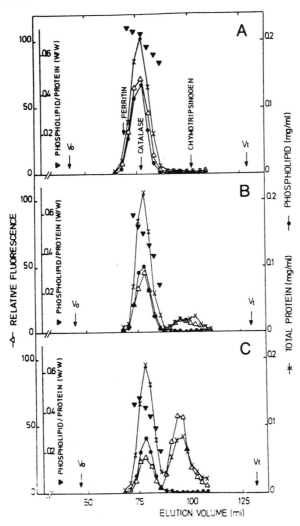

FIG. 8. Gel chromatography of native human HDL **(A)** and HDL incubated for 3 hr at 25°C with human apo A-II at apo A-I/A-II (wt/wt) ratios of **(B)** 0.5, **(C)** 1.

TABLE 5. *Apolipoprotein and lipid concentration of high-density lipoprotein before and after* in vitro *incubation with apolipoprotein A-II*

Added apo A-II/apo A-I (moles/moles)	Strokes radius (Å)	PL/Protein[a] (wt/wt)	apo A-I/apo A-II (moles/moles)
0[b]	56.6	0.65	1.34
0.8	57.1	0.52	0.70
1.6	56.7	0.50	0.24
2.5	57.6	0.48	0.08
3.3	58.0	0.46	0.04
3.9	58.3	0.49	0.04

[a]PL = total lipoprotein.
[b]Native high-density lipoprotein.

These data support the concept that apo A-II has a higher affinity for HDL lipids than apo A-I because of the ability of apo A-II to displace HDL from apo A-I-lipid complexes (22) as well as from native HDL (31). This process might be physiologically relevant as it could also be induced in human plasma where apo A-II displaces apo A-I from HDL in the presence of other serum proteins (25).

CONCLUSION

The experimental results summarized in this chapter indicate that the lipid and apoprotein composition of human and primate HDL can vary under a wide range of circumstances. The phospholipid composition can be modified *in vivo* by feeding saturated and polyunsaturated lecithin to animals and probably humans. The type of diet affects the distribution, amount, and degree of saturation of the HDL phospholipid. An increase of the lysolecithin content increases the fluidity of the outer layer of the particle and an increased proportion of cholesteryl esters increases the rigidity of the core. These particles might act as better carriers for cholesterol. The *in vitro* experiments have shown that twofold increases of the phospholipid content of HDL can be induced by incubation with fluid lecithin or lecithin-cholesterol vesicles. The dimensions and fluidity of the HDL are not significantly modified and its apoprotein content remains unchanged. Similar results can be obtained by incubation with unsaturated lecithin (32).

A variation of the phospholipid content of HDL must involve a rearrangement of the outer layer of the particle where apoprotein, phospholipid, and cholesterol coexist. The apo A-I and apo A-II proteins are both involved in the apoprotein-phospholipid interaction (15,30). The affinity of apo A-II for lipids is higher than that of apo A-I. This difference accounts for the displacement of apo A-I from the HDL as induced by either phospholipids (29) or apo A-II (25,31).

The stability of the apo A-I-lipid association is, therefore, dependent on the nature of the phospholipid, the presence of cholesterol, and the relative distribution of apo A-I and apo A-II on the HDL particle (31). The apo A-I protein regulates the esterification of cholesterol by the LCAT enzyme in the course of HDL synthesis. A feedback mechanism for the LCAT activation might be the displacement of apo A-I from HDL by apo A-II and by phospholipids originated during VLDL degradation (17). During this process apo A-II-rich particles are formed, which are more like HDL_3 compared to the apo A-I-rich HDL_2. The HDL_2/HDL_3 distribution in plasma might consequently be regulated by apoprotein and phospholipid transfer. Data from other laboratories (5) support this hypothesis, which requires confirmation in more physiological situations.

REFERENCES

1. Assmann, G., and Brewer, B. H. (1974): Lipid-protein interactions in high-density lipoproteins. *Proc. Natl. Acad. Sci. USA,* 71:989–993.
2. Assmann, G. (1976): LCAT, lipoprotein and phospholipid substrate specificty. In: *Phosphatidylcholine,* edited by H. Peeters, pp. 34–39. Springer-Verlag, Berlin.
3. Bell, F. P. (1976): Lipoprotein lipid exchange in biological systems. In: *Low-Density Lipoproteins,* edited by C. E. Day and R. S. Levy, pp. 111–133. Plenum Press, New York.
4. Blaton, V., Howard, A. N., Gresham, G. A., Vandamme, D., and Peeters, H. (1970): Lipid changes in the plasma lipoproteins of primates given an atherogenic diet. *Atherosclerosis,* 11:497–503.
5. Chung, J., Abano, D. A., Fless, G. M., and Scanu, A. M. (1979): Isolation, properties and mechanism of in vitro action of lecithin:cholesterol acyl transferase from human plasma. *J. Biol. Chem.,* 254:7456–7464.
6. Edelstein, C., Kézdy, F. J., Scanu, A. M., and Shen, B. W. (1979): Apolipoproteins and the structural organization of plasma lipoproteins; human plasma high-density lipoproteins—3. *J. Lipid Res.,* 20:143–153.
7. Fox, J. M. (1976): A glossary of essential phospholipids and lipoproteins. In: *Phosphatidylcholine,* edited by H. Peeters, pp. 1–7. Springer-Verlag, Berlin.
8. Glomset, J. A. (1968): The plasma lecithin–cholesterol acyl transferase reaction. *J. Lipid Res.,* 9:155–167.
9. Jackson, R. L., and Gotto, A. M. (1974): The phospholipids in biology and medicine. *N. Engl. J. Med.,* 290:24–29, 87–93.
10. Jackson, R. L., Stein, O., Gotto, A., and Stein, Y. (1975): A comparative study on the removal of cellular lipids from Landschütz ascites cells by human plasma apolipoproteins. *J. Biol. Chem.,* 250:7204–7209.
11. Jackson, R. L., Morrisett, J. D., and Gotto, A. M. (1976): Lipoprotein structure and metabolism. *Physiol. Rev.,* 56:259–316.
12. Jonas, A. (1979): Interaction of bovine serum high density lipoprotein with mixed vesicles of phosphatidylcholine and cholesterol. *J. Lipid Res.,* 20:817–824.
13. Lange, Y., and D'Alessandro, J. S. (1977): Characterization of mechanisms for transfer of cholesterol between human erythrocytes and plasma. *Biochemistry,* 16:4339–4343.
14. Lowry, O. H., Rosebrough, W. J., Farr, A. L., and Randall, R. J. (1951): Protein measurements with the Folin phenol reagent. *J. Biol. Chem.,* 193:265–275.
15. Rosseneu, M., Soetewey, F., Middelhoff, G., Peeters, H., and Brown W. V. (1976): Studies of the lipid binding characteristics of the apolipoproteins from human high density lipoproteins. Calorimetry of the binding of apo AI and apo AII with phospholipid. *Biochim. Biophys. Acta,* 441:68–80.
16. Morrisett, J. D., Pownall, H. J., Jackson, R. L., Segura, R., Gotto, A. M., and Taunton, J. D. (1976): Effects of polyunsaturated and saturated fat diets on the chemical composition and thermotropic properties of human plasma lipoproteins. In: *The Chemistry and Biochemistry of Polyunsaturated Fatty Acids,* edited by N. Kanau and R. Holman, pp. 149–157. Am Oil Chem. Soc., Champaign, Illinois.
17. Patsch, J. R., Gotto, A. M., Olivecrona, T., and Eisenberg, S. (1978): Formation of high-density lipoprotein 2 live particles during lipolysis of very low density lipoproteins in vitro. *Proc. Natl. Acad. Sci. USA,* 75:4519–4523.

18. Rosseneu, M., Soetewey, F., Vercaemst, R., Lievens, M., and Peeters, H. (1977): Microviscolity of plasma lipoproteins and lipids. In: *Protides of the Biological Fluids*, edited by H. Peeters, pp. 47–51. Pergamon Press, Oxford.
19. Rosseneu, M. (1978): Reassembly of lipids and apoproteins. In: *The Lipoprotein Molecule*, edited by H. Peeters, pp. 129–154. Plenum Press, New York.
20. Rosseneu, M., Declercq, B., Vandamme, D., Vercaemst, R., Soetewey, F., Peeters, H., and Blaton, V. (1979): Influence of oral polyunsaturated and saturated phospholipid treatment on the lipid composition and fatty and profile of chimpanzee lipoproteins. *Atherosclerosis*, 32:141–153.
21. Rosseneu, M., Vercaemst, R., Van Tornout, P., Caster, H., Lievens, M. J., and Herbert, P. N. (1979): Fluorescence depolarization studies of the fluidity and phase transition in human apoprotein –phospholipid complexes. *Eur. J. Biochem.*, 96:357–362.
22. Rosseneu, M., Van Tornout, P., Lievens, M. J., and Assmann, G. (1981): Displacement of human apo AI by human apo AII protein from apo AI–lecithin–cholesterol complexes. *Eur. J. Biochem. (in press).*
23. Rosseneu, M., Vercaemst, R., Vinaimont, N., Van Tornout, P., Henderson, L. O., and Herbert, P. N. (1981): Quantitative determination of human plasma apolipoprotein by immunoneplelometry. *Clin. Chem. (in press).*
24. Rosseneu, M., Vinaimont, N., and Herbert, P. N. (1981): Quantitation of human plasma apolipoprotein AII by immunonephelometry. *Clin. Chem. (in press).*
25. Rosseneu, M., Caster, H., Vinaimont, N., Lievens, M. J., and Assmann, G. (1981): Displacement of apolipoprotein AI by apolipoprotein AII from HDL, in human plasma. *Biochim. Biophys. Acta (in press).*
26. Scherphof, G., Roerdink, F., Waite, M., and Parks, J. (1978): Disintegration of phosphatidyl Cholineliposomes in plasma as a result of interaction with high-denisty lipoproteins. *Biochim. Biophys. Acta*, 542:296–307.
27. Stein, Y., Glangeaud, M. C., Fainaru, M., and Stein, O. (1975): The removal of cholesterol from aortic-smooth muscle cells in culture and Landschütz ascites cells by fraction of human high-denstiy lipoproteins. *Biochim. Biophys. Acta*, 380:106–118.
28. Tall, A. R., Hogan, V., Askinazi, L., and Small, D. M. (1978): Interaction of plasma high density lipoproteins with dimyristoyl lecithin multi-lamellar liposomes. *Biochemistry*, 17:322–326.
29. Tall, A. (1980): Studies on the transfer of phosphatidyl choline from unilamellar vesicles into plasma high density lipoproteins in the rat. *J. Lipid Res.*, 21:354–363.
30. Van Tornout, P., Vercaemst, R., Lievens, M. J., Caster, H., Rosseneu, M., and Assmann, G. (1980): Reassembly of human apoproteins AI and AII with unilamellar phosphatidylcholine–cholesterol liposomes: Association kinetics and characterization of the complexes. *Biochim. Biophys. Acta*, 601:509–523.
31. Van Tornout, P., Caster, H., Lievens, M. J., Rosseneu, M., and Assmann, G. (1981): In vitro interaction of human HDL with human apolipoprotein AII: Synthesis of apo AII-rich HDL. *Biochim. Biophys. Acta*, 663:630–636.
32. Zierenberg, O., Assmann, G., Rosseneu, M., Schmitz, G., and Meirits, N. (1981): Effect of polyenephosphatidylcholine on cholesterol uptake by human high density lipoprotein. *Atherosclerosis*, 39:527.

Phospholipids and Atherosclerosis, edited by
P. Avogaro, M. Mancini, G. Ricci, and
R. Paoletti. Raven Press, New York © 1983.

Clinical and Biochemical Studies of the Transport of Polyenephosphatidylcholine in Human Serum and Its Physiological Impact on Cholesterol Distribution Between Serum Lipoproteins

Ottfried Zierenberg

A. Nattermann & Cie. GmbH, Abt. Biochemie, Köln, West Germany

LeKim and Betzing (7) were able to show that following oral administration of polyenephosphatidylcholine (PPC) to rats, 50% of the PPC molecules was hydrolyzed by phospholipase A_2 to lyso-PC which in turn was reacylated to PC in the mucosa cells (see also Fox et al., *this volume*). Thus far, no data of PPC absorption that could support the metabolic fate of PPC in man are available. Results of a recent clinical study (13) of the absorption and serum transport of PPC will, therefore, be discussed in this chapter.

Knowledge of the absorption mechanism of PPC, its transport to peripheral cells by lipoproteins, and its effect on lipoprotein composition is of major importance when discussing the pharmacological effect of PPC as an antiatherosclerotic drug. There is some histological evidence to the effect that atherosclerotic plaques were reduced when PPC was administered to hypercholesterolemic animals (1,5,9,10). A possible biochemical conclusion could be that PPC facilitates the transport of cholesterol from hypercholesterolemic cells to an acceptor particle in serum. According to epidemiological studies the acceptor molecule may be high-density lipoprotein (HDL) because HDL-cholesterol concentration and atherosclerosis were found to be negatively correlated. The hypothesis advanced to explain the antiatherosclerotic effect of PPC in animals is that PPC is incorporated into HDL after absorption and that it modifies the lipoprotein composition, thus increasing the cholesterol uptake capacity of HDL. The first part of the hypothesis was confirmed by the above-mentioned clinical study (13); the second part was ruled out by *in vitro* experiments (14). The results of both the clinical and biochemical studies will be discussed here.

METHODS

Clinical Study

Di-(1'-^{14}C-linoleoyl)-3-*sn*-phosphocholine (^{14}C-PC) (specific activity 8 mCi/mmole) and diacyl-phospho-N-(C^3H_3)-choline (specific activity 60 mCi/mmole) was synthesized according to established procedures (6,11). To obtain 1 g of labeled material, 150 μCi ^{3}H-PPC and 50 μCi ^{14}C-PC were mixed with PPC. Then 350 mg of the labeled mixture was filled into each hard-gelatine capsule for administration to patients. Five patients were hospitalized in the Special Diagnostic and Treatment Unit (metabolic ward) of the Veterans Administration Medical Center, La Jolla, California, throughout the study. Their sex, age, weight, and concentrations of plasma lipids are shown in Table 1. All of the patients had normal gastrointestinal function. Four of the five had moderate elevations in their plasma triglyceride (TG). All gave informed consent for the study.

The analytical methods are described in detail elsewhere (13). Briefly, blood was drawn after 1, 2, 3, 4, 6, 8, 12, 24, 48, 72, and 96 hr. The lipid extracts of the blood samples were analyzed for radioactivity and distribution of radioactivity between the blood lipids. The apo-B-containing lipoproteins [chylomicrons, very low-density (VLDL), and low-density lipoprotein (LDL)] were precipitated by heparin-Mn^{2+}. Stools and urine were analyzed for radioactivity for 7 days.

Biochemical Studies

Experimental details were published recently (14). The flow sheet of the incubation of ^{14}C-LDL with HDL-PPC is summarized in Fig. 1. The technical procedure of the ^{14}C-cholesterol distribution test is described in Fig. 2. Briefly, the cholesterol pools of human serum lipoproteins were labeled with ^{14}C-cholesterol. Afterwards, the incubation mixture was divided. One part served as a blank; to the other, PC liposomes were added. Both parts were incubated for a second period. The incubated serum was separated into the lipoprotein fractions by electrophoresis, and the lipoproteins were counted. Therefore, a shift of radioactivity from LDL to HDL indicated a transfer of cholesterol from one lipoprotein to another.

RESULTS

Clinical Studies

Intestinal Absorption of PPC

After oral administration of 1 g ^{3}H/^{14}C-labeled PPC, more than 90% of the radioactivity was absorbed from the intestine. The average excretion of ^{3}H and ^{14}C over a period of 7 days in feces was 2 and 4.5% of the administered dose, respectively. Six percent of ^{3}H from the choline moiety was excreted as ^3H_2O or water-soluble metabolites in urine.

TABLE 1. Sex, age, weight, and concentrations of plasma lipids (mg/dl) for the patients studied [a]

Patient	Sex	Age	Body Weight (kg)	Triglycerides				Cholesterol			
				Total	VLDL	LDL	HDL	Total	VLDL	LDL	HDL
B.C.	F	59	77	378	323	32	23	323	65	225	33
R.R.	M	53	130	178	125	26	27	226	32	159	35
W.V.	M	59	81	289	230	42	17	303	65	192	46
R.K.	M	56	79	411	360	20	31	269	55	138	76
L.D.	M	59	98	149	99	27	23	276	24	214	38

[a]VLDL = very low-density lipoprotein; LDL = low-density lipoprotein; HDL = high-density lipoprotein.

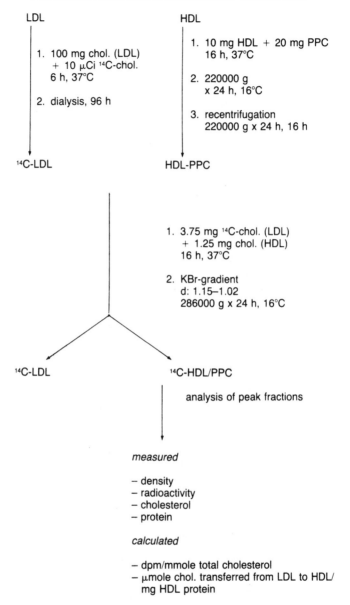

FIG. 1. Flow chart of the incubation of ^{14}C-LDL with HDL-PPC. LDL, low-density lipoprotein; HDL, high-density lipoprotein; PPC, polyenephosphatidylcholine; chol., cholesterol.

The pharmacokinetics of ^{3}H/^{14}C-PC are shown in Fig. 3. After a lag time of approximately 2 hr, labeled lipids could be measured in blood. The peak of ^{14}C was reached earlier than that of ^{3}H. The ^{14}C maximum was between 4 and 12 hr; ^{3}H peaked between 6 and 24 hr. At the peak of radioactivity in total blood, activity of ^{3}H was 19.9 $\pm$ 3.9% (SEM) of the given dose and ^{14}C was 27.9 $\pm$ 4.4%. The

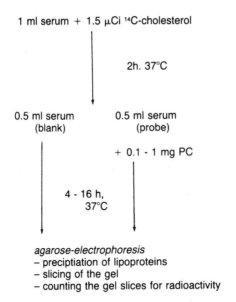

1 ml serum + 1.5 μCi ¹⁴C-cholesterol

2h. 37°C

0.5 ml serum   0.5 ml serum
    (blank)   (probe)

+ 0.1 - 1 mg PC

4 - 16 h,
  37°C

agarose-electrophoresis
– preciptiation of lipoproteins
– slicing of the gel
– counting the gel slices for radioactivity

FIG. 2.   Flow chart of the ¹⁴C-cholesterol distribution test. PC, phosphatidylcholine.

half-life of decay in radioactivity between 24 and 96 hr was 64.7 hr for ^{3}H and 37.8 hr for ^{14}C. Table 2 presents the distribution of radioactivity among the different lipids of plasma at various time intervals. Results are presented for one patient (R.K.), but the others showed essentially identical results.

Approximately 80% of ^{14}C radioactivity at the beginning of the experiment (4 hr) was in nonpolar lipids [TG and cholesteryl ester (CE)], but this percentage decreased to 40 to 50% during the peak of activity (6–24 hr). However, it increased again when the PC was metabolized over the next 4 days. Almost all of the remaining ^{14}C was found in the PC fraction. The ^{3}H/^{14}C ratios of total blood PC are given in Table 2 for the entire experiment. The pattern of change in this parameter was essentially the same in all five patients. During the first 4 hours it was only slightly above the ratio of the administered PC, but it increased progressively throughout the experiment. In 4 of 5 patients the ^{3}H/^{14}C ratio at the peak of radioactivity was nearly twice that of the oral PC. Phospholipase A_2 cleavage of the blood PC fraction of one patient suggested that the absorption mechanism of PPC in man is probably different from that in rats. In man, 39% of the ^{14}C label was present in the 1-position compared with the administered PPC which contained 50% of the ^{14}C label in that position. On the other hand, 89% of the fatty acid label was measured in the 1-position of rat blood-PC (7).

Radioactivity in Plasma Lipoproteins

To determine the distribution of radioactivity between HDL and apo-B-containing lipoproteins, heparin-Mn^{2+} percipitation was carried out immediately after obtaining blood samples in three patients (W.V., R.K., and L.D.). The data for these patients

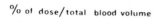

% of dose/total blood volume

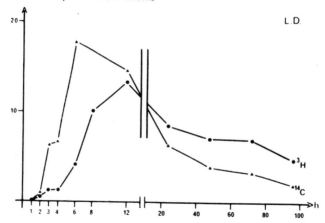

L.D.

% of dose / total blood volume

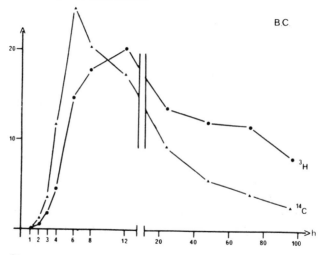

B.C

% of dose/total blood volume

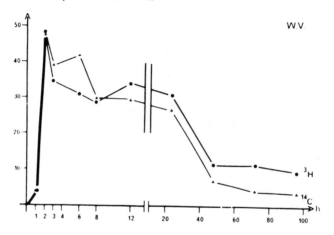

W.V.

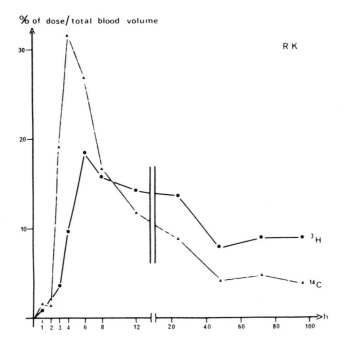

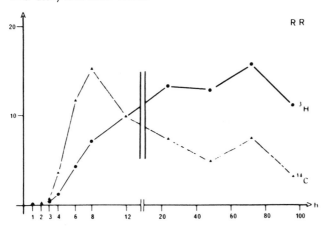

FIG. 3. Absorption kinetics of ³H and ¹⁴C following oral ingestion of ³H/¹⁴C polyenephosphatidylcholine.

are presented in Table 3. In patients W.V. and R.K. more than half the ³H activity was found in HDL; in patient L.D., approximately 40%. In contrast to the results for ³H, most of the ¹⁴C activity, which was derived from the fatty acid moieties of PC, was found in lipoproteins containing apo B. Most of ¹⁴C radioactivity was associated with nonpolar lipids (CE and TG) in apo B lipoproteins; whereas, the

TABLE 2. *Distribution of radioactivity between blood lipids after polyenephosphatidylcholine (PPC) administration for patient R.K.[a]*

Hr	Lysolecithin plus sphingomyelin		PC		TG and CE[b]		$^3H/^{14}C$ of PC
	^3H	^{14}C	^3H	^{14}C	^3H	^{14}C	
4	19	1	76	15	3	83	4.6
6	7	1	82	30	0	67	5.5
8	9	2	84	42	0	55	6.0
12	10	2	84	43	0	54	7.3
24	12	1	82	36	1	62	10.6
48	9	0	80	25	1	74	18.6
72	16	8	74	11	6	77	23.2
96	24	15	69	10	3	73	27.2

[a]PPC administered in a $^3H/^{14}C$ ratio of 3.5. Data given in percent of blood reactivity.
[b]TG, triglyceride; CE, cholesteryl ester.

TABLE 3. *Distribution of radioactivity between serum lipoproteins[a,b]*

Patient	Hr	$^3H(\%)$		$^{14}C(\%)$	
		HDL	LDL, VLDL, chylomicrons	HDL	LDL, VLDL, chylomicrons
W.V.	6	56	44	32	68
	8	63	37	10	90
	12	64	36	15	85
	24	54	46	18	82
R.K.	6	68	32	11	89
	8	80	20	26	74
	12	62	38	29	71
L.D.	8	37	63	13	87
	12	37	63	22	78
	24	37	63	25	75

[a]Plasma radioactivity = 100%.
[b]VLDL, very low-density lipoprotein; LDL, low-density lipoprotein; HDL, high-density lipoprotein.

PC of HDL had a much greater fraction of ^{14}C than did other lipid fractions. Almost all ^3H radioactivity was associated with PC of each lipoprotein. In addition, no difference was found in the $^3H/^{14}C$ ratio of PC between HDL and other lipoproteins.

The specific activities of PC in the different lipoprotein fractions as well as in total blood were measured in two patients. The results are presented in Table 4. At 6 hr in patient R.K., the specific activity of PC in HDL was about 30% of the

TABLE 4. *Specific activity of phosphatidylcholine (PC) of lipoproteins and blood[a]*

		Lipoproteins				Blood
		Specific activity of PC				
		HDL	LDL, VLDL, chylomicrons	HDL	LDL, VLDL, chylomicrons	Specific activity of PC
Patient	Hr	(dpm ^{3}H/μmole PC)		(dpm ^{14}C/μmole PC)		(dpm ^{3}H/μmole PC)
R.K.	6	8.6×10^4	2.6×10^4	2.5×10^4	5.1×10^3	1.9×10^3
	8	4.0×10^4	3.6×10^4	7.2×10^3	3.1×10^3	1.8×10^3
	12	2.1×10^4	1.3×10^4	2.6×10^3	1.4×10^3	1.9×10^3
	24	1.5×10^4	1.1×10^4	1.0×10^3	0.7×10^3	1.5×10^3
L.D.	6	—	1.6×10^3	—	5.2×10^2	4.0×10^2
	8	1.9×10^4	3.1×10^3	1.7×10^4	9.4×10^2	1.2×10^3
	12	6.5×10^3	3.8×10^3	2.0×10^3	8.6×10^2	2.0×10^3
	24	—	3.7×10^3	—	5.5×10^2	1.6×10^3
Oral PC		2.0×10^5		8.3×10^4		

[a]VLDL = very low-density lipoprotein; LDL = low-density lipoprotein; HDL = high-density lipoprotein.

administered dose, and it declined to 7 to 13% after 8 hr, and to 2 to 7% after 12 hr. In most of the plasma samples studied the ^{3}H and ^{14}C specific activities were much higher in HDL than in the apo-B-containing lipoproteins and even higher than in total blood. Hence, there had to be a specific incorporation of labeled PC into lipoproteins, especially HDL, rather than a nonspecific distribution of PC between red blood cells and lipoproteins.

Biochemical Studies

Cholesterol Transfer Between HDL-PPC and LDL

The specific incorporation of PPC into HDL, demonstrated in man and also in some animal species (15), was achieved *in vitro* by incubation of human HDL with PPC liposomes. PPC was taken up by human HDL after incubation at 37°C for 16 hr (Fig. 1). By this procedure a maximum enrichment of the HDL-PC fraction by PPC was obtained with approximately 50% PPC. LDL was labeled with ^{14}C-cholesterol. The ^{14}C-LDL, HDL-PPC, and native HDL were incubated with a ratio of cholesterol (LDL) to cholesterol (HDL) of 3:1, resembling physiological conditions of human plasma.

After incubation of ^{14}C-LDL with HDL or HDL-PPC and after separation of both lipoproteins by ultracentrifugation, part of the LDL cholesterol was shifted to HDL. Analysis of the HDL and LDL fractions is presented in Table 5 for a representative

TABLE 5. *Incubation of ^{14}C-LDL with native HDL or HDL-PPC—Calculation of cholesterol transfer from LDL to HDL*[a]

	HDL		LDL	
	Native	HDL-PPC	Native	HDL-PPC
Specific activity (dpm/mmole cholesterol) of incubated LDL			1.62 × 10^8	
Specific activity (dpm/mmole cholesterol)	2.7 × 10^7	4.6 × 10^7	1.6 × 10^8	1.76 × 10^8
Δ%		+70		
Millimoles cholesterol taken up by HDL per milligram HDL protein (analysis after incubation)	132	194		
Δ%		+47		
Millimoles cholesterol per mg LDL protein (analysis after incubation)			1,410	1,115
Δ%				−21

[a]LDL = low-density lipoprotein; HDL = high-density lipoprotein; PPC = polyenephosphatidylcholine.

experiment. The specific activity of HDL cholesterol (disintegrations per minute per millimole of total cholesterol) was significantly higher in HDL-PPC than in native HDL. Using the specific activity of ^{14}C-LDL cholesterol, it was calculated that 194 mmole cholesterol were taken up per milligram protein of HDL-PPC. On the other hand, only 132 mmole cholesterol were taken up by native HDL. HDL-PPC consequently accepted 47% more cholesterol from LDL than native HDL.

An uptake of cholesterol by HDL-PPC or HDL is likely to result in a cholesterol depletion of LDL. Owing to the different cholesterol affinities there will obviously be differences in cholesterol depletion of LDL after HDL-PPC and HDL incubation. This is also shown in Table 5. After incubation of ^{14}C-LDL with HDL-PPC, LDL had lost significantly more cholesterol per milligram protein than after incubation with native HDL. On the other hand, the specific activity of LDL cholesterol did not differ significantly between the pre- and postincubation periods; that is, there was no redistribution between the unlabeled HDL-cholesterol pool and the labeled LDL-cholesterol pool.

^{14}C-Cholesterol Distribution Test

After incubation of ^{14}C-PPC with serum (1 mg PPC/ml serum) (Fig. 2), approximately 70% of PPC was incorporated into HDL and approximately 30% into VLDL and LDL. This observation confirms those results obtained after both incubation of human serum with PPC and separation of the incubation mixture by ultracentrifugation (15). On the other hand, ^{14}C-PPC liposomes do not migrate in the electric field, enabling the separation of lipoproteins and unbound PPC liposomes by agarose electrophoresis. An example of this analysis is presented in Fig. 4.

After incubation of serum with PPC (1 mg/ml serum), the ^{14}C-cholesterol concentration in HDL was increased in comparison with the control, whereas ^{14}C-cholesterol in LDL and VLDL was decreased, resulting in a significant decrease in the ratio of ^{14}C-LDL + VLDL/^{14}C-HDL. The test was designed to study the effect of the fluidity of different PC species on the cholesterol uptake by HDL. The results plotted in Fig. 5 suggest that the cholesterol uptake capacity of HDL was limited by the composition of the HDL lipid phase. After incubation of serum with PPC, more cholesterol was shifted from LDL and VLDL to HDL than after incubation with more saturated PC species. The uptake of cholesterol by HDL decreased in the order PPC > egg-PC > saturated PC (Fig. 5). As a result of the cholesterol uptake by HDL, the ratio of LDL + VLDL/HDL decreased with increasing unsaturation of the PC species.

Whether or not serum enzymes might be limiting factors for cholesterol uptake in HDL was investigated. Heat-inactivated serum was employed to eliminate enzymatic activities. No significant difference in the lipoprotein/cholesterol ratio was

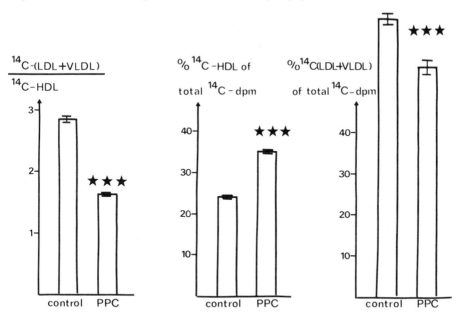

FIG. 4. ^{14}C-cholesterol distribution test. Conditions: 1 mg PPC/ml serum; first incubation: 2 hr, 37°C; second incubation: 16 hr, 37°C; $N = 7$; ***$p = 0.001$. VLDL, very low-density lipoprotein; LDL, low-density lipoprotein; HDL, high-density lipoprotein; PPC, polyenephosphatidylcholine.

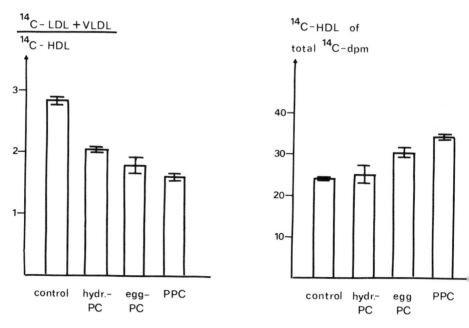

FIG. 5. ^{14}C-cholesterol distribution test. Cholesterol uptake by HDL after incubation of serum with PPC, egg-PC, hydrogenated PC (for conditions, see Fig. 4 legend).

found between normal and heat-inactivated serum. In particular, no effect of lecithin-cholesterol acyltransferase (LCAT) on the cholesterol uptake into HDL was observed by selective inhibition of its enzymatic activity with 5,5-dithio-*bis*-2-nitrobenzoic acid (DTNB).

DISCUSSION

More than 90% of the polyenephosphatidylcholine (PPC) was absorbed from the intestine into the mucosa cells. With the data now available the possible absorption mechanism can be described. According to radiochemical analysis the absorbed labeled PC lost one labeled fatty acid, and the resulting lyso-PC was reesterified to PC with an unlabeled fatty acid. The $^3H/^{14}C$ ratio of the absorbed PC was approximately doubled in the peak maximum. So far, the results concur with those obtained by LeKim and Betzing (7) in rats. A difference was found, however, with regard to the fatty acid composition of the absorbed labeled PC. In rats, the remaining labeled fatty acids were exclusively contained in the 1-position of PC, and it was assumed that a specified reesterification of the 2-position with unlabeled linoleic acid had taken place.

In man, the labeled linoleic acids were distributed equally between the 1- and 2-positions; that is, a nonspecific hydrolysis of the 1- or 2-position occurred before PPC was absorbed via lyso-PC into the mucosa cell. The labeled lyso-PC was reesterified with an unlabeled fatty acid to PC. These findings show that, after oral administration in man, the PC species absorbed from the intestine contained an unsaturated linoleic acid in the 1-position of the molecule. This species is different from physiological PC which has a saturated fatty acid in the 1-position. Furthermore, as has been shown recently, the 1-linoleoyl-2-acyl-PC species was not synthesized in man following administration of linoleic acid (8). Consequently, administration of unsaturated triglycerides, e.g., safflower oil which is hydrolyzed to linoleic acids and glycerol in the intestine, will not produce 1,2-linoleoyl-PC after absorption.

The experimental design of measuring PPC concentrations in blood did not allow calculation of the total amount of PPC absorbed because a first-pass effect might have been involved. This was demonstrated, for example, by LeKim and Betzing (7) who measured 50% of the administered PPC dose in the lymph chylomicrons of rats, but only 4% in the total blood compartment. Using the radiochemical data, the present authors were able to calculate a maximum PC blood concentration in man of 8% of the administered dose; the total concentration of absorbed PPC was likely to be from four to six times this amout. The absorbed PPC was metabolized by hydrolysis of the fatty acids. The resulting lyso-PC or glycerophosphocholine was used for PC resynthesis and was not further degraded to smaller molecules. The reesterified PC was again shunted into the blood stream. A recent clinical study by Beil and Grundy (3) has shown that the absorbed PPC is incorporated into chylomicrons, thereby increasing the surface-to-coat ratio and decreasing particle

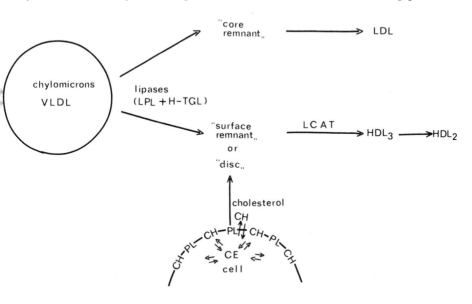

FIG. 6. Interconversion of lipoproteins. VLDL, very low-density lipoprotein; LDL, low-density lipoprotein; HDL, high-density lipoprotein; LPL, lipoprotein lipase; TGL, hepatic triglyceride lipace; LCAT, lecithin-cholesterol acyltransferase; CH, cholesterol; PL, phospholipids; CE, cholesteryl ester.

diameter. It was now possible to follow-up the transport of PPC after degradation of the triglyceride-rich particles and measure a specified uptake of PPC into HDL. The specific activity of PC in HDL was higher than in apo-B-containing lipoproteins or in red blood cells. The same results were obtained in dogs, rabbits, and rats after oral administration of PPC (15).

As it was of interest to study the physiological effect of an enhanced PPC uptake by HDL on the cholesterol-acceptor function of HDL, HDL-PPC was prepared *in vitro*. This preparation had a lower density than native HDL owing to an increased PPC concentration in the particle of about 50%. LDL labeled with ¹⁴C-cholesterol was used as a cholesterol donor. After incubation of HDL-PPC and native HDL with labeled LDL, HDL-PPC increased its uptake of cholesterol by approximately 50% compared with native HDL. The ¹⁴C-cholesterol distribution test was developed to determine whether the increased PC concentration in HDL-PPC or the substitution of native PC for highly fluid PPC regulate the cholesterol uptake capacity of HDL-PPC. In this test cholesterol transfer from LDL to HDL depended, apart from other factors, on the fluidity of the PC species used: transfer was optimal for PPC, whereas cholesterol transfer declined with increasing fatty acid saturation of the PC species. The transfer was not dependent on LCAT activity. Hence, the surface properties of HDL, rather than the ability of LCAT to remove cholesterol from the surface, were responsible for limiting the cholesterol uptake. These findings show that the composition of HDL can regulate its cholesterol-acceptor function: the more fluid the surface of the particle, the higher its affinity for cholesterol. The clinical and biochemical results discussed complement each other, providing a description of some pharmacodynamic properties of PPC, which are depicted in Fig. 6.

Orally ingested PPC formed HDL-PPC particles after degradation of the chylomicrons. HDL-PPC had a high affinity for cholesterol and might be a good acceptor for membrane cholesterol and for lipoproteins with a pathological PC/cholesterol ratio. In addition, as was shown by Desreumaux et al. (4), PPC increased lipoprotein lipase activity. Therefore, the generation of HDL particles might be increased. Cholesterol from the surface of HDL is shifted to its core after LCAT transesterification. This enzymatic activity is also enhanced by PPC (2,12). Increased HDL-particle generation and increased cholesterol uptake by these particles should have a favorable effect on cholesterol excretion via bile acids and thus on the regression of atherosclerosis. These questions are now the subject of further clinical investigation.

REFERENCES

1. Adams, C. W. M., Abdulla, Y. H., Bayliss, O. B. and Morgan, R. S. (1967): Modification of aortic atheroma and fatty liver in cholesterol-fed rabbits by i.v. injection of saturated and polyunsaturated lecithins. *J. Pathol. Bacteriol.*, 94:77.
2. Assmann, G., Schmitz, G., Donath, N., and LeKim, D. (1978): Phosphatidylcholine substrate specificity of LCAT. *Scand. J. Clin. Lab. Invest.*, 38:16.
3. Beil, F. U., and Grundy, S. M. (1980): Studies of plasma lipoproteins during absorption of exogenous lecithin in man. *J. Lipid Res.*, 21:525.

 4. Desreumaux, C., Dedonder, E., Dewailly, P., Sezille, G., and Fruchart, J. C. (1979): Effects of unsaturated fatty acids in phospholipids on the in vitro activation of the lipoprotein lipase and the triglyceride lipase. *Drug Res.*, 29:1581.
 5. Howard, A. N., Patelski, J., Bowyer, D. E., and Gresham, G. A. (1971): Atherosclerosis induced in hypercholesterolaemic baboons by immunological injury, and the effects of i.v. polyunsaturated phosphatidylcholine. *Atherosclerosis*, 14:17.
 6. LeKim, D., and Betzing, H. (1974): Der Einbau von EPL-Substanz in Organe von gesunden und durch Galaktosamin geschädigte Ratten. *Drug. Res.*, 24:1217.
 7. LeKim, D., and Betzing, H. (1976): Intestinal absorption of PPC in the rat. *Hoppe Seylers Z. Physiol. Chem.*, 357:1321.
 8. Mercuti, O., De Thomas, M. E., and Travella, M. (1980): Linoleic acid enrichment of serum PC in humans by low doses of sodium linoleate. *Atherosclerosis*, 37:169.
 9. Samochowiec, L., Kadlubowska, D., and Rozewicka, L. (1976): Investigations in experimental atherosclerosis, Part 1 (The effects of phosphatidylcholine (EPL) on experimental atherosclerosis in withe rats). *Atherosclerosis*, 23:305.
10. Stafford, W. W., and Day, C. E. (1975): Regression of atherosclerosis effected by i.v. phospholipids. *Artery*, 1:106.
11. Stoffel, W., LeKim, D., and Tschung, T. (1971): A simple chemical method for labelling phosphatidylcholine and sphingomyeline in the choline moiety. *Hoppe Seylers Z. Physiol. Chem.*, 352:1058.
12. Wallentin, L. (1977): Influence of i.v. and oral administration of phospholipids on LCAT acyltransfer rate in plasma. *Artery*, 3:40.
13. Zierenberg, O., and Grundy, S. M. (1982): Intestinal absorption of PPC in man. *J. Lipid Res.*, 23:1136.
14. Zierenberg, O., Assmann, G., Schmitz, G., and Rosseneu, M. (1981): Effect of PPC on cholesterol uptake by human HDL. *Atherosclerosis*, 39:527.
15. Zierenberg, O., Odenthal, H., and Betzing, H. (1979): Incorporation of PPC into serum lipoproteins after oral or i.v. administration. *Atherosclerosis*, 34:259.

Phospholipids and Atherosclerosis, edited by
P. Avogaro, M. Mancini, G. Ricci, and
R. Paoletti. Raven Press, New York © 1983.

Determination of High-Density Lipoprotein Phospholipids

G. Assmann and H. Schriewer

Zentrallaboratorium der Medizinischen Einrichtungen der Westfälischen Wilhems-Universität, D-4400 Münster/Westfälischen, West Germany

The analysis of high-density lipoprotein (HDL) as an indicator of the risk of coronary heart disease has gained considerable importance in recent years (1,2). The hitherto most widely used procedure of quantitatively assaying HDL is based on the determination of cholesterol in the supernatant fraction of serum after precipitation of apolipoprotein-B-containing lipoproteins with a solution of polyanions and divalent cations. However, since HDLs form a heterogeneous group of compounds (differences in composition, physicochemical properties, and metabolism), it is not possible to establish a simple correlation between the HDL cholesterol fraction and HDL mass.

HDL particles are composed of approximately 50% proteins, 25 to 30% phospholipids, 10 to 20% cholesterol and its esters, and 3 to 5% triglycerides. Although the phospholipid content of HDL particles is higher than their cholesterol content, the assay of the total HDL phospholipids or of the individual phospholipid fractions is quite complicated, so that it has not yet become a routine procedure. Studies by Weisweiler et al. (6) and Telesforo et al. (5) have shown that there is a close correlation between HDL cholesterol and total HDL phospholipids in normal serum. If one assumes that the composition of HDL particles can vary considerably (especially in hyperlipidemic sera), then it appears likely that a more detailed analysis of the phospholipid fraction of these particles would improve the early diagnosis of coronary heart disease and allow a more reliable prognosis.

Assays of phosphatidylcholine (lecithin) and sphingomyelin have hitherto been based on the time-consuming, laborious separation of these phospholipids by thin-layer chromatography (TLC) or column chromatography, with subsequent elution and determination of phosphate in the eluates. However, the recent commercial availability of specific phospholipases and recent development of sensitive analytical methods for choline have made it possible to assay phosphatidylcholine and sphingomyelin relatively quickly and easily. A procedure has been developed for deter-

191

TABLE 1. *Lecithin and sphingomyelin in apolipoprotein-B-free supernatant after precipitation of apolipoprotein B with MgCl₂-phosphotungstic acid*[a]

	Women	Men
Sphingomyelin	$\bar{x}$ = 12.85 mg/dl s = 3.85 mg/dl N = 37	$\bar{x}$ = 12.04 mg/dl s = 4.88 mg/dl N = 44
Lecithin	$\bar{x}$ = 106.71 mg/dl s = 31.15 mg/dl N = 37	$\bar{x}$ = 97.82 mg/dl s = 34.97 mg/dl N = 44
Sphingomyelin/lecithin	r = 0.5748 y = 0.0729x + 5.573 N = 37	r = 0.653 y = 0.09x + 3.12 N = 44
apolipoprotein A-I/lecithin	r = 0.67 y = 0.415x + 9.962 N = 35	r = 0.74 y = 1.33x + 92.78 N = 30
HDL-Chol./lecithin[b]	r = 0.79 y = 0.415x + 9,962 N = 37	r = 0.76 y = 0.406x + 6.16 N = 44
HDL-Chol./sphingomyelin	r = 0.54 y = 2.37x + 22.64 N = 37	r = 0.76 y = 3.36x + 11.25 N = 44
Sphingomyelin/apolipoprotein A-I	r = 0.62 y = 0.04x + 2.31 N = 33	r = 0.79 y = 0.06x − 3.27 N = 30

[a]Prospective study on employees in Westphalia, West Germany, with the aim of improving early diagnosis of coronary heart disease.
[b]HDL-Chol. = high-density lipoprotein cholesterol.

I. phosphatidylcholine $\xrightarrow{\text{phospholipase C}}$ phosphorylcholine + diglyceride;

II. sphingomyelin $\xrightarrow{\text{sphingomyelinase}}$ phosphorylcholine + N-acylsphingosine

phosphorylcholine $\xrightarrow{\text{alkaline phosphatase}}$ choline + phosphate

choline + ATP $\xrightarrow{\text{choline kinase}}$ phosphorylcholine + ADP

ADP + phosphoenolpyruvate $\xrightarrow{\text{pyruvate kinase}}$ pyruvate + ATP

pyruvate + NADH₂ $\xrightarrow{\text{lactate dehydrogenase}}$ lactate + NAD⁺

FIG. 1. Enzymatic determination of phosphatidylcholine and sphingomyelin.

mination of these two parameters in HDL that is suitable for screening purposes and is presented here. It entails precipitation of apolipoprotein-B-containing lipoproteins from native serum with MgCl₂-phosphotungstic acid and subsequent specific enzymatic determination of the individual phospholipids in the supernatant.

The assay of phosphatidylcholine makes use of the phospholipase-C-catalyzed cleavage of phosphatidylcholine into diglycerides and phosphorylcholine (Fig. 1). Phospholipase C from *B. cereus* (Boehringer Mannheim, Cat. No. 241 709) cleaves phosphatidylcholine, phosphatidylethanolamine, and phosphatidylserine, but not sphingomyelin, lysophosphatidylcholine, or phosphatidylinositol. The phosphorylcholine liberated from phosphatidylcholine is hydrolyzed to phosphate and choline by alkaline phosphatase, and the choline is then determined enzymatically with choline kinase and adenosine triphosphate (ATP).

The ADP formed in the latter reaction is transformed to pyruvate in the presence of phosphoenolpyruvate (PEP) and pyruvate kinase (PK), and the pyruvate formed is finally reduced to lactate by $NADH_2$ and lactate dehydrogenase (LDH). The concentrations in the test (3) are:

REAGENTS

1. Buffer	glycine	200 mmole/liter
	$MgSO_4 \times 7H_2O$	10 mmole/liter
	sodium dodecylsulfate	0.1 g/liter
	pH	8.00
2.	Phospholipase-C	80 U/ml
	Alkaline phosphatase	100 U/ml
3.	$NADH_2$	4 mmole/liter
	ATP	20 mmole/liter
	PEP	7 mmole/liter
	Glucose	45 mmole/liter
4.	PK	300 U/ml
	LDH	300 U/ml
5.	Choline kinase	2.0 U/ml

HYDROLYSIS OF PHOSPHATIDYLCHOLINE

Pipette into Eppendorf vials:

	Sample	Reagent blank
Buffer	0.5 ml	0.5 ml
Sample	0.020 ml	—
0.9% NaCl	0.980 ml	1.000 ml
Suspension 2	0.050 ml	0.050 ml

The reaction mixture is mixed thoroughly, incubated at 37°C for 30 min, and then heated to 95°C for 15 min. The denatured proteins are centrifuged out after the suspension has cooled down to room temperature.

CHOLINE ASSAY

Pipette into cuvettes:

	Sample	Reagent blank
Supernatant	1.000 ml	1.000 ml
Coenzyme solution	0.050 ml	0.050 ml
PK/LDH	0.020 ml	0.020 ml

Mix, incubate at 37°C for 10 min, then read A_1 against water at 366 nm. Add:

	Sample	Reagent blank
Choline kinase	0.025 ml	0.025 ml

Again mix the reaction mixture thoroughly and incubate at 37°C for 7 min, then read A_2. Read A_3 after a further 7 min.

PHOSPHATIDYLCHOLINE CONCENTRATION

$$\Delta A \text{ (sample, blank)} = (A_1 - A_2) - (A_2 - A_3)$$
$$\Delta A = \Delta A_{\text{sample}} - \Delta A_{\text{blank}}$$
$$\text{Concentration } (C) = \Delta A \times \text{factor}$$

where the factor equals 2111.2 mg/dl or 27.31 mmole/liter. The mean concentration of phosphatidylcholine in HDL was found to be 106.71 mg/dl for men and 97.82 mg/dl for women. Linear regression analysis of the values obtained after precipitation with phosphotungstic acid-$MgCl_2$ (y) and after ultracentrifugation ($d = 1.063 - 1.21$ kg/liter) (x) disclosed a good correlation of these data ($y = 0.93x + 8.5$; $r = 0.93$, $N = 25$) (3).

Sphingomyelin is determined according to the same principle as phoshpatidylcholine (4), being split into phosphorylcholine and N-acylsphingosine by sphingomyelinase from B. cereus (Boehringer Mannheim, Cat. No. 396 753). This enzyme is relatively specific for sphingomyelin, exhibiting only slight contamination with phospholipase C (0.1%) and phosphatidylinositol phosphodiesterase. The procedure is given below (4):

HYDROLYSIS OF SPHINGOMYELIN

Pipette into Eppendorf vials:

	Sample	Reagent blank
Buffer	0.500 ml	0.500 ml
Sample	0.100 ml	—
0.9% NaCl	0.900 ml	1.000 ml
Sphingomyelinase (100 U/ml)	0.020 ml	0.020 ml
Alkaline phosphatase (650 U/liter)	0.010 ml	0.010 ml

After incubation at 37°C for 30 min, the assay mixture is heated to 95°C for 10 min, and the amount of choline is determined as in the phosphatidylcholine assay.

SPHINGOMYELIN CONCENTRATION

$$C = \Delta A \times \text{factor}$$

where the factor equals 410.19 mg/dl or 5.307 mmole/liter. The mean sphingomyelin concentration in HDL was 12.85 mg/dl for women and 12.04 mg/dl for men. The sphingomyelin values obtained by ultracentrifugation (d = 1.063 – 1.21 kg/liter) (x) correlated well with those found in the supernatant after precipitation of apo-B-containing lipoproteins (y): y = 1.06x – 3.1; r = 0.900, N = 32 (4).

REFERENCES

1. Assmann, G., and Schriewer, H. (1981): Möglichkeiten und Grenzen der Analytik des HDL-Cholesterins. *J. Clin. Chem. Clin. Biochem.*, 19:1–6.
2. Assmann, G., Schriewer, H., and Funke, H. (1981): Zur Richtigkeit der HDL-Cholesterin- und HDL-Apolipoprotein A-I-Bestimmung nach Phosphorwolframsäure/MgCl₂ Präzipitation Apolipoprotein B-haltiger Lipoproteine. *J. Clin. Chem. Clin. Biochem.*, 19:273–278.
3. Schriewer, H., Jabs, H.-U., J. Günnewig, V., and Assmann, G.: Determination of HDL phosphatidylcholine by an enzymatic method. *J. Clin. Chem. Clin. Biochem. (in press)*.
4. Schriewer, H., Jabs, H.-U., and Assmann, G. (1982): Zur enzymatischen Analytik des HDL Sphingomyelin. *J. Clin. Chem. Clin. Biochem. (in press)*.
5. Telesforo, P., Salino, L., and D'Errico, A. (1981): HDL-cholesterol or HDL-phospholipids? *Clin. Chem.*, 27:354–255.
6. Weisweiler, P., Sperl, B., and Schwandt, P. (1981): Determination of high density lipoproteins: Comparison of HDL cholesterol, HDL phospholipids, and HDL apolipoprotein A-I. *Clin. Chem.*, 27:348.

Phospholipids and Atherosclerosis, edited by
P. Avogaro, M. Mancini, G. Ricci, and
R. Paoletti. Raven Press, New York © 1983.

Phospholipids, Atherosclerosis, and Aging

Cesare R. Sirtori

*Center E. Grossi Paoletti and Chemotherapy Chair,
University of Milano, 20129 Milano, Italy*

The impact of various nutrients, e.g., lipids, carbohydrates, ethanol, trace elements, has received considerable attention in the past few years in the evaluation of the dietary origin of atherosclerosis and aging (37). Among the different lipids, phospholipids—particularly lecithin—have been the object of numerous studies, both in view of their postulated activity in lipid metabolism and in experimental atherosclerosis (34,41), and also because lecithin may be a precursor of choline, a substrate for the central neurotransmitter biosynthesis (31).

The activity of phospholipids (PL) on the different metabolic steps linked to the development of atherosclerosis was evaluated in many experiments with the aim of establishing the mode of action of different PL, notably the lecithin of vegetable origin. The experimental studies in several animal models will be reviewed together with the more recent investigations on the central effect of oral lecithin in conditions of impaired brain function because of the regressive changes secondary to aging.

PREVENTION AND REGRESSION OF ATHEROSCLEROSIS IN DIFFERENT ANIMAL MODELS

The prevention of diet-induced atherosclerosis or the regression of established lesions, or both, with PL have been shown in many animal models. The most widely applied model has been the dietary-induced hypercholesterolemic rabbit. Rats, quails, and baboons have also been studied, both with the objective of confirming the rabbit data and for specific studies on the mechanism of action. Essential phospholipids (EPL), i.e. highly polyunsaturated lecithin extracted from soybeans, have been used in most experiments.

Rabbits

A prompt elevation of plasma cholesterol levels, following sustained infusions of different phosphatides, was noted as early as 1955 by Friedman and Byers (25). The suggestion that the plasma cholesterol rise might be due to sterols already present in extravascular tissues (14) was later supported by a regression experiment.

Rabbits were fed a cholesterol-enriched diet for 3 months and brought back for 1 month to the normal pellet diet. Then they received, in paired experiments, either crude brain phosphatide or soybean phosphatides from different sources (15). Both brain and vegetable phosphatides induced a prompt rise of plasma PL and cholesterol levels; the plasma lipid elevation usually vanishing from 24 to 48 hr after each infusion. However, a marked decrease in the severity of the atherosclerotic lesions in rabbits repeatedly infused with the phosphatide suspensions was noticeable, whether they were derived from animal or vegetable sources (Table 1). Within the same experiment, aortic segments were implanted into the anterior eye chamber of rabbit pairs. The effect of PL infusions was insignificant when atherosclerotic segments were implanted; however, when normal tissue was placed into the eye chamber of rabbits treated with cholesterol plus phosphatide, lipid infiltration was more marked than in rabbits fed only cholesterol.

These early findings suggested that the antiatherosclerotic mechanism of PL infusions could be related to a direct transport of cholesterol out of extrahepatic tissues into plasma, possibly after tissue cholesterol solubilization. The mechanism appeared to be direct, in view of the negligible activity on corneally implanted aortic tissue. Further evidence for this hypothesis was provided by Adams et al. (1), who studied cholesterol resorption from subcutaneous implants. Resorption of cholesterol amounted to 11% 1 week after the implant. With the administration of a purified PL from soybean, 95% of the implanted cholesterol was reabsorbed. Later studies by the same authors showed that cholesterol implants induced an inflammatory response, ameliorated by PL administration. Cholesterol arachidonate was the least sclerogenic of all the esters tested, and egg lecithin was less effective in inducing resorption than EPL (3). EPL might enhance the formation of poly-unsaturated cholesteryl esters, less sclerogenic and more easily dispersed, possibly via the action of tissue lecithin-cholesterol acyltransferase (LCAT) (4). The same authors could later confirm that in a rabbit model of hypercholesterolemia, both aortic atheroma and fatty liver could be prevented by intravenous injection of polyunsaturated lecithins; a lesser activity was displayed by saturated lecithins (2).

In other studies in rabbits, on a cholesterol-enriched (0.5%) diet, PL extracted from the bovine heart and EPL (both 25 mg/kg i.v. 6 days/week) were compared with oral metformin (75 or 135 mg/kg per day), a drug known to markedly decrease cholesterol atherosclerosis in rabbits (46). The atherogenic diet lasted 16 weeks, with the three different treatments being administered during the last 8 weeks. Both bovine PL and EPL significantly increased total serum cholesterol at the end of the schedule, whereas the 75 mg/kg dose of metformin did not affect cholesterolemia and the 135 mg/kg dose significantly decreased it (9). As shown in Fig. 1, EPL markedly reduced aortic atherosclerosis, to a similar degree as elicited by the low- and high-dose metformin. A similar effect was noted with bovine PL.

TABLE 1. *Plasma cholesterol changes and aortic atherosclerosis regression in rabbits infused with different phosphatides (mean values)[a]*

	N	Plasma cholesterol (mg/dl)		No. of infusions	Aorta	
		During cholesterol feeding	One month after feeding[b]		Atherosclerosis score (0–5)	Cholesterol (g/100 g)
		Rabbits infused with soybean phosphatides (prep. S-W)[c]				
Infused	7	585	203	13	2.7	4.18
Controls	7	568	187	0	4.5	5.31
		Rabbits infused with soybean phosphatides (prep. C)[c]				
Infused	6	909	68	12	2.3	5.04
Controls	6	908	72	0	4.0	6.49
		Rabbits infused with crude phosphatides (from brain)[c]				
Infused	6	995	167	8	3.3	6.69
Controls	6	958	213	8[d]	4.8	12.8

[a]Data adapted from Byers and Friedman (15).
[b]Rabbits were infused twice weekly for 1 month after the end of cholesterol feeding.
[c]Five percent phosphatide suspensions. S-W, Sterling Winthrop; C, Cutter.
[d]Five percent dextrose.

Other Animal Species

In rats, the administration of EPL (50–1,800 mg/kg per day) to animals receiving a diet enriched with cholesterol and cholic acid determines a dose-related plasma total cholesterol decrease, statistically significant with the high EPL dose (36). In other experiments, when EPL were given orally (280–2,800 mg/kg per day) to rats on an atherogenic diet, significant effects on the development of the atherosclerotic lesions were detected (43). Both when given together with the diet or following it, EPL significantly reduced the size and extent of aortic lesions.

In minipigs, similar studies were carried out with EPL (dosage 28–280 mg/kg per day). Also in these studies, EPL protected the animals from the development of the arterial lesions induced by the cholesterol plus cholic acid diet (44). An interesting preventive effect on the changes induced by the diet on retinal vessels was also noted (42).

Quails were treated for 3 months with an atherogenic diet. Then the diet was coupled with a weekly intravenous injection of an EPL solution (0.8 ml per animal of Lipostabil). After 3 months of this atherogenic diet plus EPL infusions, arterial cholesterol was markedly reduced, as were the degree and extent of arterial lesions

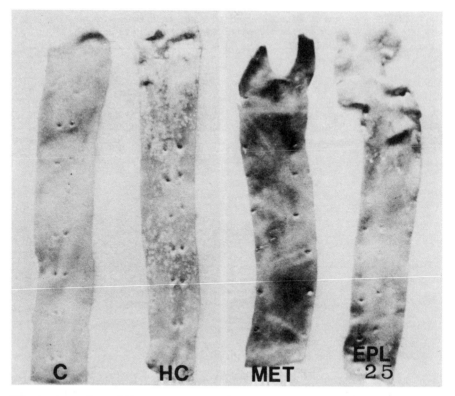

FIG. 1. Aortas from rabbits on a normal diet (C), following cholesterol feeding (HC: 16 weeks on a 0.5% cholesterol–enriched diet) and after addition, during the last 8 weeks of the dietary regimen, of metformin (MET: 75 mg/kg/day or of essential phospholipids (EPL: 25 mg/kg i.v. 6 days per week). A remarkable reduction of the atheromatous lesions is noted with both combined treatments. (From Bauer et al. ref. 9, with permission.)

(47). Quails may be the animal species most sensitive to atherosclerosis regression induced by PL.

In baboons, atherosclerosis was induced by a 6-month treatment with an atherogenic diet. In the last 90 days five i.v. injections of bovine serum albumin (BSA) were given at 16-day intervals. One group of monkeys concomitantly received thrice weekly injections of 1 g of EPL. Baboons with the diet plus BSA have severe atherosclrosis with increased aortic lipase activity and no change in cholesterylesterase. EPL treatment significantly reduced atherosclerosis; lipase activity was unchanged; and esterase increased 50% (32). Cholesterol esterification and hydrolysis in the arterial wall may be a balanced process; if EPL enhances cholesteryl ester hydrolysis, free cholesterol may be easily transported across cell membranes, with ensuing atherosclerosis regression (33). More recently, excess membrane cholesterol has been indicated as a cause of altered membrane permeability and of changes in enzyme activities (39). These effects may be prevented by membrane enrichment with polyunsaturated lecithin (30).

STUDIES ON THE MECHANISM OF THE ANTIATHEROSCLEROTIC EFFECT OF PHOSPHOLIPIDS

Some of the suggested hypotheses for the antiatherosclerotic effect of PL have been indicated in the previous chapter. Among these are the formation of less sclerogenic cholesteryl esters and an enhanced hydrolysis of cholesteryl esters in the arterial wall via a stimulation of cholesterylesterase activity, and so forth. Three sites of activity of EPL, in particular, will be analyzed here. EPL may markedly modify the arterial wall metabolism, both by reducing plasma membrane PL and by inhibiting arterial wall lipid biosynthesis. They may also interact with the binding of atherogenic lipoprotein fractions with the arterial wall polyanions. A second site of action of PL may be at the level of plasma LCAT, thus allowing cholesterol removal from tissues. Finally, several recent cholesterol balance studies have suggested that neutral fecal steroid elimination may be enhanced following EPL treatment.

Arterial Wall Metabolism and Interaction with Plasma Lipoproteins

Significant changes in lipid metabolism of the arterial wall occur during the infusion of PL, particularly EPL. A significant reduction of lysolecithin, phosphatidylserine, and phophatidylethanolamine are detected following arterial EPL perfusion, suggesting that micelle suspensions of polar EPL in plasma may withdraw PL from the arterial wall (13). In the same experiment a significant reduction in the arterial free fatty acid biosynthesis was noted; moreover, newly synthetized free fatty acids were removed to a greater extent in the presence of EPL. A reduction, although not statistically significant, of arterial cholesteryl esters, is noted following perfusion with EPL (Fig. 2).

Arterial lipid changes may be also related to the different affinity of plasma lipoproteins for arterial wall binding factors. Low-density lipoproteins (LDL) may bind with high affinity to arterial wall polyanions (16), and the LDL-polyanion interaction may be the basic mechanism for LDL deposition in arteries (21). *In vitro* studies on LDL precipitation induced with amylopectin sulfate indicated that PL, and particularly phosphatidylinositol, may greatly inhibit complex precipitation at micromolar concentrations (18).

Lecithin-Cholesterol Acyltransterase (LCAT)

Contrasting reports, coming from clinical and experimental studies, have been provided on the changes of LCAT activity following EPL administration. Day et al. (19) in cholesterol-fed rabbits administered EPL (200 mg i.v. three times per week) showed, as expected, acute plasma cholesterol and PL increases following each treatment. Only plasma free cholesterol increased in the hypercholesterolemic animals. No variations in LCAT activity were found at the different time intervals in both acute and chronic studies. According to these authors, an increased cholesterol removal by way of plasma esterification is probably not operative in the

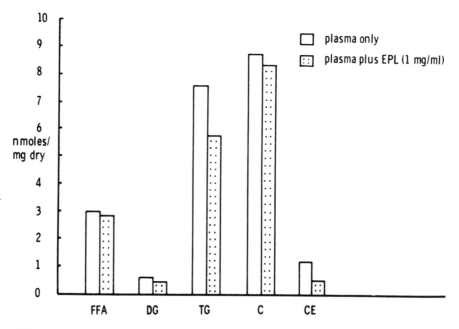

FIG. 2. Changes in aortic lipid composition following perfusion with essential phospholipids: a reduction particularly of the aortic triglyceride (TG) and cholesteryl ester (CE) content is noted. (From Bowyer and Davies ref. 13, with permission.)

rabbit model; free cholesterol may be complexed with the injected PL, thus being raised in plasma. It may be noted that in the reported study the discontinuous administration of EPL might have influenced the results.

Somewhat different findings were reported by Wallentin (49) in humans, following i.v. administration of a large EPL dose. Increase of both plasma total and HDL-PL, as well as of free cholesterol, were noted up to 4 hr from EPL administration. The LCAT rate increased approximately 30%, with this rise also lasting approximately 4 hr. The observation of an increased LCAT rate, not separating the influences of substrate and enzyme, and paralleling the increase of plasma PL, suggests that LCAT may be stimulated by the excess PL of substrate lipoproteins. These findings do not, of course, indicate the ultimate fate of newly synthetized cholesteryl esters. The reported antiatherosclerotic activity of EPL, as well as their hypolipidemic action in humans (see below), support the hypothesis that increased tissue cholesterol removal may follow their administration.

Cholesterol Balance

Data indicating that EPL may induce a significant cholesterol removal from tissues need to be substantiated by the demonstration of clear changes in the cholesterol input-output mechanisms. Cholesterol balance studies, i.e., investigations on cholesterol absorption and elimination in humans, may offer the opportunity of studying this mechanism of action of oral PL.

The effect of oral lecithin (dosage 4.5–30 g/day) was studied in normo- and hyperlipidemic patients, some of whom were also treated with clofibrate (45). In approximately half of the cases, lecithin induced some decrease (10–12%) of total cholesterolemia. Fecal steroid excretion was approximately doubled in all subjects, whether responding with a plasma cholesterol drop or not. An inconsistent effect on bile acid elimination was observed; a rise was mostly shown. The combination of lecithin with clofibrate further reduced plasma cholesterol, with variable effects on fecal steroid elimination. Clofibrate tended, in general, to raise neutral steroids, as expected from previous investigations (29). The reported findings are consistent with an increased endogenous cholesterol synthesis, accompanied by enhanced elimination. In responding patients, a reduction of cholesterolemia, and possibly of atheromatous lesions, may occur. The concomitant administration of clofibrate may favor a more significant plasma cholesterol drop.

More recently, Greten et al. (27) administered polyunsaturated lecithin (dosage 18 g/day) orally to normo- and hypercholesterolemic subjects. As in the previous study, a considerable increase in the fecal excretion of neutral steroids, and not of bile acids, was detected. Plasma cholesterol changes were minimal.

The mechanism of the increased neutral steroid elimination following EPL administration is a subject of debate. Increased cholesterol biosynthesis and, in some subjects, enhanced tissue sterol mobilization may be found. Some interesting effects on intestinal sterol absorption were recently described following infusions of EPL (150 mg/kg per hour) into the duodenum of healthy subjects, as compared to a similar administration of safflower oil (100 mg/kg per hour) (10). Cholesterol was reduced approximately 45% during EPL infusion. Significant lipoprotein changes were also detected, specifically an increase of very low-density lipoprotein (VLDL) (chylomicrons are mostly increased by the safflower oil infusion) with a lower cholesterol/triglyceride ratio than at preinfusion. These newly formed lipoproteins, most likely of gut origin, may be considered as "small chylomicrons" floating in the VLDL density range. EPL infusion may thus modulate lipoprotein biosynthesis, possibly affecting secondarily the metabolism of other lipoproteins, i.e., HDL, derived from the surface components of triglyceride-rich lipoproteins (40). By this mechanism, a mobilization of tissue cholesterol may take place together with a reduced absorption.

EPL TREATMENT IN HUMAN HYPERLIPIDEMIAS

Studies on the effects of chronic EPL treatment in hyperlipoproteinemias have been numerous [see references in Blaton et al. (11)]. The basic mechanisms of a possible lipid-lowering activity of EPL may be related to the above-quoted changes of intestinal lipoprotein secretory pattern (10) or to modifications of lipoprotein composition, favoring changes in LCAT rate (49), increasing lipoprotein turnover, and so on.

EPL may be effective on hyperlipoproteinemias characterized by excess triglycerides (a) by inhibiting carbohydrate-induced hypertriglyceridemia and (b) by stimulating lipoprotein and hepatic lipase activities. The addition of large amounts of sucrose (240 g/day) and skim milk powder to a normal diet significantly raises plasma triglyceride levels, particularly in VLDL. Concomitant administration of EPL (3 g/day) reduced the maximal triglyceride rise approximately 50% (20). An interesting rise in HDL-cholesterol levels following EPL administration was also noted. Studies on the activity of EPL on tissue lipolysis *in vitro* have shown a significant antagonism of norepinephrine-induced lipolysis in epididymal adipose tissue (48). In the same study, the i.p. injection of EPL in rats (750 mg/kg either 120 or 240 min before sacrifice) increased plasma free fatty acid levels; also in this condition, however, norepinephrine lipolysis was counteracted by EPL.

A systematic study on hyperlipidemic patients was carried out by a combined regimen of i.v. EPL given for 14 days (2 × 500 mg EPL per day), followed by 46 days of oral treatment (3 × 100 mg EPL per day) (11). A significant decrease of plasma cholesterol, and particularly of cholesteryl esters, was noted after the i.v. treatment; these changes were partially maintained after the oral regimen (Fig. 3). Interesting increases were noted in the linoleate content of plasma cholesteryl esters and PL. These findings could support the hypothesis (33) that the rate of cholesteryl ester hydrolysis is increased in the presence of polyunsaturated fatty acids, thus accelerating plasma cholesterol removal.

ORAL LECITHIN, CEREBRAL FUNCTION, AND AGING

The degeneration of acetylcholine (ACh) containing neurons and the deficiency of the choline acetyltransferase enzyme have both been described in the brains of aged subjects (12), particularly in cases with Alzheimer disease. These findings, related to regressive neuronal changes consequent to aging, have suggested that some form of replacement therapy should be administered to sustain the inadequate synthesis of the main mediator of neuronal function.

Two lines of research have been aimed at the development of treatment strategies for cerebral degeneration. One relies on drugs inhibiting ACh breakdown; the other, on the administration of choline itself or of choline-containing precursors, in particular, lecithin.

The use of drugs that affect the central cholinergic mechanisms has shown interesting effects in both primate and human experiments. Administration of scopolamine, which blocks central cholinergic mechanisms, induces an amnesia in young monkeys and humans, resembling that naturally occurring in aged subjects (8). Conversely, administration of the anticholinesterase physostigmine reduces scopolamine-induced amnesia (22). The administration of progressive doses of physostigmine in young and aged monkeys *(Macaca mulatta)* by the use of an automated device, objectively evaluating recent memory, resulted in minimal changes in memory retention in the young subjects (7). Conversely, in more than half of the aged monkeys, physostigmine administration (between 0.025 and 0.04 mg/kg) clearly showed a significant positive effect on memory. These findings suggest that the administration of agents increasing neuronal ACh content may positively affect some of the cognitive decline associated with aging; moreover, they provide, at

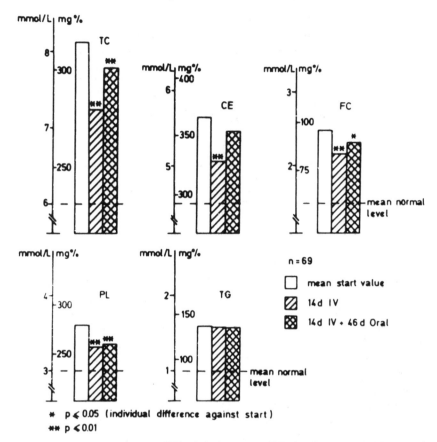

FIG. 3. Plasma total cholesterol (TC), cholesterol ester (CE), free cholesterol (FC), phospholipid (PL) and triglyceride (TG) levels in type II hyperlipoproteinemic patients treated for 14 days with i.v. essential phospholipids (EPL: 2 × 500 mg/day), followed by 46 days of oral treatment (3 × 100 mg EPL per day). (From Blaton et al. ref. 11, with permission.)

least, circumstantial evidence for an important cholinergic role in age-related memory impairment.

Phospholipid Administration and Neuronal Function

The observed deficiency of ACh in the whole brain of aged subjects or animals suggested that lecithin administration might beneficially affect brain ACh content, as well as behavioral changes related to aging. Hirsch and Wurtman (31) gave lecithin to normal rats in single or repeated oral administrations. With both types of feedings, lecithin significantly increased both brain (Table 2) and adrenal choline and ACh contents, thus showing that exogenously administered lecithin might provide a precursor for brain ACh. From this and other experimental studies, many trials have been planned in order to evaluate the efficacy of lecithin administration in patients with impaired neuronal function caused by aging or degenerative disorders (6).

TABLE 2. *Effect of lecithin administration on choline and acetylcholine (ACh) levels in rat brain*[a]

	N	Choline (nmole/g)	ACh (nmole/g)
		Exp. 1 (single meal)[b]	
Control	21	36.5 ± 2.9	21.5 ± 0.8
Lecithin	22	54.3 ± 3.8[c]	25.6 ± 1.0[c]
		Exp. 2 (3 days)	
Control	8	38.5 ± 4.6	21.5 ± 0.8
Lecithin	12	66.1 ± 7.1[d]	25.6 ± 1.0[d]

[a]Data taken from Hirsch and Wurtman (31).
[b]Lecithin dry granules were given as 50% of the dry weight of food; daily choline administration was around 220 mg/kg.
[c]$p < 0.02$.
[d]$p < 0.01$.

The administration of cholinergic drugs or diets may exert a variety of actions on the central nervous system: from increasing the turnover of striatal dopaminergic neurons to stimulating guanylate cyclase and raising cyclic guanine monophosphate (cGMP) levels in the cerebellum (35). These may result in changes in sleep habits, motor behavior, improved learning, and memory, as well as facilitative effects on mating, copulatory, and erectile behavior (38). Experimental and clinical studies have been related to the posssiblity of exerting one or more of these changes within the nervous system.

The more significant positive effects of oral lecithin have been recorded on tardive dyskinesia. This neurological disorder, characterized by abnormal, involuntary choreoathetotic movements that involve the tongue, face, extremities, and even the trunk (17), occurs typically after years of therapy with antipsychotic drugs. It may also result from degenerative brain changes owing to aging. Administration of choline (10–20 g/day) or of lecithin (50–100 g/day) significantly improves motor changes in the extremities (26). Significant effects may also be noted in the face and jaw (28). Other movement disorders positively affected by lecithin treatment are Friedreich's ataxia and, to a lesser extent, Huntington's chorea; lesser benefits are noted in Gilles de la Tourette's disease and in spastic ataxia (5).

Psychological and cognitive changes related to lecithin treatment in presenile dementia have been less extensively quantitated. It appears that some patients, following lecithin treatment (25–100 g per day in progressive doses) which raises plasma choline levels from 10.9 ± 0.6 to 38.7 ± 3.2 nmole/ml, show improvement in learning and visual retention tests (23).

These clinical observations are mostly derived from noncontrolled studies. They are, however, probably reliable in view of the very careful observation of the patients, and they clearly indicate that high doses of lecithin may be beneficial in some disorders related to degenerative brain changes. Experience with EPL administration in these cases is still limited. It appears, however, from animal studies that EPL which contains a higher percentage of choline as compared to the standard lecithin used for treatment (usually 3.7% of choline by weight), may reach the central nervous system in a higher percentage (24). EPL may thus provide a simpler way to administer the ACh precursor to patients.

REFERENCES

1. Adams, C. W. M., Bayliss, O. B., Ibrahim, M. Z.M., and Webster, M. W. Jr. (1963): Phospholipids in atherosclerosis: The modification of the cholesterol granuloma by phospholipid. *J. Pathol. Bacteriol.*, 86:431–436.
2. Adams, C. W., Abdulla, Y., Bayliss, O., and Morgan, R. S. (1967): Modifications of aortic atheroma and fatty liver in cholesterol-fed rabbits by intravenous injection of saturated and polyunsaturated lecithins. *J. Pathol. Bacteriol.*, 94:77–87.
3. Adams, C. W. M., and Morgan, R. S. (1967): The effect of saturated and polyunsaturated lecithins on the resorption of 4-^{14}C-cholesterol from subcutaneous implants. *J. Pathol. Bacteriol.*, 94:73–76.
4. Adams, C. W. M., and Abdulla, Y. H. (1972): Polyunsaturated phospholipids and experimental atherosclerosis. In: *Phospholipids, Biochemistry, Experimentation, Clinical Application*, edited by G. Schettler, pp. 44–49. Georg Thieme Verlag, Stuttgart, West Germany.
5. Barbeau, A. (1979): Lecithin in movement disorders. In: *Nutrition and the Brain*, Vol. 5, edited by A. Barbeau, J. M. Growdon, and R. J. Wurtman, pp. 263–271. Raven Press, New York.
6. Barbeau, A., Growdon, J. H., and Wurtman, R. J., eds. (1979): *Nutrition and the Brain.* Raven Press, New York.
7. Bartus, R. T. V. (1979): Physostigmine and recent memory: Effects in young and aged primates. *Science*, 206:1087–1089.
8. Bartus, R. T., and Johnson, H. R. (1976): Short term memory in the rhesus monkey: Disruption with the anticholinergic scopolamine. *Pharmacol. Biochem. Behav.*, 5:39–40.
9. Bauer, R., Servida, E., Nazarri, M. G., and Torlaschi, G. (1978): Biochemical pharmacological investigations on the antiatherogenic effects of heart phospholipids. In: *International Conference on Atherosclerosis*, edited by L. A. Carlson, R. Paoletti, C. R. Sirtori, and G. Weber, pp. 513–520. Raven Press, New York.
10. Beil, F. U., and Grundy, S. M. (1980): Studies on plasma lipoproteins during absorption of exogenous lecithin in man. *J. Lipid Res.*, 21:525–536.
11. Blaton, V., Soeteway, F., Vandanne, D., Declercq, B., and Peeters, H. (1976): Effect of polyunsaturated phosphatidylcholine on human types II and IV hyperlipoproteinemias. *Artery*, 2:309–325.
12. Bowen, D. M., White, P., Spillane, J. A., Goodhardt, M. J., Curzon, G., Iwangoff, P., Meier-Ruge, W., and Davison, A. N. (1979): Accelerated ageing and selective neuronal loss as an important cause of dementia. *Lancet*, i:11–14.
13. Bowyer, D. E., and Davies, P. F. (1976): Effect of EPL on the metabolism of lipids in the arterial wall. In: *Phosphatidylcholine*, edited by H. Peeters, pp. 160–186. Springer-Verlag, New York.
14. Byers, S. O., and Friedman, M. V. (1956): Independence of phosphatide induced hypercholesterolemia and hepatic function. *Proc. Soc. Exp. Biol. Med.*, 92:459–462.
15. Byers, S. O., and Friedman, M. V. (1960): Effect of infusions of phosphatides upon the atherosclerotic aorta *in situ* and as an ocular atherosclerotic implant. *J. Lipid Res.*, 1:343–348.
16. Camejo, G., Lopez, A., Vegas, H., and Paoli (1975): The participation of aortic proteins in the formation of complexes between low density lipoproteins and intima-media extracts. *Atherosclerosis*, 21:77–91.
17. Crane, G. E. (1968): Tardive dyskinesia in patients with major neuroleptics, a review of the literature. *Am. J. Psychiatry*, 124(Suppl.):40–54.
18. Day, C. E., and Levy, R. S. (1975): Control of the precipitation reaction between low density lipoproteins and polyions. *Artery*, 1:150–164.
19. Day, A. J., Horsch, A., and Hudson, K. (1976): Effect of polyunsaturated lecithin on serum and aortic lipids in normal and cholesterol fed rabbits. *Artery*, 2:400–422.
20. Ditschuneit, H., Klör, H-U., and Ditschuneit, H. H. (1976): Effects of essential phospholipids on the carbohydrate-induced hypertriglyceridemia. In: *Phosphatidylcholine*, edited by H. Peeters, pp. 98–114. Springer-Verlag, New York.

21. Donnelly, P. V., Di Ferrante, N., and Jackson, R. L. (1978): The interaction of human plasma glycosaminoglycans with plasma lipoproteins. II. Hemoagglutination studies. *Circ. Res.*, 43:234–238.

22. Drachman, D. A. (1977): Memory and cognition function in man: Does the cholinergic system have a specific role? *Neurology*, 27:783–790.

23. Etienne, P., Gauthier, S., Dastor, D., Collier, B., and Retner, J. (1979): Alzheimer's disease: Clinical effect of lecithin treatment. In: *Nutrition and the Brain*, Vol. 5, edited by A. Barbeau, J. M. Growdon, and R. J. Wurtman, pp. 389–396. Raven Press, New York.

24. Fox, J. M., Betzing, H., and LeKim, D. (1979): Pharmacokinetics of orally ingested phosphatidylcholine. In: *Nutrition and the Brain*, Vol. 5, edited by A. Barbeau, J. M. Growdon, and R. J. Wurtman, pp. 95–108. Raven Press, New York.

25. Friedman, M., and Byers, S. O. (1955): Role of hyperlipemia in the genesis of hypercholesterolemia. *Proc. Soc. Exp. Biol. Med.*, 90:496–499.

26. Gelenberg, A. J., Doller, J., Wojcɛκ, J., and Growdon, J. H. (1979): Lecithin for the treatment of tardive dyskinesia. In: *Nutrition and the Brain*, Vol. 5, edited by A. Barbeau, J. M. Growdon, and R. J. Wurtman, pp. 285–303. Raven Press, New York.

27. Greten, H., Raetzer, H., Stichl, A., and Schettler, G. (1980): The effect of polyunsaturated phosphatidylcholine on plasma lipids and fecal sterol excretion. *Atherosclerosis*, 36:81–88.

28. Growdon, J. H., Gelenberg, A. J., Doller, J., Hirsch, H. J., and Wurtman, R. J. (1978): Lecithin can suppress tardive dyskinesia. *N. Engl. J. Med.*, 298:1029–1030.

29. Grundy, S. M., Ahrens, E. H., Jr., and Salen, P. H. (1969): Mode of action of Atromid S' on cholesterol metabolism in men. *J. Clin. Invest.*, 48:330–340.

30. Hegner, K. (1976): Effect of essential phospholipids on the ATPases and on the fluidity of liver plasma membranes. In: *Phosphatidylcholine*, edited by H. Peeters, pp. 87–96. Springer-Verlag, New York.

31. Hirsch, M. J., and Wurtman, R. J. (1978): Lecithin consumption elevates acetylcholine concentrations in rat brain and adrenal gland. *Science*, 202:223–225.

32. Howard, A. N., Patelski, J., Bowyer, D. E., and Gresham, G. A. (1971): Atherosclerosis induced in hypercholesterolemic baboons by immunological injury, and the effects of intravenous polyunsaturated phosphatidylcholine. *Atherosclerosis*, 14:17–29.

33. Howard, A. N., and Patelski, J. (1974): Hydrolysis and synthesis of aortic cholesterol esters in atherosclerotic baboons. *Atherosclerosis*, 20:225–232.

34. Howard, A. N., and Patelski, J. (1976): Effect of EPL on the lipid metabolism of the arterial wall and other tissues. In: *Phosphatidylcholine*, edited by H. Peeters, pp. 187–200. Springer-Verlag, New York.

35. Karczmar, A. G. (1979): Overview: Cholinergic drugs and behaviour—What effects may be expected from a "Cholinergic Diet"? In: *Nutrition and the Brain*, Vol. 5, edited by A. Barbeau, J. M. Growdon, and R. J. Wurtman, pp. 141–175. Raven Press, New York.

36. Leuschener, F., Wagener, H. H., and Neumann, B. (1976): Die antihyperlipämísche und antiatherogene Wirksamkeit der "essentiellen" Phospholipide (EPL) in pharmakologischen Versuch. *Arzneim Forsch. (Drug Res.)*, 26:1743–1772.

37. Lewis, B. (1980): Dietary prevention of ischaemic heart disease—A policy for the 80's. *Br. Med. J.*, 281:177–180.

38. Lindstrom, L. H. (1973): Further studies on cholinergic behavior in the female rat. *J. Endocrinol.*, 56:275–278.

39. Papahadjopoulos, D. (1974): Cholesterol and cell membrane function: A hypothesis concerning the etiology of atherosclerosis. *J. Theor. Biol.*, 43:329–337.

40. Patsch, J. R., Gotto, A. M., Jr., Olivecrona, T., and Eisenberg, S. (1978): Formation of high density lipoprotein-like particles during lipolysis of very low density lipoproteins. *Proc. Natl. Acad. Sci. USA*, 75:4519–4523.

41. Peeters, H. (1976): The biological significance of plasma phospholipids. In: *Phosphatidylcholine*, edited by H. Peeters, pp. 10–33. Springer-Verlag, New York.

42. Samochowiec, L. (1976): On the action of essential phospholipids in experimental atherosclerosis. In: *Phosphatidylcholine*, edited by H. Peeters, pp. 211–226. Springer-Verlag, New York.

43. Samochowiec, L., Kadlubowska, D., and Rozewicka, L. (1976): Investigations in experimental atherosclerosis. I. The effects of phosphatidylcholine (EPL) on experimental atherosclerosis in white rats. *Atherosclerosis*, 23:305–317.

44. Samochowiec, L., Kadlubowska, D., Rozewicka, L., Kuzma, W., and Szyszka, K. (1976): Investigations in experimental atherosclerosis. II. The effect of phosphatidylcholine (EPL) on experimental atherosclerotic changes in miniature pigs. *Atherosclerosis*, 23:319–331.

45. Simons, L. A. (1978): The effect of oral lecithin and clofibrate on cholesterol metabolism. *Artery*, 4:167–182.
46. Sirtori, C. R., Catapano, A., Ghiselli, G. C., Innocenti, A. L., and Rodriguez, J. (1977): Metformin: An anti-atherosclerotic agent modifying very low density lipoproteins in rabbits. *Atherosclerosis*, 26:79–89.
47. Stafford, W. W., and Day, C. E. (1975): Regression of atherosclerosis effected by intravenous phospholipid. *Artery*, 1:106–114.
48. Szyszka, K. (1976): Influence of EPL on lipolysis *in vitro* and *in vivo*. In: *Phosphatidylcholine*, edited by H. Peeters, pp. 115–124. Springer-Verlag, New York.
49. Wallentin, L. (1977): Influence of intravenous and oral administration of phospholipids on lecithin: cholesteryl acyl transfer rate in plasma. *Artery*, 3:40–51.

Phospholipids and Atherosclerosis, edited by
P. Avogaro, M. Mancini, G. Ricci, and
R. Paoletti. Raven Press, New York © 1983.

Phospholipids in Human Atherosclerosis

Pietro Avogaro

Regional General Hospital, Venice, Italy

Phospholipids are universal cellular components. They are essential for the structure and function of biologic membranes although they do not represent a major energy source. Membrane phospholipids show a bilayer structure with their hydrophilic groups exposed to the aqueous environment of the cells and the hydrophobic group oriented toward the interior face of the bilayer. The specific functions of phospholipids are not clearly understood. Present knowledge however stresses a relevant role for phospholipids in various enzyme membrane systems. Their role has been established for the cytochrome oxidase reaction (14), and beta-hydroxybutyrate dehydrogenase, Na^+,K^+-ATPase (11) and adenyl cyclase (4). Phosphatidylcholine (PC) plays an important role in the activation of both lipoprotein-lipase and lecithin-cholesterol acyltransferase (LCAT) activity (8). As the other major plasma lipids, the phospholipids are constituents of plasma lipoproteins. Free cholesterol, proteins, and phospholipids are components of the lipoprotein surface; esterified cholesterol and triglycerides are components of the core.

Phospholipid (PL) and protein are major components of high-density lipoprotein (HDL) ($d < 1.063$). PL is able to reassociate with apoprotein, and seems necessary for the binding by the apoprotein of cholesteryl esters and triglycerides.

Studies performed through microcalorimetry and gradient ultracentrifugation have shown that within the native HDL, apo A-I and apo A-II are associated, at least in the presence of lipids, and that the binding of PL to these peptides is strongly cooperative (8). Binding of phospholipids to either apo A-I, apo A-II, or to a mixture of both, is not a random process but is determined by the apoprotein structure (8). Recently, it has been stressed that lysophosphatidylcholine is an important factor in determining the egress of cholesterol from cultured human skin fibroblasts (12). Lysophosphatidylcholine accounts for 55 to 60% of all phospholipids of $d > 1.25$ infranate; it is bound to albumin and to a lipoprotein having pre-alpha mobility. Although incubation of ^{3}H-cholesterol-enriched fibroblasts with delipidated albumin resulted in a limited efflux of cholesterol from the cells, the efflux could be doubled in presence of lyso-PC. Cholesterol egress can be further enhanced by addition of 1 pM apo A-I and the effect observed is more than additive (12). As apo A-I binds lipids readily only in monomeric form, it seems possible that lyso-PC, which forms stable complexes with apo A-I, could enhance cholesterol release by inhibiting polymer formation of the dissociate apoprotein (12). When the effect of the fatty acid chain length of the lyso-PC was compared, it could be seen that the capacity for cholesterol removal increases markedly with the chain length of the fatty acid above C_{14} (12).

PLs are accumulated together with cholesterol and cholesteryl esters in the arterial plaque; the PL from the arterial lesion has a greater content of saturated fatty acids than the PL in the plasma. During the development of the arterial plaque there is a relative increase in the content of sphingomyelin (SM) while PC and phosphatidylethanolamine (PE) decrease (6). This is especially true for microsomal membranes and for the cell membrane of smooth-muscle cells (9,10).

It has been postulated that the initial net increase in the arterial concentration of PL rich in saturated fatty acids may be the real early step in atherogenesis (5). The increase in content of saturated fatty acyl groups in the smooth-muscle cell membrane can decrease the fluidity of the membrane and interfere with membrane-associated enzymes and functions. To restore the membrane fluidity and to keep constant the sphingomyelin/cholesterol ratio of the cell membrane, more cholesterol

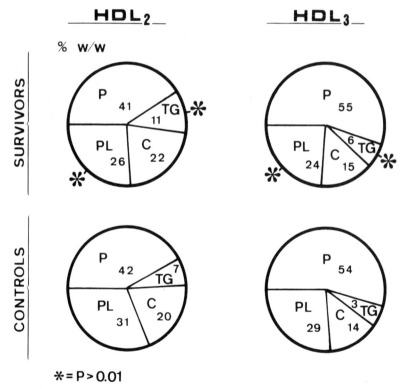

FIG. 1. Chemical percentage composition of high-density lipoproteins HDL₂ and HDL₃ in survivors of myocardial infarction and in controls. Phospholipid (PL) decreases significantly and triglyceride (TG) increases. C, cholesterol; P protein. *$p > 0.01$.

would be required. In this "alternative hypothesis" for plaque formation, cholesterol accumulation appears, therefore, as a secondary phenomenon (5).

PLs are a major component of plasma lipids and lipoproteins. In man, the cholesterol/phospholipid (C/PL) ratio is around 0.8 in normal patients, slightly above 1.0 in type II hyperlipoproteinemia and low or nearly normal in type IV hyperlipoproteinemia (8). Sphingomyelin/phosphatidylcholine (SM/PC) ratio is 0.25 in normals, 0.32 in type IIA, 0.30 in type IIB, and 0.20 in type IV (8). Mills et al. (7) noted that the lecithin/sphingomyelin ratio is abnormally low in familial hypercholesterolemia homozygotes. LDL of patients affected by FH show an increased ratio of C/PL and a decreased lecithin/sphingomyelin ratio (6). Since this abnormal composition of LDL returns to normal following plasma exchange, it has been suggested that the abnormal composition of LDL in FH is due to hypocatabolism and then to the aging of LDL (6). The chemical percentage composition has been studied in the major lipoprotein classes in survivors of myocardial infarction and in controls (1). In both HDL_2 and HDL_3 a significant decrease of PL and protein has been recorded with a triglyceride (TG) increase (Fig. 1). The chemical composition of a narrow segment of ultracentrifugally obtained LDL ($d = 1.040–1.050$) has been analyzed from survivors of myocardial infarction and from controls (Table 1). The LDL of survivors are characterized by a higher content of TG and apo B, and by a lower content of PL. From these studies it appears, therefore, that the decrease in PL content is an important feature of the deranged structure of lipoproteins in patients with clinical atherosclerosis. Despite this relevant information concerning the deep involvement of PL in lipid homeostasis, in cellular life, and in atherogenesis, little attention has been paid to the therapeutical effects of PL. The main contribution comes from Blaton et al. (2). In this study a large cohort of subjects presenting type II and type IV hyperlipoproteinemia were given 1,000 mg polyunsaturated PC intravenously for 14 days and then 1,800 mg/day for 106 days. A significant decrease of both cholesterol and PL was recorded while a slight increase of TG was observed. The C/PL ratio and the esterified to free cholesterol

TABLE 1. *Chemical composition of low-density lipoprotein (d = 1.040–1.050)[a]*

	LDL (mg/dl)	C (%)	TG (%)	PL (%)	P (%)	apo B (%)	apo B/P ratio
Controls	283.0	40.0	12.2	24.0	23.8	20.4	0.86
	66.2	2.6	0.8	1.1	0.9	0.4	0.03
MI survivors	361.0	39.8	16.9[b]	17.1[c]	26.2[b]	24.5[c]	0.93[c]
	56.3	4.7	4.3	0.5	1.2	0.7	0.02

[a]LDL = low-density lipoprotein; C = cholesterol; TG = triglyceride; PL = phospholipid; P, protein; MI = myocardial infarction.
[b]$p < 0.05$.
[c]$p < 0.01$.

ratio remained unchanged; however, the C/PL ratio increased in alpha-lipoprotein and decreased in beta-lipoprotein. The prolonged therapy was particularly characterized by a decrease of plasma saturated and monounsaturated fatty acids, especially cholesterol palmitate and oleate, and an increase of cholesterol linoleate. The daily oral administration of lecithin linoleate (1,700 mg) to five patients with hypertriglyceridemia caused (a) an increase of alpha-cholesterol, (b) an increase in the linoleic content of alpha-phosphoglycerides, and (c) a decrease of triglycerides (13). It has been suggested that the beneficial effect of linoleic acid and lecithin linoleate might be mediated through an increase of alpha-lipoprotein lecithin linoleic acid, a substrate for LCAT reaction.

REFERENCES

1. Avogaro, P., Cazzolato, G., Bittolo Bon, G., and Belussi, F. (1979): Levels and chemical composition of HDL$_2$, HDL$_3$ and other major lipoprotein classes in survivors of myocardial infarction. *Artery*, 5:495.
2. Blaton, V., Deqlercq, B, Vandamme, D., Soetewey, F., and Peeters, H. (1976): The human plasma lipids and lipoprotein under influence of EPL-therapy. In: *Phosphatidylcholine*, edited by H. Peeters, p. 125. Springer-Verlag, Berlin.
3. Böttcher, C. J. F., and Van Gent, C. M. (1961): Change in the composition of phospholipids and of phospholipid fatty acids associated with atherosclerosis in the human aortic wall. *J. Atheroscler. Res.*, 1:36–46.
4. Goldman, S. S., and Albers, R. W. (1973): Sodium potassium activated adenosine triphosphatase. IX. The role of phospholipids. *J. Biol. Chem.*, 248:867–874.
5. Jackson, R. L., and Gotto, A. M., Jr. (1974): Phospholipids in biology and medicine. *N. Engl. J. Med.*, 290:24–29, 87–93.
6. Jadhav, A. V., and Thompson, G. R. (1979): Reversible abnormalities of low density lipoprotein composition in familial hyper cholesterolaemia. *Eur. J. Clin. Invest.*, 9:63–67.
7. Mills, G. L., Taylaur, C. E., and Chapman, M. J. (1976): Low density lipoproteins in patients homozygous for familial hyperbetalipoproteinaemia. *Clin. Sci. Mol. Med.*, 51:221–231.
8. Peeters, H. (1976): The biological significance of the plasma phospholipids. In: *Phosphatidylcholine*, edited by H. Peeters, p. 10. Springer-Verlag, Berlin.
9. Portman, O. W. (1969): Atherosclerosis in nonhuman primates: sequences and possible mechanisms of change in phospholipid composition and metabolism. *Ann. N.Y. Acad. Sci.*, 162:120–136.
10. Portman, O. W., Alexander, M., and Maruffo, C. A. (1967): Composition of subcellular constituents of aortic intima plus inner media isolated by differential and density gradient centrifugation. *Arch. Biochem. Biophys.*, 122:344–353.
11. Sekuzu, I., Jurtshuk, P., Jr., and Green, D. E. (1963): Studies on the electron transfer system. LI: isolation and characterization of the D-( )-B-hydroxybutyric apodehydrogenase from beef heart mitochondria. *J. Biol. Chem.*, 238:975–982.
12. Stein, O., Fainaru, M., and Stein, Y. (1979): The role of lysophosphatidylcholine and apolipoprotein A-I in the cholesterol-removing capacity of lipoprotein-deficient serum in tissue culture. *Biochim. Biophys. Acta*, 574:495–504.
13. Svanberg, U., Gustafson, A., and Ohlson, R. (1974): Polyunsaturated fatty acids in hyperlipoproteinemia. II. Administration of essential phospholipids in hypertriglyceridemia. *Nutr. Metabol.*, 17:338–246.
14. Zahler, W. L., and Flescher, S. (1971): Kinetic studies of the lipid requirement of mitochondrial cytochrome C oxidase. *J. Bioenerg.*, 2:209–215.

Phospholipids and Atherosclerosis, edited by
P. Avogaro, M. Mancini, G. Ricci, and
R. Paoletti. Raven Press, New York © 1983.

Phospholipids and Platelets: A Second Link Between Lipoprotein Disorders and Atherosclerosis

Jürgen Schneider

Department of Internal Medicine, Philipps-University, 355 Marburg, West Germany

Exogenous risk factors in atherogenesis have been evaluated in the past decades with hyperlipoproteinemia, hypertension, inhalative cigarette smoking, and diabetes being identified as the major and primary ones in human atherogenesis. Hyperlipoproteinemia (HLP) has played a predominant role and this chapter will present only this factor.

The underlying theoretical base of the lipid hypothesis was affirmed in the 1950s and 1960s, mainly in long-term follow-up studies. The consecutive considerations had to be preventive or therapeutical ones. Thus the combined risk factor model of atherogenesis as well as interventive approaches are the substantial content of what is called "lipid hypothesis" in this chapter. Most approaches against atherosclerosis and dependent disorders have attempted to eliminate these risk factors with equivocal results. In particular, lipid-lowering drug treatment has been subject to severe contradiction. Besides poor adherence some other processes may have contributed to such failings. One of them is a certain independence from the initial promoters of atherogenesis during a process which takes decades. A further progression then reaches a still unknown degree of disease where the process becomes self-dynamic and independent of the pertinence of HLP.

The "lipid hypothesis" in the sense used here is a general formula and does not include furthergoing pathogenetical assumptions, although it is often referred to in connection with the lipid infiltration mechanism. Altered filtration of plasma lipoproteins within the vessel wall, metabolic changes in enzymatic equipment of vessel walls, and changes in platelet behavior and plasmatic coagulation may play important roles in a still unknown sequence, or in parallel. Uncertainty in this area is demonstrated by some recent findings. Preventive studies using clofibrate have shown beneficial effects irrespective of significant changes in total cholesterol or triglyceride levels. This points out the importance of other supplementary antiatherogenic effects of the drug, attributable to effects on coagulation and thrombogenesis.

This chapter's focus is on the platelet's role in the relationship between HLP and atherosclerosis. In some regards the reaction of the vessel wall as the second part of a balanced system needs to be included, mainly in a discussion of the prostaglandin system.

PHOSPHOLIPIDS IN LIPOPROTEINS

At the end of a decade which had seen the detection of a high-affinity low-density lipoprotein (LDL) cholesterol receptor, the elucidation of catabolic processes within the plasma lipoproteins, and considerable progress in the knowledge about structure and function of the apoproteins, the phospholipid moiety had lost a great deal of its scientific attractiveness. On the other hand, the phospholipids in the plasma are essential parts of the different lipoprotein classes and may contribute in a significant amount to pathomechanisms which arise from hyper- or dyslipoproteinemic conditions and lead to premature or clinically significant atherosclerosis. One of these probable mechanisms is the ability of phospholipids to (re)combine with cholesterol. The knowledge of an antiatherogenic predictive value of the lipoprotein class with the highest phospholipid content, the alpha-lipoprotein, has had a tremendous renaissance in the past decade.

The content of phospholipids (PL) in total plasma and in lipoprotein subclasses is often expressed in relation to the accompanying cholesterol concentration (C/PL). The total C/PL ratio in normolipemic subjects is about 0.8. In hypercholesterolemia the total PL content varies to a much lower degree than the C/PL ratio, reflecting increases in cholesterol with relatively stable phospholipid content. In hypertriglyceridemia the total C/PL ratio is usually unaltered. A comprehensive study on phospholipids in human lipoproteins and hyperlipoproteinemia has been performed by Peeters (39). In that study total phospholipid content and C/PL ratios were observed. The results showed that total phospholipids do not differ significantly between different types of HLP, but that the C/PL ratio is increased in all hypercholesterolemic types.

The accessibility of different phospholipids as well as special fatty acid patterns in phospholipids for the action of (phospho)lipases is not entirely understood at present. This makes speculation impossible on the primary functional role of the distribution of different phospholipids and different fatty acid patterns in phospholipids in the lipoprotein subclasses. The main phospholipids in human plasma are phosphatidylcholine (PC) and sphingomyelin (SM). Their distribution varies widely between different lipoprotein density classes: the SM/PC ratio is 0.38 in low-density lipoprotein (LDL) and 0.15 in high-density lipoprotein (HDL); both were derived from normolipemic subjects. HDL contains the highest percentage of PL. High total PL/C ratios, suggested to be an antiatherogenic indicator 30 years ago, may reflect a relatively high HDL content in modern terminology (46). One reason why this has been neglected may be methodological difficulties. Phospholipid measurements are not applicable to large-scale specimens of epidemiological studies. The observation of a relative increase in total phospholipids in octo- and nonagenarians without clinical manifestation of vascular diseases has not been affirmed by others but is explained by the HDL-cholesterol values found in such patients (48,49).

With regard to the platelet as a linkage between dys- and hyperlipoproteinemia and atherogenesis, the phospholipids in normal subjects and in those with HLP should be examined in detail to determine (a) if they can alter platelet behavior by exchange between lipoproteins and platelets and (b) if they can provide precursors for thrombogenic and antithrombogenic compounds or induce a dysequilibrium between them. A major difficulty is to provide platelets from hyper- or dyslipoproteinemic patients without thromboembolic or atherosclerotic disorders which may influence the sensitivity of platelets, i.e., to isolate platelets influenced by the lipoprotein abnormality alone.

PLATELETS IN NORMAL STATE AND IN HLP

One of the links between different forms of HLP and atherogenesis, proven in experimental as well as practical medicine, is the hyperaggregability of platelets. Recent results in prostaglandin research have revitalized this idea. The promoting effects of beta-lipoproteins on platelet aggregation and adhesiveness were early recognized by Fabriszewski and co-workers (15,16).

Platelets of patients with type IIa HLP are more sensitive to aggregating agents than those of normolipoproteinemics (9,58). Since early in this century the crucial role of PL in the conversion of prothrombin to thrombin is a well-known fact (10,30). The platelet lipid composition in the normal state was studied extensively by Douste-Blazy et al. (13). They found a cholesterol/phospholipid ratio in platelet membranes of 0.53. Furthermore, a high thrombotic tendency in experimental animals has been shown to be related to an increase in the saturated + monounsaturated/polyunsaturated fatty acid ratio in platelets, as observed in patients recovering from acute myocardial infarction (44). The crucial role of linoleic acid was recently affirmed in dietary experiments in rats (29).

Three mechanisms have been discussed to explain the changes of platelet reactivity in hypercholesterolemia:

1. Changes in the platelet membrane composition leading to altered fluidity and reactibility,
2. Coating of platelet surface area by excess lipoproteins, and
3. Variations in the supply of precursors for the synthesis of thromboactive substances (prostaglandins).

Nordoy and Rodset (37) found an increased phospholipid content in hypercholesterolemic patients with unchanged fatty acid pattern. This increase was not affected by effective cholesterol lowering with diet or drug treatment despite the sophisticated methods applied. On the other hand, the platelet dysfunction observed in hyper β-lipoproteinemia was normalized after treatment (37). Miettinen (31) found only weak correlations between platelet cholesterol content and the levels of total plasma cholesterol in normocholesterolemic and obviously low degree hypercholesterolemic patients without giving data of the related phospholipid content. In β-lipoprotei-nemia and in lecithin-cholesterol acetyltransferase (LCAT) deficiency, conditions with very low plasma cholesterol values, no alteration in cholesterol content in platelets was found (12,34). As was pointed out earlier, ratios of C/PL may be more important than absolute values of one component, and data covering only one of these fractions may provide false conclusions. The observations by Nordoy and Rodset (37) confirmed this.

At the present time two conclusions can be drawn. The environment exerts effects on the platelet function even without altering their biochemical composition. However, it cannot be excluded that the linking biochemical changes are in a range within the accuracy of the methods applied.

Under in vitro conditions platelets are highly susceptible to their cholesterol and phospholipid environment. An enrichment of the medium by cholesterol-rich liposomes (C/PL ratio = 2.2) resulted in an excess cholesterol content of +39.2% with a 35-fold increase in sensitivity to epinephrine-induced aggregation and a 15-fold increase in ADP-induced aggregation (54). In vivo the free cholesterol compound can be exchanged only, with less than 1% of platelet cholesterol being esterified. The comparably modest biochemical changes seen in platelets derived from hyper-β-lipoproteinemic patients can be explained by the much lower imbalance in the C/PL ratios of lipoproteins referred to earlier. In view of this the experiments of Shattil and co-workers (54) demonstrate the principle of susceptibility, but their artificial experiments do not reflect situations within the (patho)physiological range. In a recent study (55) elevated C/PL ratios in platelets were accompanied by increased sensitivity to agonists [adenosine diphosphate (ADP), epinephrine] and were followed by increased aggregation and secretion. This increased sensitivity to epinephrine is not due to a change in either the number or the affinity of epinephrine receptors (21). Furthermore, it should be kept in mind that the trigger mechanism of the release reaction is the minimal hydrolysis of phospholipids near or at the active site of receptor on the platelet surface. It has been shown that phospholipase A and Ca^{2+} are necessary, with phosphatidyl choline being a better substrate than sphingomyelin (47).

The structure of the phospholipids in the platelet membranes is of great importance for their role in coagulation (platelet factor 3). It explains why the same amount of extracted phospholipids as that of phospholipids that are part of intact platelet vesicles give extremely different answers in clotting time measurements (27). As the platelet is highly organized to react on surface properties, minimal alterations in the platelet membrane itself can modify the reaction to a considerable amount. One of the main determinants of membrane fluidity is the C/PL ratio. So far, the discussion on the relationship between lipoproteins and platelets has been confined to the quantitative aspects of cholesterol and phospholipid contents. However, it is well known that functional changes occur when membrane properties change following alterations in fatty acid patterns of membrane constituents.

In most investigations of platelet lipids and platelet function, hypercholesterolemia was the model preferred. Less is known about the influence of elevated levels of very low-density lipoproteins (VLDL) on these parameters. An actual decrease in platelet adhesiveness in hyper-pre-β-lipoproteinemia induced by carbohydrate-rich diets was observed and explained by partial coating of the platelets (23). In patients with different types of HLP Schneider et al. found higher spontaneous aggregability. In these patients atherosclerosis in an asymptomatic degree could not be excluded. In some of these patients with persistent HLP of types IV and IIb, high degrees of spontaneous aggregation could be demonstrated irrespective of the total cholesterol or β-lipoprotein concentration (50).

Even if the assumption is right that increased platelet aggregability may act in later phases of the atherogenic process, i.e., in the presence of altered endothelium, difficulties in the experimental design of human *in vivo* studies may occur in the way that make early lesions difficult to detect. Therefore, the vascular condition may be the real but hidden reason for changes in the thrombogenic potential of platelets and clotting factors. Increased platelet activity has been observed in hyper- or dyslipoproteinemia as well as after dietetic or other modifications in the system. However, since the practical importance of this activity seems not to depend on time or clinical degree of atherosclerosis, antiatherogenic approaches in this field seem to lack primary preventive character. The first and second mechanisms listed earlier have been dealt with up to this point. The discussion of the third one, which will follow, concerns the inner vessel wall.

The transformation of cyclic endoperoxides into compounds with thrombogenic and antithrombogenic properties seems to be one important factor in the relation between dietary fats, HLP, and atherosclerosis, but it is not the whole story for significant progress in understanding prostaglandins has been made in other areas. It was demonstrated that the conversion of cyclic endoperoxides to TXA_2 is not a prerequisite for induction of platelet aggregation and vasoconstricting effects are not associated with platelet-aggregating properties (41). Arachidonic acid has been of interest in recent years because it serves as a direct precursor for cyclization and oxidation. Arachidonic acid is one of the most abundant fatty acids in platelet membranes, granules, and soluble fractions; the bulk is esterified in PL and only traces exist free (26). Also, the availability of arachidonic acid for cyclooxygenation is greatly facilitated when the acid is being released from phospholipids (57). The arachidonic acid content in different platelet phospholipids was studied with un-equivocal results in different species of animals. It seems to be concentrated in phosphatidylethanolamine and phosphatidylinositol and underrepresented in the main phospholipid, phosphatidylcholine (3,5,26). The major hydrolyzing enzyme phos-pholipase A_2 is a constituent of the platelet, and its activity is markedly increased by thrombin (3).

Under the action of thrombin, arachidonic acid is released from platelet surface phospholipids. Liberation of arachidonic acid under the influence of thrombin takes place from distinct phospholipids, altering the distribution of the acid before and after release (24). Finally, the release of arachidonic acid by thrombin is greater from intact platelets than from prepared membranes (40). All these findings suggest that arachidonic acid, esterified in distinct phospholipids at distinct sites of the platelet surface, is an extremely susceptible substrate for thrombin-activated phospholipase to provide cyclic endoperoxides and thromboxanes, important mediators of secondary hemostasis. It has been argued that arachidonic acid, as well as cyclic endoperoxides released from platelets, could be transformed into $PG-I_2$ (prostacyclin) in the intima of blood vessels; however, the results of Needleman and co-workers rule out this possibility (33).

The significant influence of hypercholesterolemia was affirmed in studies on prostaglandin metabolism of platelets. The production of TXB_2 from labeled arachidonic acid was found increased in platelets that were derived from hypercholesterolemic patients (2,56).

DIETARY MODIFICATIONS

Modifications have been mentioned only indirectly when pathological situations of platelet function and prostaglandin metabolism were discussed in connection with HLP; the dietetic treatment of HLP includes modification of such situations. Dietary modifications will be discussed here in a more generalized view, irrespective of the existence or improvement of HLP. Two observations mark the wide range of relationships between dietary fatty acids and coagulation/thrombosis. The first one is the observation of Burr and Burr in 1929 (6) and in 1930 (7) that a depletion in linoleic acid leads to deficiency diseases and that the most common cause of death in such animals was hemorrhage and hemorrhagic renal necrosis. (Essential fatty acids have been linked with coagulation and platelets since the first studies.) The second may be the recent reports of Dyerberg and co-workers on Eskimos. These will be referred to in detail after the following discussion of the effects of acute fat ingestion on platelets and coagulation.

Various investigators have demonstrated that experimental modifications in total fat intake and in the fatty acid pattern of food fat influence platelet function and platelet-dependent (platelet factor 3 dependent) coagulation in man. Over all, long-chain saturated fatty acids and large amounts of food fat directed the platelet function toward a higher susceptibility to, or higher degrees of, spontaneous aggregation (20,22,36,38). Acute effects of large fat meals on heparin-thrombin clotting time have been observed with different results when ingesting saturated or highly unsaturated fat: saturated fatty acids shortened and unsaturated fatty acids prolonged the heparin-thrombin clotting time (38). Antithrombin clotting time and radial immunodiffusional determinations of antithrombin III after ingestion of saturated or unsaturated fat showed similar changes (38). Comparable observations in animals are numerous: in dogs (11), rabbits (28), rats (18,19,35,42,43), and pigs (32).

This effect of fat ingestion was mediated by a change in the fatty acid pattern of platelet phospholipids (17,44). Therefore, as Renaud et al. pointed out, at least in human subjects with rather normal serum cholesterol concentrations, the main link between premature and severe atherosclerotic complications might not be their actual lipoprotein content but dietetically altered platelet behavior (45). Indeed, those authors were able to show that some populations at high or low risk of coronary heart disease (CHD) differ significantly in their food fat ingestion, as well as platelet function and platelet factor 3 release, irrespective of their total HDL-cholesterol serum levels. Modifications in fat consumption in otherwise free-living farmers for 1 year affirmed this concept. Unfortunately, the effects of the one year long experiment with increased supply of unsaturated fatty acids on total and lipoprotein cholesterol contents are not given in their most recent paper (45). In that report, it was pointed out that in a pilot study two areas of Scotland with high and low incidence of CHD differed in fat consumption as well as in platelet function. However, the mean HDL-cholesterol values of 62.5 and 65.9 mg/dl, declared as similar, may reach significant difference in the range of many other epidemiologic studies when the number of participants is increased from the 43 studied at the time of first publication.

As stated earlier, the link between dietary and platelet changes are the platelet phospholipids with plasma lipoproteins being involved, at least as a temporary transport system. Until now, it has been unclear whether the density subclasses develop different rates of phospholipid exchange with platelets and whether HDL with its high content of phospholipids has a corresponding role in this transfer. Additional differences in the action on the functional system of vessel wall and platelets have been found among highly unsaturated fatty acids themselves.

Dyerberg and Bang (14), studied the content of eicosatetraenoic (arachidonic) and eicosapentaenoic acid in Eskimos and Danes. All members of the eicosa-acid family are substrates of cycloxygenase. Their fates are different. All can be transformed (in the vessel wall) to prostacyclins (PG-I$_2$ and -I$_3$) which dilate blood vessels and prevent platelet aggregation to similar degrees. However, when being transformed to thromboxanes (within the platelet), only TXA$_2$, the derivative of arachidonic acid, is a potent aggregating compound; TXA$_3$ has been found to be rather ineffective (41). An increase in nutritional supply and tissue storage of eicosatrienoic and eicosapentaenoic acid at the cost of arachidonic acid would result in a predominance of antiaggregating products.

The findings of Dyerberg and Bang (14) of increased levels of eicosapentaenoic acid in eskimo seafood nutrients and plasma lipid fractions as well as their findings of a parallel low incidence of coronary heart disease and delayed atherosclerosis culminate in the conclusion of increased bleeding times because of impaired secondary hemostasis. Their findings and interpretation is persuasive for it provides a basis for future practical use. In every case their work is a splendid demonstration of the possibility to intervene in an important mechanism of atherogenesis by external (dietetic) modification, and thus by a relatively simple method.

POLYUNSATURATED PHOSPHATIDYLCHOLINE

Polyunsaturated phosphatidylcholine (PUPC), a natural product from soybean oil, has aroused the interest of many investigators especially since it has been shown that considerable amounts of the molecule were rediscovered in plasma after oral intake (25). Experimental research with PUPC in isolated cells has been performed mainly in erythrocytes and observations on the effects of PUPC in biological membranes were done in red blood cells as well (52). PUPC has also been tried in patients with HLP and normal or abnormal platelet function. The method used was to measure the spontaneous aggregation by microscopy of platelet-rich plasma after rotation. This method has been developed and standardized by Breddin (4) (Fig. 1). Significant decreases in platelet aggregation have been found mainly in cases with increased initial values after an oral intake of 3.0 g/day of PUPC after 8 weeks. This result persisted for the whole time of the study with a mean duration of 3.5 months. No changes in the parameters of a standard check of coagulation were observed (50) (Table 1). In a second study in which 1.8 g of PUPC were used in combination with 1.2 g of clofibrate, a significant difference from clofibrate alone was not obtained, which can be explained by the lower dose, a superposition of clofibrate effects, or both (51,53).

As mentioned before, a significant reduction in plasma cholesterol and phospholipids by nicotinic acid and clofibrate treatment was disappointing with respect to a normalization of the phospholipid content of platelets, but not to normalized platelet factor 3 activity and availability (37). The antiaggregating properties of PUPC were affirmed by Cafiero and co-workers (8).

The effect of PUPC on platelet aggregation, particularly in cases with spontaneously increased aggregability, seems to be dependent on the plasma concentrations achieved, as was shown for lyso-forms of the same compound (1). It is obvious as

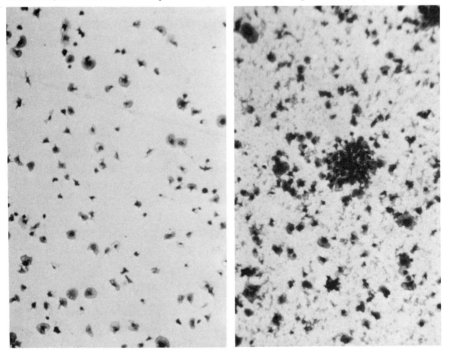

FIG. 1. Degrees of spontaneous platelet aggregation (PAT I). **Left:** degree 1. **Right:** degree 3.

TABLE 1. *PAT I values in hyperlipoproteinemia before and during oral treatment with 3 g/day of polyunsaturated phosphatidylcholine*

Time	N	PAT ± SEM	α
Initial	12	2.79 ± 0.45	
4 wk	11	3.32 ± 0.78	7.3
8 wk	11	1.68 ± 0.40	0.0
End (mean/15 wk)	10	1.75 ± 0.49	0.0

Significant for $\alpha < 5$ (Mann-Whitney test).

well that the specific fatty acid pattern in the 1- and 2-positions of this compound contributes to the effects observed which cannot be explained by the absolute amounts of $C_{18:2}$ and $C_{18:3}$ fatty acids given per day, which are small compared to experiments with dietary modifications.

To conclude, studies on phospholipids have been stimulated by recent advances in prostaglandin research, which has allowed more conclusive interpretations. It seems necessary in order to perform further work in the prevention of atherosclerosis to keep two areas in mind: lipoprotein alterations and, by no means less important, platelet and intima changes in biochemical, structural, and functional aspects.

REFERENCES

1. Besterman, E. M. M., and Gillett, M. P. T. (1972): A comparison of the effects of saturated and polyunsaturated lysolecithin fractions on platelet aggregation and erythrocyte sedimentation. *Atherosclerosis*, 16:89–94.
2. Bizios, R., Wong, L. K., Vallaincourt, R., Lees, R. S., and Carvalho, A. C. (1977): Platelet prostaglandin peroxides formation in hyperlipidemias. *Thromb. Haemostasis*, 38:228.
3. Blackwell, G. J., Duncombe, W. G., Flower, R. J., Parsons, M. F., and Vane, J. R. (1977): The distribution and metabolism of arachidonic acid in rabbit platelets during aggregation and its modification by drugs. *Br. J. Pharmacol.*, 59:353–366.
4. Breddin, K. (1968): Experimental and clinical investigations on the adhesion and aggregation of human platelets. In: *Platelets in Hemostasis Experimental Biology and Medicine*, edited by E. Hagen, W. Wechsler, and S. Zilliken, p. 14. Karger, Basel, New York.
5. Broekman, M. J., Handin, R. I. Derksen, A., and Cohen, P. (1976): Distribution of phospholipids, fatty acids, and platelet factor 3 activity among subcellular fractions of human platelets. *Blood*, 47:963–971.
6. Burr, G. O., and Burr, M. M. (1929): A new deficiency disease produced by the rigid exclusion of fat from the diet. *J. Biol. Chem.*, 82:345–367.
7. Burr, G. O., and Burr, M. M. (1930): On the nature and role of the fatty acids essential in nutrition. *J. Biol. Chem.*, 86:587–621.
8. Cafiero, M., Buono, G., Rocca, G., and Sensale, P. (1975): Klinischer Beitrag zur Wirksamkeit zweier Pharmaka mit aggregationshemmender Wirkung auf Thrombozyten. *Clin. Ter.*, 72:563–576.
9. Carvalho, A. C. A., Colman, R. W., and Lees, R. S. (1974): Platelet function in hyperlipoproteinemia. *N. Engl. J. Med.*, 290:434–438.
10. Chargaff, E. (1944): The thromboplastic activity of tissue phosphatides. *J. Biol. Chem.*, 155:387–399.
11. Connor, W. E., Hoak, J. C., and Warner, E. D. (1965): The effects of fatty acids on blood coagulation and thrombosis. *Thromb. Diath. Haemorrh.*, 13:89–96.

12. Cooper, R. A., and Guldbransen, C. L. (1970): Lecithin: cholesterol acyl transferase (LCAT) deficiency in abetalipoproteinemia. *Blood*, 36:840(Abstr.).
13. Douste-Blazy, L., Chap, H., and Gautheron, P. (1973/4): Platelet lipid composition. *Haemostasis*, 2:85–91.
14. Dyerberg, J., and Bang, H. O. (1979): Lipid metabolism, atherogenesis, and haemostasis in eskimos: The role of the prostaglandin-3-family. *Haemostasis*, 8:227–233.
15. Fabriszewski, R., and Worowski, K. (1968): Enhancement of platelet aggregation and adhesiveness by betalipoprotein. *J. Atheroscler. Res.*, 8:988–995.
16. Fabriszewski, R., and Worowski, K. (1969): The effect of modified β-lipoproteins on adhesiveness and on aggregation of blood platelets. *J. Atheroscl. Res.*, 9:339–344.
17. Gautheron, P., and Renaud, S. (1972): Hyperlipemia induced hypercoagulable state in rat. Role of an increased activity of platelet phosphatidyl serine in response to certain dietary fatty acids. *Thromb. Res.*, 1:353–359.
18. Hartroft, W. S. (1958): Abnormal fat transport. *Diabetes*, 7:221–227.
19. Hornstra, G. (1974): Dietary fats and arterial thrombosis. *Haemostasis*, 2:21–30.
20. Hornstra, G., and Vendelmans-Starrenburg (1973): Induction of experimental occlusive thrombi in rats. *Atherosclerosis*, 17:369–375.
21. Insel, P. A., Nirenberg, P., Turnbull, J., and Shattil, S. J. (1978): Relationship between membrane cholesterol, α-adrenergic receptors, and platelet function. *Biochemistry*, 17:5269–5274.
22. Iacono, J. M., Binder, R. A., Marschall, M. W., Schoeme, N. W., Jencks, J. A., and Mackin, J. F. (1975): Decreased susceptibility to thrombin and collagen platelet aggregation in man fed a low fat diet. *Haemostasis*, 3:306–318.
23. Korsan-Bengtson, K., Gustavsson, A., Sjöström, L., and Bjorntorp, P. (1972): Effect of carbohydrate feeding on blood coagulation, fibrinolysis and platelet adhesiveness. Relation to serum lipids and lipoproteins. *Thromb. Res.*, 114:407–413.
24. Lapetina, E. G., Schmitges, C. J., Chandrabose, K., and Cuatrecasas, P. (1977): Cyclic adenosine 3',5'-monophosphate and prostacyclin inhibit membrane phospholipase activity in platelets. *Biochem. Biophys. Res. Commun.*, 76:828–835.
25. LeKim, D. (1976): On the pharmacokinetics of orally applied essential phospholipids (EPL). In: *Phosphatidylcholine*, edited by H. Peeters, pp. 48–65. Springer-Verlag, Berlin.
26. Marcus, A. J., Ullmann, H. L., and Safier, L. B. (1969): Lipid composition of subcellular particles of human blood platelets. *J. Lipid Res.*, 10:108–114.
27. Marcus, A. J., Zucker-Franklin, D., Safier, L. B., and Ullmann, H. L. (1966): Studies on human platelet granules and membranes. *J. Clin. Invest.*, 45:14–28.
28. Mathues, J. K., Wolff, C. E., Cevallos, W. H., and Holmes, W. L. (1968): Platelet adhesiveness and thrombosis in rabbits on an atherogenic diet. *Med. Exp.*, 18:121–127.
29. McGregor, L., Morazain, R., and Renaud, S. (1980): Effect of dietary linoleic acid on platelet function in the rat. *Thromb. Res.*, 20:499–507.
30. McLean, J. (1917): The relation between the thromboplastic action of cephalin and its degree of unsaturation. *Am. J. Physiol.*, 43:586–596.
31. Miettinen, T. A. (1974): Hyperlipoproteinemia relation to platelet lipids, platelet function and tendency to thrombosis. *Thromb. Res.*, 4:41–47.
32. Mustard, J. F., Rowsell, H. C., Murphy, E. A., and Downie, H. G. (1963): Diet and thrombus formation: Quantitative studies using an extracorporeal circulation in pigs. *J. Clin. Invest.*, 42:1783–1789.
33. Needleman, P., Wyche, A., and Raz, A. (1979): Platelet and blood vessel arachidonate metabolism and interaction. *J. Clin. Invest.*, 63:345–349.
34. Nordoy, A., and Gjone, E. (1971): Familial plasma lecithin: cholesterol acyltransferase deficiency. A study of the platelets. *Scand. J. Clin. Lab. Invest.*, 27:263–268.
35. Nordoy, A., Hamlin, J. T., Chandler, A. B., and Vewland, H. (1968): The influence of dietary fats on plasma and platelet lipids and ADP induced platelet thrombosis in the rat. *Scand. J. Haemat.*, 5:458–473.
36. Nordoy, A., and Rodset, J. M. (1971): The influence of dietary fats on platelets in man. *Acta Med. Scand.*, 190:27–34.
37. Nordoy, A., and Rodset, J. M. (1971); Platelet function and platelet phospholipids in patients with hyperbetalipoproteinemia. *Acta Med. Scand.*, 189:385–389.
38. O'Brien, J. R., Etherington, M. D., and Jamieson, S. (1976): Acute platelet changes after large meals of saturated and unsaturated fats. *Lancet*, i:878–880.

39. Peeters, H. (1976): The biological significance of plasma phospholipids. In: *Phosphatidylcholine*, edited by H. Peeters, pp. 10–33. Springer, Berlin.

40. Pickett, W. C., Jesse, R. L., and Cohen, P. (1976): Trypsin-induced phospholipase activity in human platelets. *Biochem. J.*, 160:405–408.

41. Raz, A., Minkes, M. S., and Needleman, P. (1977): Endoperoxides and thromboxanes: structural determinants for platelet aggregation and vasoconstriction. *Biochim. Biophys. Acta*, 488:305–311.

42. Renaud, S. (1969): Thrombotic, atherosclerotic and lipemic effects of dietary fats in the rat. *Angiology*, 20:657.

43. Renaud, S. (1968): Thrombogenicity and atherogenicity of dietary fatty acids in rats. *J. Atheroscler. Res.*, 8:625–630.

44. Renaud, S., Kuba, K., Goulet, C., Lemire, Y., and Allard, C. (1970): Relationship between fatty-acid composition of platelets and platelet aggregation in rat and man. Relation to thrombosis. *Circ. Res.*, 26:552–559.

45. Renaud, S., Morazain, R., McGregor, L., and Baudier, F. (1979): Dietary fats and platelet functions in relation to atherosclerosis and coronary heart disease. *Hemostasis*, 8:234–251.

46. Schettler, G. (1961): *Arteriosklerose Ätiologie, Pathologie, Klinik und Therapie*. Thieme, Stuttgart, West Germany.

47. Schick, P. K., and Yu, B. B. (1974): The role of platelet membrane phospholipids in the platelet release reaction. *J. Clin. Invest.*, 54:1032–1039.

48. Schneider, J. (1980): High-density lipoproteins and peripheral vascular disease in octo- and nonagenarians. *J. Am. Geriatr. Soc.*, 28:215–219.

49. Schneider, J., Boldt, J., Leyhe, A., and Kaffarnik, H. (1980): HDL cholesterol, peripheral and coronary vascular disease in high age groups. *Atherosclerosis*, 35:487–489.

50. Schneider, J., Fuchs, G., Mühlfellner, G., and Kaffarnik, H. (1975): Der Einfluss von hochungesättigtem Phosphatidylcholin auf Gerinnung und Thrombozytenaggregation bei verschiedenen Hyperlipoproteinämien. *Folia Angiol.*, 6:230–235.

51. Schneider, J., Fuchs, G., Kaffarnik, H., Schubotz, R., Hausmann, L., Mühlfellner, G., Mühlfellner, O., and Zöfel, P. (1977): Serum lipids and lipoproteins, blood coagulation and platelets during a double-blind trial of clofibrate/clofibrate-EPL in hyperlipoproteinemia. In: *Atherosclerosis*, Vol. 4, edited by G. Schettler, Y. Goto, Y. Hata, and G. Klose, p. 557. Springer-Verlag, Berlin.

52. Schneider, J., Goebel, K. M., and Schubotz, R. (1978): Modification of red cell membrane phospholipids by phosphatidylcholine-rich serum dispersions. Abstract from the 12th FEBS meeting, Dresden.

53. Schneider, J., Müller, R., Buberl, W., Kaffarnik, H., Schubotz, R., Hausmann, L., Mühlfellner, G., and Mühlfellner, O. (1979): Effect of polyenyl phosphatidyl choline on clofibrate-induced increase in LDL cholesterol. *Eur. J. Clin. Pharmacol.*, 15:15–19.

54. Shattil, S. J., Anaya-Galindo, R., Bennett, J., Colman, R. W., and Cooper, R. A. (1975): Platelet hypersensitivity induced by cholesterol incorporation. *J. Clin. Invest.*, 55:636–643.

55. Stuart, M. J., Gerrard, J. M., and White, J. G. (1980): Effect of cholesterol on production of thromboxane B_2 Bz by platelets in vitro. *N. Engl. J. Med.*, 302:6–10.

56. Tremoli, E., Folco, G., Agradi, E., and Galli, C. (1979): Platelet thromboxanes and serum cholesterol. *Lancet*, i:107–108.

57. Vonkeman, H., and van Dorp, D. A. (1968): The action of prostaglandin synthetase on 2-arachidonyl-lecithin. *Biochim. Biophys. Acta*, 164:430–432.

58. Zakari, J., Betteridge, J. D., Jones, N. A. G., Gatton, D. J., and Kakkar, V. V. (1981): Enhanced in vivo platelet release reaction and malonyldialdehyde formation in patients with hyperlipidemia. *Am. J. Med.*, 70:59–64.

Phospholipids and Atherosclerosis, edited by
P. Avogaro, M. Mancini, G. Ricci, and
R. Paoletti. Raven Press, New York © 1983.

Altered Pulmonary Function in Hyperlipidemias

G. Enzi, A. Baritussio, R. Carraro, L. Bellina,
L. Favaretto, and E. Monico

*Department of Internal Medicine, Division of Gerontology and Metabolic Diseases,
University of Padua, Italy*

Several studies in animal models and in man demonstrate the possible influence of circulating lipids on pulmonary functions.

First in 1957, Kuo et al. (10) reported the observation of a decrease in arterial oxygen tension in dogs rendered hyperlipidemics by infusion of fat emulsions. A further study by the same authors (11) in humans confirmed a derangement in pulmonary gas exchange in primary hyperlipemias that was responsible for decreased oxygen tension in arterial blood. Joiner et al. (8) observed that in patients with severe coronary artery disease, hyperlipemia following a large fat meal precipitated attacks of angina pectoris, which were relieved by intravenous injection of heparin. The heparin-induced changes of plasma turbidity were followed by an increase in the skin oxygen tension without significant changes in blood flow.

Further indications of a relationship between elevated levels of circulating lipids and disturbances in pulmonary function in normal man emerge from the observations of Greene et al. (6). The infusion of fat in normal man causes a decrease in pulmonary membrane diffusion, relieved after heparin administration as a consequence of the clearing effect on plasma lipids.

Furthermore, a decrease in pulmonary diffusing capacity for carbon monoxide during lipid infusion in normal subjects was demonstrated by Sundström et al. (14). An i.v. infusion of a soybean oil emulsion induced a decrease in pulmonary diffusing capacity for carbon monoxide and an increase in alveolar-arteriolar difference in oxygen tension. The effects of lipemia on arterial oxygen tension have been enhanced by exposure to (simulated) high altitudes (13).

In order to explain these findings, several hypotheses have been advanced. Functional and histopathological studies have shown that the lung participates in the removal of lipid particles from the blood stream (4). Fat embolism could be the basis of altered lung function in hyperlipidemias. However, although fat globules were present in the lung capillaries after fat infusion, there is no evidence of fat microembolism in human hyperlipidemias. An alteration in microvascular rheology

TABLE 1. *Plasma triglycerides (TG), diffusing capacity*
for carbon monoxide (DLCO), arterial oxygen tension in
hyperlipidemic type IV patients (mean ± SEM)[a]

	Age	TG (mg/dl)	DLCO (ml/min/mm Hg)	PO$_2$ (mm Hg)
Controls	41	84	21.0	90.3
(N = 15)	±4.0	±28	±2.0	±1
Type IV	39.5	1960[c]	14.8[b]	80.7[c]
(N = 10)	±3	±547	±1.0	±3

[a]Statistical analysis carried out using the Student's *t*-test: [b]$p < 0.05$. [c]$p < 0.01$.

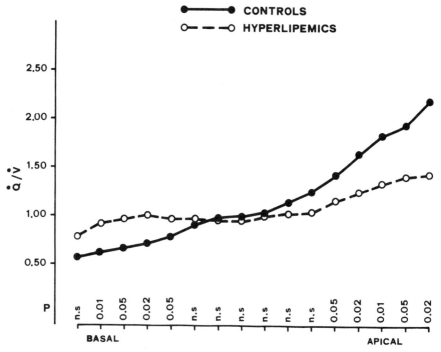

FIG. 1. Distribution of the ventilation/perfusion ratios (V̇/Q̇) in hyperlipemic patients and in controls, studied with xenon 133. (From Enzi et al., ref. 3, with permission.)

at the pulmonary level can be expected when the number of lipoproteic particles in plasma are elevated. By using the pancreas chamber technique, Kroeger et al. (9) were able to demonstrate in rabbits a reduction in the corpuscular blood flow following an intravenous injection of cottonseed-oil emulsion. Alterations in the erythrocyte-membrane lipid composition can be another possible cause of reduced oxygen tension in arterial blood (1). Recent observations demonstrate an effect of insulin on phospholipids and cholesterol subcellular fractions in rat lungs, suggesting direct influences of circulating hormones, namely insulin, on tensioactive lipoprotein synthesis and turnover (7).

Moving from these observations, a study was planned in order to evaluate the lung function in hyperlipidemic patients and to elucidate the mechanisms responsible for altered gas exchange in primary hyperlipidemias in man and in diet-induced hyperlipidemias in the rat. The results are presented in this chapter.

HUMAN HYPERLIPIDEMIAS

A previous study on the carbon monoxide diffusing capacity in hyperlipidemic patients (12) demonstrated alterations in pulmonary gas exchange that were related to the plasma triglyceride levels. Therefore, in selected groups of hyperlipidemic patients, nonsmokers without a history of pulmonary diseases, carbon monoxide diffusing capacity (DLCO), arterial blood gases at rest and during exercise, and the distribution of the ventilation/perfusion ratio ($\dot{V}/\dot{Q}$) using xenon 133 were analyzed.

Patients with Fredrickson's type IV hyperlipidemia were found to have significantly lower DLCO values than controls (Table 1). Furthermore, a negative correlation existed between DLCO and plasma triglyceride values; the DLCO and plasma cholesterol values did not correlate. Insulin levels in hyperlipemic patients were significantly higher than in controls, but no relation was found between DLCO or arterial oxygen tension (PO_2) values and plasma insulin levels. These patients had a significant reduction in PO_2 (Table 1) that became normal after exercise. In hyperlipemic patients the ventilation appeared normally distributed, increasing from the bases toward the apex of the lung, but the distribution of the regional perfusion was abnormal. As shown in Fig. 1, $\dot{V}/\dot{Q}$ ratio progressively increased from the basal to the apical segments of the lungs. The reduced DLCO, the loss of $\dot{V}/\dot{Q}$ gradients, and the reduced PO_2 which normalize after exercise, suggest an alveolar maldistribution, improved by exercise-induced deep breathing.

The possible hematological effects of constantly lower PO_2 levels in hyperlipemic patients were then evaluated on 36 type IV subjects, compared to 40 presumably healthy, normolipemic subjects; nonsmoker subjects without signs of pulmonary or cardiovascular diseases were admitted to the study. As shown in Table 2, significantly lower mean values of PO_2, corrected by exercise, were confirmed in hyperlipemic patients when compared to the controls. In the same patients, significantly higher values of red blood cell (RBC) counts, hemoglobin, hematocrit, and red cell volumes were found (Table 2). The possible relationship between the increase in RBC counts and the decrease in arterial oxygen tension was then evaluated by means of regression analysis. For this study, a further selection was made, excluding patients with a daily alcohol intake over 100 ml. In this group of 29 patients, in which a reduction in PO_2 was confirmed, no correlations emerged between the values of PO_2 and the values of RBC counts, hemoglobin, and hematocrit.

TABLE 2. Total cholesterol (TC), triglycerides (TG), red blood cell count (RBC), hemoglobin (Hg), hematocrit (Ht), diffusing capacity for carbon monoxide (DLCO), and arterial oxygen tension (Po_2) before and after exercise in hyperlipidemic type IV patients (mean ± SEM)[a]

	Age (yr)	TC (mg/dl)	TG (mg/dl)	RBC (× 10⁶)	Hb (g/liter)	Ht (%)	DLCO (ml/min/mm Hg)	Po_2 (mm Hg)	
								Before exercise	After exercise
Controls	42.8 ±1.8	192 ±12.8	82 ±40	4.55 ±0.07	13.40 ±0.2	40.6 ±0.8	19.8 ±1.6	90.3 ±1.0	91.1 ±1.2
Type IV	43.5 ±1.7	263[d] ±10.0	483[d] ±49	4.83[d] ±0.07	14.40[c] ±0.2	43.0[b] ±0.7	15.1[c] ±1.0	77.4[d] ±2.5	90.4 ±1.2

[a]Statistical analysis carried out using the Student's t test: [b]$p < 0.05$, [c]$p < 0.01$, [d]$p < 0.001$.

TABLE 3. *Body weight, lung wet weight, and circulating levels of glucose, glycerol, cholesterol, triglycerides, free fatty acids, and insulin in controls and treated rats*[a]

	Control diet (N = 15)	Glycerol-rich diet (N = 15)	Hydrogenated coconut oil/cholesterol/ saccharose-rich diet (N = 15)
Body weight (g)	289 ± 12	326[b] ± 11	357[c] ± 6
Lung weight (g)	1.48 ± 0.09	1.53 ± 0.08	1.45 ± 0.09
Glucose (mg/100 ml)	118 ± 12	182 ± 30	169[c] ± 6
Glycerol (μM/liter)	44 ± 5	69[b] ± 9	36 ± 6
Cholesterol (mg/100 ml)	67 ± 6	60 ± 5	188[b] ± 20
Triglyceride (mg/100 ml)	63 ± 6	285[c] ± 33	150[c] ± 22
FFA (μEq/liter)	230 ± 29	522[c] ± 70	567[c] ± 65
IRI (μU/ml)	61 ± 12	78 ± 13	92 ± 15

[a]Values expressed as mean ± SEM. FFA, free fatty acid; IRI, immunoreactive insulin.
[b]$p < 0.05$ (treated vs control).
[c]$p < 0.01$ (treated vs control).

From all these observations, an alteration in gas exchange, related to elevated levels of circulating triglycerides, was presumed. Capillary obstructions by fat or rheological changes in pulmonary microcirculation seem to represent the more conventional explanation of this finding. Nevertheless, the observation that in hyperlipemic patients PO_2 rises above normal values after exercise is not consistent with the hypothesis of a restricted pulmonary microcirculation and suggests an alveolar maldistribution, which improves by deep breathing. The alterations in gas exchange in hyperlipidemic patients, reported above, could be fully explained by modifications in the alveolar surfactant activity, which is responsible for alterations in the elastic properties of the lung. To verify this hypothesis, the elastic properties of the lungs and the composition of the alveolar wash were studied in rats rendered hyperlipemic by suitable diet.

DIET-INDUCED HYPERLIPIDEMIAS IN RATS

Preliminary studies (2) demonstrated that rats rendered hyperlipidemic by a diet rich in glycerol display an increase in lung distensibility and a higher index of alveolar stability, and that these modifications are related to changes in the properties of the alveolar surfactant. However, it is unclear if these observations were due to changes in the absolute amount of surfactant present in the alveoli or to changes in its composition.

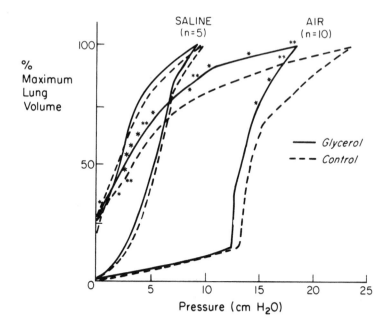

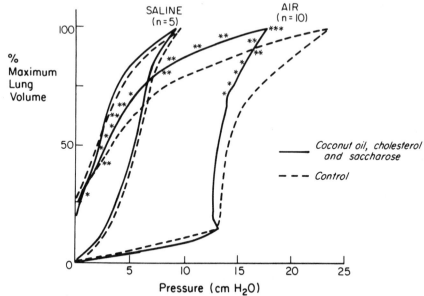

FIG. 2. Pressure/volume curves obtained by inflating isolated lungs of control and treated rats with air or with saline. The parentheses indicate the number of experiments. Statistical analysis (Student's *t*-test) was performed by comparing, at corresponding values of volume, the airway pressure recorded in controls versus that recorded in treated rats. *$p < 0.05$, **$p < 0.01$, ***$p < 0.001$ (treated vs control). (From Baritussio et al., *Metabolism*, 29:503–510, 1980, with permission.)

TABLE 4. *Phospholipid composition of lung wash in control and treated rats[a]*

Phospholipid	Control diet (N = 15)	Glycerol-rich diet (N = 15)	Hydrogenated coconut oil/cholesterol/ saccharose-rich diet (N = 15)
bis-(Monoacylglycerol) phosphate	2.0 ± 0.3	1.8 ± 0.5	1.7 ± 0.3
Phosphatidylglycerol phosphate	Trace	Trace	Trace
Phosphatidylglycerol	7.8 ± 0.7	11.7 ± 0.5[b]	11.8 ± 0.7[b]
Phosphatidylethanolamine	3.1 ± 0.5	1.3 ± 0.3[c]	1.7 ± 0.4[d]
Phosphatidylcholine	80.7 ± 1.4	78.9 ± 1.6	80.2 ± 2.0
Sphingomyelin	2.8 ± 0.5	4.7 ± 0.9	3.4 ± 1.6
Lysophosphatidylcholine	2.9 ± 0.7	1.3 ± 0.5	1.3 ± 0.5

[a]Values are expressed as mean ± SEM.
[b]$p < 0.001$ (treated vs control), [c]$p < 0.01$ (treated vs control), [d]$p < 0.05$ (treated vs control).

In order to answer this question, the present authors studied, in rats with diet-induced hyperlipidemia, the pressure/volume relationship in isolated lungs, the amount of phospholipid composition of surfactant present in the alveolar spaces, and the fatty acid composition of alveolar phosphatidylcholine, which is thought to play the most important role in lowering surface tension (5). A hyperlipidemic state was induced by feeding a group of rats with a diet rich in glycerol for one month. A second group was fed with a diet rich in glycerol, cholesterol, and coconut oil. The first group had an increase of the serum levels of glycerol, triglycerides, and free fatty acids (FFA). The second group had an increase of the serum levels of glucose, cholesterol, triglyceride, and FFA (Table 3).

Isolated lungs of rats from both groups displayed an increased distensibility at maximal inflation with air and a higher degree of alveolar stability during deflation (Fig. 2). These alterations were seen only when the lungs were inflated with air. A conclusion is that they are related to some modifications of the properties of alveolar surfactant.

Lung lavage fluid obtained from hyperlipidemic rats revealed an increase in the percent content of phosphatidylglycerol and a decrease of phosphatidylethanolamine; the levels of total and saturated (not shown) phosphatidylcholine did not show significant changes (Table 4). The percentage of phosphatidylglycerol correlates with the circulating levels of FFA (Fig. 3) but the circulating levels of glucose, glycerol, triglyceride, cholesterol, and immunoreactive insulin (IRI) do not correlate with the phospholipid composition of lung lavage (3). The FFA might affect the activity of enzymes operating in lung phospholipid synthesis, and the reported increase in surfactant phosphatidylglycerol might explain the increment of alveolar stability observed in hyperlipidemic rats.

In conclusion, an increase in lung distensibility and a higher degree of alveolar stability was demonstrated in diet-induced hyperlipemic rats. The increase in alveolar stability was related to the higher levels of alveolar phosphatidilglycerol, which in turn relates to the levels of circulating FFA. So far, it is not possible to

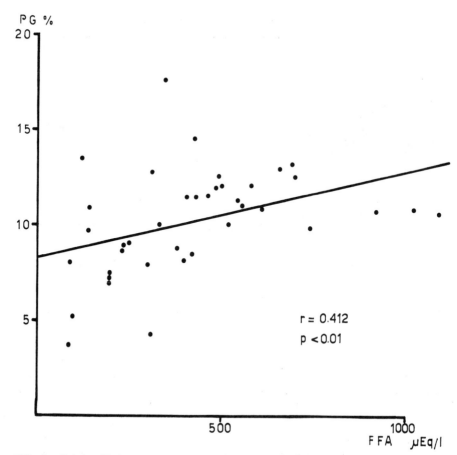

FIG. 3. Relationship between circulating levels of free fatty acids (μEq/liter) and percent content of phosphatidylglycerol in lung wash. (From Baritussio et al., *Metabolism* 29:503–510, 1980, with permission.)

say if changes in lung distensibility, as observed in hyperlipemic rats, play a role in the pathogenesis of the respiratory disturbances observed in human hyperlipidemias.

REFERENCES

1. Bagdade, J. D., and Ways, P. O. (1970): Erythrocyte membrane lipid composition in exogenous and endogenous hypertriglyceridemia. *J. Lab. Med.*, 75:53–61.
2. Baritussio, A., Enzi, G., Schiavon, M., De Biasi, F., Allegra, L., and Inelmen, E. M. (1978): Elastic properties of the lung in hyperlipoproteinemias. In: *Diabetes, Obesity, Hyperlipidemias*, edited by G. Crepaldi, P. Lefébvre, K. G. M. M. Alberti. pp. 325–329. Academic Press, London.
3. Enzi, G., Bevilacqua, M., and Crepaldi, G. (1976): Disturbances in pulmonary gaseous exchange in primary hyperlipoproteinemias. *Bull. Eur. Physiopathol. Respir.*, 12:433–442.
4. Gigon, P., von Enderlin, F., and Scheidegger, S. (1966): Über das Schicksal infundierter. *Schweiz. Med. Wochenschr.*, 96:71–75.
5. Goerke, J. (1974): Lung surfactant. *Biochem. Biophys. Acta*, 344:241–261.

6. Greene, H. L., Hazlett, D., and Demeree, R. (1976): Relationship between intralipid-induced hyperlipemia and pulmonary function. *Am. J. Clin. Nutr.*, 29:127–135.
7. Hadjiivanova, N., Koumanou, K., Mincheva, R., Dimitrov, G., and Georgiev, G. (1981): Insulin effect on lung subcellular fraction phospholipids and cholesterol. *Bull. Eur. Physiopathol. Respir.*, 17:53–64.
8. Joiner, C. R., Horwitz, O., and Williams, P. G. (1960): The effect of lipaemia upon tissue oxygen tension in man. *Circulation*, 22:901–907.
9. Kroeger, A., Heisig, N., and Hardes, H. (1970): Rheologische Aspekte der Blutströmung in Capillaren bei lipämie. *Klin. Wochenschr.*, 48:723–728.
10. Kuo, P. T., Whereat, A. F., Altman, A. A. (1957): Effects of intravenous fat infusion on the blood oxygen exchange and coronary. *Circulation*, 16:902 (Abstr.).
11. Kuo, P. T., Whereat, A. F., and Horwitz, O. (1959): The effect of lipaemia upon coronary and peripheral arterial circulation in patients with essential hyperlipaemia. *Am. J. Med.*, 26:68–75.
12. Reggiani, A., Crepaldi, G., Enzi, G., and Avogaro, P. (1968): Comportement du transfert du CO dans les hyperlipémies essentielles. *Bull. Eur. Physiopathol. Respir.*, 4:833–837.
13. Stutman, L. J., Kriewaldt, F. H., Doerr, V., and George, M. (1959): Effect of lipemia on arterial oxygen at high altitude. *J. Appl. Physiol.*, 34:894–896.
14. Sundström, G., Zauner, C. V., and Arborelius, M., Jr. (1973): Decrease in pulmonary diffusing capacity during lipid infusion in healthy man. *J. Appl. Physiol.*, 34:816–820.

Phospholipids and Atherosclerosis, edited by
P. Avogaro, M. Mancini, G. Ricci, and
R. Paoletti. Raven Press, New York © 1983.

Relationship Between Linoleic Acid Intake, Plasma Phospholipids, and Prostaglandin Formation in Man[1]

Olaf Adam, Günther Wolfram, and Nepomuk Zöllner

*Forschergruppe Ernährung, Medizinische Poliklinik der Universität München,
West Germany*

Linoleic acid is an abundant, essential fatty acid in human nutrition. Its dietary supply influences plasma lipid levels—well known to lower those of plasma cholesterol, triglycerides, and phospholipids. The lipid-lowering effect of linoleic acid is most pronounced in low-density lipoproteins (LDL). LDL are formed by the degradation of triglyceride-rich lipoproteins, transporting triglycerides formed in the liver. Hence, LDL provide for the transport of cholesterol and phospholipid to peripheral cells (11,28,29). High-density lipoproteins (HDL) are rich in phospholipids and cholesterylesters (32,51). HDL originate as discoidal particles from the liver (23). They take up lipids (and apoproteins) from peripheral tissues and transport them to the liver (6,23,30,33). Linoleic acid intake, by lowering plasma lipoprotein levels, may diminish the capacity of the plasma for fatty acid transport to and from peripheral cells. Moreover, linoleic acid has a variety of cellular effects, e.g., on the fluidity of membranes, the activity of membrane-bound and fatty acid metabolizing enzymes. Membrane fluidity tends to be lower with the incorporation of polyunsaturated fatty acids and higher with saturated fatty acids (7). The activity of lecithin-cholesterol acyltransferase (LCAT) is decreased by linoleic acid intake (18), but an increase is found for Na^+-,K^+-ATPase. In animals ingestion of linoleic acid decreases the activity of desaturating enzymes (24,42). As a consequence the more desaturated fatty acids, derived from linoleic acid, occur at a lower concentration. Furthermore, a dose-dependent inhibition on prostaglandin synthesis by linoleic and linolenic acid *in vitro* has been reported (41). From this data a very complex interrelationship between linoleic acid intake and prostaglandin formation might be expected in man.

Linoleic and α-linolenic acid are, after chain elongation and desaturation, precursors of prostaglandins (Fig. 1). Availability of precursor substances is a limiting

[1]Supported by a grant from the Deutsche Forschungsgemeinschaft.

237

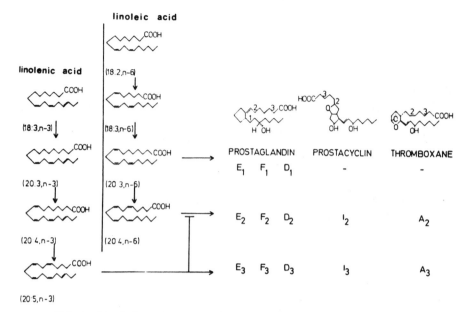

FIG. 1. Metabolism of linoleic and linolenic acid and prostaglandin formation.

factor for prostaglandin synthesis. This observation has been made for arachidonic (45) and dihomo-γ-linolenic acid (39) *in vitro* (13), in isolated perfused organs (35), and *in vivo* in animal (10) and man (45). The concentration of linoleic acid in the lipids of plasma and membranes is determined by the daily intake. Yet, linoleic acid concentration differs in certain tissues and, especially concerning prostaglandin formation, little is known about the meaning of these differences.

Prostaglandins are not stored in particular compartments of the body, but have to be synthesized when and where required. They are formed in microsomes, and so far more than 20 different metabolites of polyunsaturated fatty acids are known, leading to a wide spectrum of effects and cellular functions. Their inactivation within from 3 to 5 min, mostly by pulmonary transit, comprises dehydration, reduction, β- and ω-hydroxylation, and excretion with the urine (Fig. 2). Many different breakdown products of prostaglandin metabolism have been identified in urine, but knowledge about their origin and the reason of their variety is very limited. For turnover studies, therefore, a wide spectrum of prostaglandin metabolites has to be measured. Recently, methods have been developed to transform many prostaglandin metabolites into one joint derivative, tetranorprostanedioic acid (TNPDA), thus allowing studies on prostaglandin formation.

According to the investigations of the last 10 years prostaglandins seem to be involved in many fundamental responses of cells like thrombocytes, leukocytes, endothelial cells, in organs like the lung, intestinum, spleen, and in the genitourinary tract. Yet their clinical importance is still far from being understood, and little is known about the daily need of prostaglandins. Information about daily prostaglandin formation and its variation by linoleic acid intake would provide a better understanding of the physiological role of essential fatty acids in human nutrition.

URINARY METABOLITES OF PROSTAGLANDINS

E AND F IN MAN

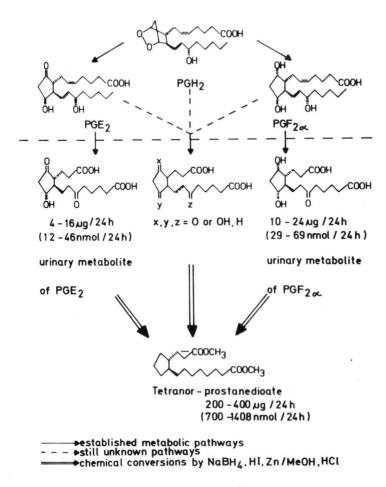

FIG. 2. Biosynthesis of prostaglandins from endoperoxides (PG-H$_2$), their degradation to main urinary metabolites, and the chemical conversion of the different polar metabolites into stable tetranorprostanedioic acid.

To study the effects of linoleic acid intake on phospholipid concentration and prostaglandin formation a constant linoleic acid supply was mandatory. Therefore, the present authors performed nutrition experiments with formula diets, allowing a constant and defined linoleic acid supply. In detail, the effect of linoleic acid intake was investigated on the

1. Phospholipid concentration in the plasma and HDL;
2. Concentration of phospholipid fractions in plasma, VLDL, LDL, and HDL;
3. Fatty acid composition of lecithin and cholesteryl esters in plasma, LDL, and HDL;

4. Prostaglandin biosynthesis; and
5. Fatty acid composition and aggregation tendency of platelets.

INFLUENCE OF LINOLEIC ACID INTAKE ON PLASMA PHOSPHOLIPID CONCENTRATIONS

Phospholipids, and especially lecithin, are the precursor pool from which phospholipase A_2 liberates essential fatty acids, mostly arachidonic acid, for prostaglandin synthesis. Cell cultures and cultures using isolated organs revealed an exchange of fatty acids and phospholipids between tissues and lipoproteins (11,28). The metabolic pathway by which linoleic acid lowers plasma phospholipid levels is not understood. Reports in the literature indicate that by ingestion of a diet rich in polyunsaturated fatty acids the ratio of cholesterol/phospholipids is not changed (49). Grundy (21) showed that an increased dietary supply of polyunsaturated fatty acids augmented sterol excretion with the bile. This was confirmed by the results of Redinger et al. (43) and Wood et al. (52). Phospholipid excretion with the bile also increases with linoleic acid intake (43). Until now, it had not been fully established if the metabolic effect of linoleic acid on both plasma lipids is similar.

Adam et al. investigated the effect of different dietary fats on the plasma levels of cholesterol, phospholipids, and phospholipid fractions (2). Total fat amounted to 25, 33, or 36% of energy intake with formula diets, and cholesterol intake was 0.6 g/day. With each amount of fat the composition of the fat was varied to give p/s ratios (ratio of polyunsaturated/saturated fatty acids) of 0.3, 0.3, or 1.8. The composition of fat and formula diets is given in Fig. 3. Each concentration of fat was given to healthy volunteers for 6 weeks and every 2 weeks the composition of fat was changed. Two persons started with one of the three fat compositions and changed after 2 weeks to the next. After 6 weeks every person had been on each composition of fat for 2 weeks.

The results given in Table 1 demonstrate determinations at the end of the 2-week periods. The expected similarity in the changes of cholesterol and phospholipid values was found, expressed by the fairly constant ratio of these two plasma lipids. The separation and quantitation of phospholipid fractions by tubular thin-layer

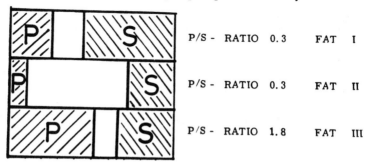

FIG. 3. Composition of formula diets providing a fat supply of 25, 33, or 36% of the energy intake. With each fat supply the same three variations of fat composition (I, II, and III) were given for 2 weeks each.

TABLE 1. *Ratios of plasma cholesterol and total phospholipids or lecithin in six healthy experimental subjects on liquid formula diets providing a fat supply of 25, 33 and 36% of the energy intake*[a]

	Conventional diet	Formula diets		
		I	II	III
p/s ratio	0.3	0.3	0.3	1.8
Fat intake (% energy)	40	25	25	25
Cholesterol/phospholipids	0.98	1.00	0.95	0.99
Cholesterol/lecithin	1.31	1.35	1.25	1.35
Fat intake (% energy)	40	33	33	33
Cholesterol/phospholipids	1.00	0.92	0.91	0.89
Cholesterol/lecithin	1.26	1.21	1.16	1.18
Fat intake (% energy)	40	36	36	36
Cholesterol/phospholipids	0.89	0.87	0.90	0.89
Cholesterol/lecithin	1.20	1.18	1.23	1.22

[a]The variation of the fat composition (p/s ratio: 0.3, 0.3, and 1.8) was the same with each formula diet. The given values are determinations at the end of 2-week formula diet periods.

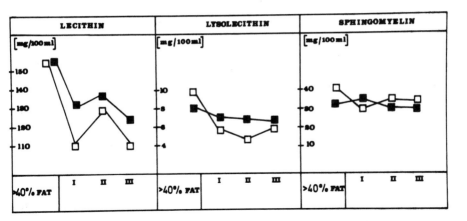

FIG. 4. Phospholipid fractions (lecithin, lysolecithin, and sphingomyelin) in the plasma of six healthy volunteers. The given values (means) are determinations on free diet (40% fat) and formula diets providing a fat supply of 25% (□) or 33% (■) of energy intake. Determinations were made at the end of 2-week periods of formula diets with fat I, II and III (see Fig. 3).

chromatography (1) showed also that the ratio cholesterol/lecithin was not appreciably influenced, neither by the amount nor by the composition of fat in the diet. Therefore, a close relationship between the changes of lecithin and phospholipids was obvious.

In fact, lecithin was responsible for phospholipid changes as could be shown by comparison of the phospholipid fractions under the influence of different dietary fats. An example (fat providing 25% and 33% of energy intake) is given in Fig. 4. The reduction of dietary fat in the formula diets resulted in a decrease of plasma phospholipid concentrations, which was effected by the decrease of lecithin. The decrease was more pronounced with the fat supply that produced 25 energy %. Only with a fat supply of 33% of energy, the changes initiated by the different compositions of fat (I, II, III) were statistically significant. This is in good agreement with the results of Bierenbaum et al. (5), who reported that the p/s ratio has little effect on plasma cholesterol levels with a nutritional fat supply of 28 energy % and lower. Lysolecithin levels, too, decreased with the reduction of dietary fat. In contrast, the plasma levels of sphingomyelin did not change, neither with the amount nor with the composition of dietary fat.

INFLUENCE OF LINOLEIC ACID INTAKE ON PHOSPHOLIPID AND CHOLESTEROL LEVELS IN HIGH-DENSITY LIPOPROTEINS

In vivo and in vitro experiments, as well as numerous epidemiological studies and the clinical experience with patients suffering from familial hypercholesterolemia, provide evidence that increased VLDL and LDL plasma levels show a high risk for atherosclerotic vascular disease. HDL cholesterol levels are inversely correlated to the risk for myocardial infarction. So a diet resulting in a decrease of HDL-lipid levels may augment the risk for atherosclerotic vascular disease.

In the nutrition experiment described above (see Fig. 3) the influence of the amount (25,33, and 36% of energy) and the composition of fat (I, III) on lipid composition of HLD were investigated. With a fat intake of 25, 33, and even 36%, cholesterol and phospholipid levels in HDL were significantly lowered compared to conventional diet, and the variation of the p/s ratio was without discernible effect (Fig. 5).

INFLUENCE OF LINOLEIC ACID INTAKE ON DIFFERENT PHOSPHOLIPIDS IN LIPOPROTEIN FRACTIONS

The proven effect of dietary changes on plasma lecithin and the known difference in HDL and LDL metabolism prompted an investigation of the influence of linoleic acid intake on different phospholipids in lipoprotein fractions. Using the same experimental design as described above, changes of lecithin, lysolecithin, and sphingomyelin were investigated in the lipoprotein fractions of six healthy females being given formula diets, providing a linoleic acid supply of 0, 4, and 20% of energy (LFD IV, V, and VI). These formula diets were given to the experimental subjects for 2 weeks each, always two persons starting with one of the formula diets, as previously described. The composition of conventional diet and formula diets is shown in Table 2.

At the end of a 2-week period without dietary fat (formula diet IV), a reduction of phospholipids was observed in LDL caused by a decrease of sphingomyelin and lecithin. The same occured with phospholipid fractions in HDL, but in VLDL sphingomyelin and lecithin were virtually unchanged. With a fat intake of 30 energy % (formula diet V) levels of lecithin and sphingomyelin increased in LDL and HDL, but decreased in VLDL. With high linoleic acid intake (formula diet VI) the

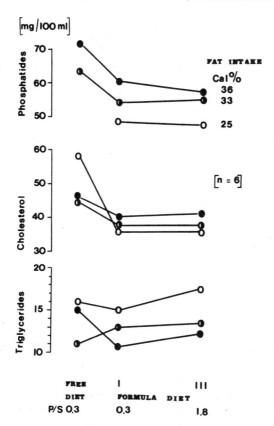

FIG. 5. Influence of different amounts (25, 33, or 36% of energy) and p/s ratios of fat supply with formula diets on phospholipids, cholesterol, and triglycerides in HDL (means) of healthy volunteers.

phospholipid fractions decreased in LDL and HDL, inversely to the increasing levels in VLDL (Fig. 6).

Total elimination of fat in the diet (formula diet IV) caused a decrease of sphingomyelin levels in HDL by 33% and in LDL by 23%. High linoleic acid intake affected sphingomyelin levels most in LDL, but in HDL only minor changes were noted (formula diets V and VI). Lecithin accounted for the greatest portion of phospholipid changes in lipoprotein fractions similar to the findings in total plasma. Changes were similar in HDL and LDL, but VLDL showed great individual differences under the influence of the different formula diets (Table 3).

INFLUENCE OF LINOLEIC ACID INTAKE ON FATTY ACID PATTERN OF LECITHIN IN LDL AND HDL AND OF CHOLESTERYL ESTERS IN PLASMA

Most investigators agree that LDL transport cholesterol and lipid to peripheral tissues and that HDL is concerned with centripedal transport to the liver. Therefore,

TABLE 2. *Composition of conventional diet and formula diets IV, V, and VI, providing a linoleic acid supply of 0, 4, and 20% of energy intake*

	Conventional diet	Formula diet		
		IV	V	VI
		(energy %)		
Protein	14	15	15	15
Carbohydrates	46	85	55	55
Fat	37	0	30	30
Linoleic acid	8	0	4	20
Alcohol	3	0	0	0
Composition of fat				
(g/3,000 Cal % of liquid				
formula diet)				
Safflower oil		0	13	97
71 g linoleic acid per 100 g)			(9.6)	(68.2)
Butter fat		0	64	0
(3.6 g linoleic acid per 100 g)			(2.3)	
Olive oil		0	20	0
(8.2 g linoleic acid per 100 g)			(1.6)	

their fatty acid pattern may be related to that of tissues. In HDL, cholesteryl esters are formed by the activity of LCAT. So a similarity between fatty acid composition of lecithin in HLD and cholesteryl esters in plasma may be expected.

To get a better understanding of the sequelae of linoleic acid supply for prostaglandin precursor availability, the fatty acid pattern of lecithin in LDL and HDL and of cholesteryl esters in plasma was determined. Experimental conditions were the same as described above (Table 2). Fatty acids were determined by gas chromatography, and their quantitation was achieved by calculating the percentage of the fatty acid content in the individual lipid. Determinations were done at the end of 2-week formula diet periods, providing a linoleic acid supply of 0, 4, and 20% of energy.

At the end of the fat-free formula diet period all subjects demonstrated the lowest linoleic acid content in the lecithin of LDL and HDL and in the cholesteryl esters of their plasma. The data of the period with 4 and 20 energy % linoleic acid intake showed the expected increase in the percentage of linoleic acid present, which was found to be similar in the three lipids examined (Figs. 7–12).

Quantitation of the amount of linoleic acid of the average present in LDL lecithin, showed a decrease with a linoleic acid intake of 20 energy %, compared to the values at the end of formula diet V (4% energy linoleic acid intake). This decrease was traceable to the reduction of LDL lecithin in the plasma. The absolute amount of linoleic acid in HDL lecithin increased slightly (Fig. 10), but in the cholesteryl esters of plasma no further increment was found (Fig. 12).

Formula diets contained no arachidonic acid. Therefore, neither the percentage nor the absolute amount of this fatty acid changed in LDL lecithin under these

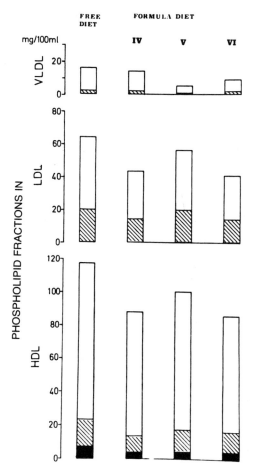

FIG. 6. Phospholipid fractions [mean values of lecithin (▭), lysolecithin (◼), and sphingomyelin (▨)] in the lipoprotein fractions (VLDL < 1.006, LDL 1.006–1.063, HDL > 1.063) of six healthy females at the end of 2-week periods of formula diets providing a linoleic acid supply of 0, 4, and 20 energy % (IV, V, VI), and the corresponding values under free diet.

experimental conditions (Figs. 7 and 8). In contrast, the percentage as well as the absolute amount of arachidonic acid in HDL lecithin and in the cholesteryl esters of the plasma decreased (Figs. 9–12) with high linoleic acid intake. This observation is compatible with a reduction of the activity of desaturating enzymes in the liver and in peripheral tissues, which transform linoleic acid to arachidonic acid.

INFLUENCE OF LINOLEIC ACID ON PROSTAGLANDIN FORMATION IN MAN

Linoleic acid intake has, according to the above results, two important effects on plasma lipids, i.e., phospholipids are lowered and the concentration of arachidonic acid in HDL and in cholesteryl esters of plasma is decreased. Both factors

TABLE 3. Phospholipids (mg/100 ml) in lipoproteins [$\bar{x}$ ± SD or range (*)] of six healthy females under a free diet and under formula diets IV, V, VI[a]

Phospholipid	Lipoprotein	Free diet	Formula diet		
			IV	V	VI
Lecithin	VLDL*	11.0 (2–23)	12.0 (5–21)	4.0 (0.8–8)	6.0 (0.9–16)
	LDL	43.0 ± 9.8	27 ± 6.9	35.0 ± 6.70	25.0 ± 10.70
	HDL	95.0 ± 26.2	75.0 ± 6.6	81.0 ± 7.50	67.0 ± 9.80
Sphingomyelin	VLDL*	2.0 (1–4)	2.0 (1–4)	0.8 (0.1–1.4)	1.5 (0.1–4)
	LDL	18.0 ± 7.2	14.0 ± 3.1	18.0 ± 3.70	13.0 ± 3.90
	HDL	15.0 ± 4.2	10.0 ± 1.9	13.0 ± 3.30	12.0 ± 3.30
Lysolecithin	VLDL*	0.3 (0.04–0.4)	0.2 (0.1–0.3)	0.05 (0.02–0.1)	0.1 (0.03–0.2)
	LDL*	0.6 (0.3–1.8)	0.2 (0.1–0.6)	0.55 (0.4–0.9)	0.4 (0.2–0.6)
	HDL*	6.0 (2.9–12)	4.0 (2.1–7.4)	4.0 (2.1–6.4)	4.0 (1.9–6.7)
Phospholipids	VLDL*	16.0 (4–26)	14.0 (6–25)	5.1 (1–9)	8.5 (1–20)
	LDL	65.0 ± 13.3	43.5 ± 8.9	56.0 ± 9.70	40.3 ± 14.70
	HDL	117.0 ± 30.2	89.0 ± 6.2	100.0 ± 9.30	85.0 ± 13.90

[a]See Fig. 3.

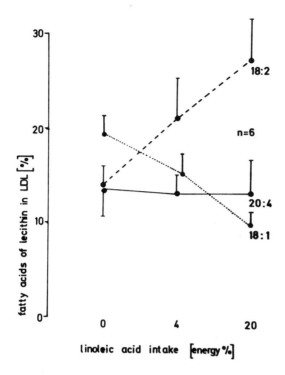

FIGS. 7–12. Influence of linoleic acid intake (0, 4, or 20% of energy) with formula diets on the percentage (Figs. 7, 9, and 11) and absolute amount (Figs. 8, 10, and 12) of linoleic acid (18:2), oleic acid (18:1), and arachidonic acid (20:4) in the lecithin of LDL and HDL and in cholesteryl esters of whole plasma in six healthy females. The given values ($\bar{x} \pm$ SD) are determinations at the end of 2-week periods of formula diets.

may influence prostaglandin metabolism, as phospholipids are the pool for precursor substances and arachidonic acid is the main precursor for prostaglandin formation.

Arachidonic acid infused intraarterially in graded doses provoked a dose-dependent increase of prostaglandin formation in isolated organs of experimental animals (14). Supplementation of arachidonic acid caused an increased biosynthesis of E prostaglandins, probably as a consequence of the enriched precursor pool (45). Infants with essential fatty acid deficiency revealed a decreased prostaglandin E (PG-E) turnover (16). There is sufficient evidence that prostaglandin turnover is related to the availability of essential fatty acids for the prostaglandin synthesizing enzymes.

Because of prostaglandins rapid formation, breakdown, and almost total excretion with the urine, the determination of urinary metabolites can give information about prostaglandin formation in the body. Monitoring one single end-product of prostaglandin metabolism may be hazardous since the individual formation of the numerous metabolites may not be equally stimulated by endocrinal, nutritional, or other factors (19,48). Therefore, the determination of a joint derivative, comprising

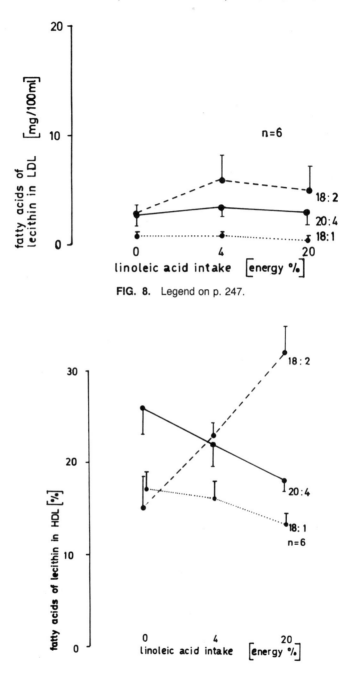

FIG. 8. Legend on p. 247.

FIG. 9. Legend on p. 247.

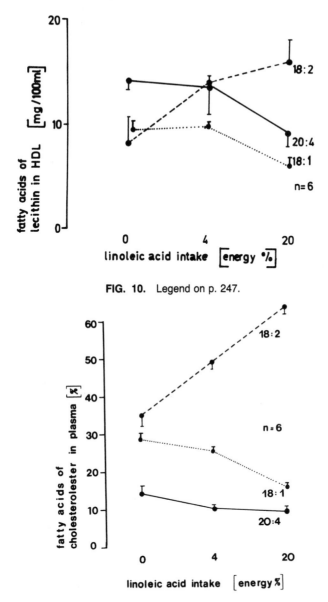

FIG. 10.   Legend on p. 247.

FIG. 11.   Legend on p. 247.

many urinary prostaglandin metabolites, seems advisable if prostaglandin formation in the body is to be measured.

The two major urinary end-products of prostaglandin E_{1+2} and F_{1+2} metabolism are derivatives of the tetranorprostanedioic acid (TNPDA). In 1975 Nugteren (37) developed a method in which these main human urinary prostaglandin metabolites are converted by chemical procedures to TNPDA (see Fig. 2). With radioimmu-

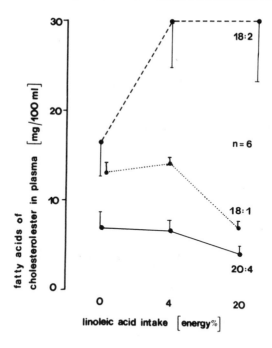

FIG. 12.   Legend on p. 247.

nological methods and with a combination of gas chromatography and mass spectrometry the quantity of the main urinary metabolites of PG-F_{1+2} has been determined with from 4 to 23 μg/day and of PG-E_{1+2} with from 2 to 35 μg/day in females (3,22). The quantity of urinary prostaglandin metabolites, which can be transformed to TNPDA, is approximately ten times higher (Fig. 2). Recently Ellis et al. (15) determined urinary metabolites of PG-D_2, which also can be converted to TNPDA. So prostaglandins of still unknown origin and function presumably contribute to urinary prostaglandin metabolites, which can be transformed to TNPDA (TNPDA-M). Not included in the determination of TNPDA-M is a small amount (~0.3 μg/day) of native prostaglandins in the urine originating from the kidney and of those prostaglandins formed in the seminal vesicles of males, as well as the small percentage (less than 5%) of prostaglandins and TNPDA-M which are excreted in the intestinal tract. Prostaglandin formation, measured as TNPDA-M in 24-hr urine, was investigated during the already described nutrition experiment (Table 2).

The six healthy females (age 22–27 years) with normal body weight recorded their diets for a period of 8 days. Afterwards, they were put on the isoenergetic formula diets, providing a linoleic acid supply of 0% (diet IV), 4% (diet V), or 20% (diet VI) of energy intake. Each of the different formula diets was given to every subject in a different order for periods of 2 weeks. Samples were taken from every 24-hr urine and were deep-frozen at −20°C until the analysis of TNPDA was done. TNPDA in urine was determined by gas-liquid chromatography on two columns with liquid phases of different polarity (37). Determinations at the end of the three formula diet periods showed a close correlation between linoleic acid intake, linoleic acid content of cholesteryl esters, and TNPDA-M in the 24-hr urine (Fig. 13). During 6 days on conventional diet, in the urine of the six female volunteers, an average of 306 μg TNPDA per day could be determined, the values ranging from 220 to 460 μg. During the two weeks under the influence of the diets with a linoleic acid supply of 0, 4, or 20% of energy, 123 ± 5.2 μg (mean ± SE) 175 ± 7.0 μg, and 352 ± 10.8 μg, TNPDA per day, respectively, were excreted.

If the linoleic acid supply was lowered, a decrease of urinary TNPDA-M resulted within 24 hr. During the period without a linoleic acid supply, TNPDA was lowest, the values ranging from 59 to 210 μg per day (Fig. 14). With a linoleic acid supply of 4 energy %, TNPDA-M increased, but not to the same extent in all experimental

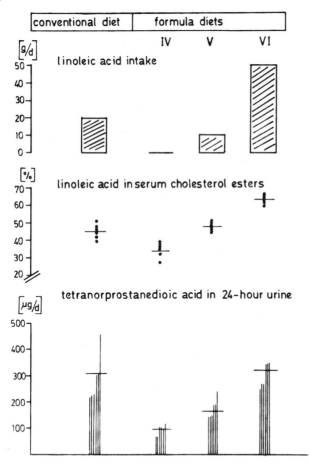

FIG. 13. Correlation between linoleic acid in serum cholesteryl esters and tetranorprostane-dioic acid in 24-hr urine of six healthy females at the end of 2-week periods of formula diets, providing a linoleic acid supply of 0% (IV), 4% (V), or 20% (VI) of energy intake. (From Zöllner et al., ref. 53, with permission.)

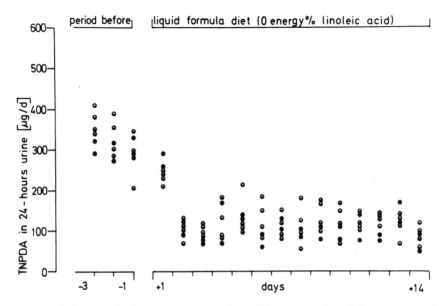

FIG. 14. Daily determination of the amount of TNPDA in 24-hr urine of six healthy female volunteers being given a linoleic acid supply of 0% of energy for 2 weeks with a liquid formula diet. The symbols indicate subjects coming from the liquid formula diet VI (◐) providing a linoleic acid supply of 20 energy % and subjects coming from a conventional diet with a linoleic acid intake of about 8 energy % (●).

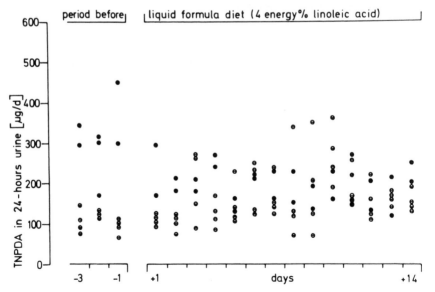

FIG. 15. Linoleic acid supply of 4 energy %: subjects coming from the linoleic acid deficient liquid formula diet (⊖); subjects coming from the conventional diet (●). (See Fig. 2.)

subjects. Although one person had up to 350 μg TNPDA in urine on several days, the increase in the other subjects was modest (Fig. 15). If linoleic acid intake was augmented from lower intakes to 20% energy, an increase of urinary TNPDA-M was found after 3 or 4 days. During the next 5 days the highest values of the period were determined, which decreased somewhat toward the end of those periods with high linoleic acid intake in 5 out of 6 persons (Fig. 16).

Two persons, after being on a conventional diet, were started on a liquid formula diet with 20 energy % linoleic acid. In these two persons the increase of TNPDA-M was less than in the other persons, changing from the formula diet V (4% energy linoleic acid) to the highest linoleic acid intake (Fig. 16). After 2 weeks of high linoleic acid intake the excretion of prostaglandin metabolites in all subjects was within the same range (Fig. 16).

In the nutrition experiment above, an increased prostaglandin turnover could be detected after 3 to 4 days of high linoleic acid intake. In contrast ethylarachidonate administered orally to healthy male volunteers in a dosage of 6 mg/day for 2- to 3-week periods resulted in an immediate increase of urinary PG-E metabolites (45). Experiments using isolated organs have shown that arachidonic acid can mimic the effect of prostaglandins, obviously because arachidonic acid is very rapidly metabolized to different cyclooxygenase products; linoleic acid is ineffective in these systems (14). Linoleic acid has to undergo a chain elongation and desaturation until it becomes arachidonic acid and is then available for prostaglandin synthesis. Experiments of Nichaman et al. (34) showed that it takes about 2 days until significant amounts of labeled linoleic acid are transformed to arachidonic acid and incorporated in phospholipids. These data correspond very well to those reported by Mead and Fillerup (31) for injected linoleic acid in rats, by Dittmer and Hanahan (12) for fed linoleate in rats, and by Ormsby et al. (40) for injected radioactive linoleic acid in humans. All these data suggest that the delayed increase of TNPDA-M in urine

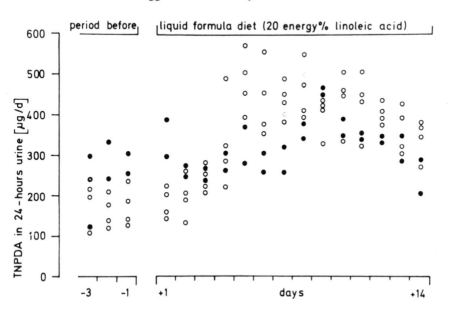

FIG. 16. Linoleic acid supply of 20 energy %: subjects coming from the conventional diet (●); subjects coming from the liquid formula diet with 4% energy linoleic acid intake (○). (See Fig. 2.)

TABLE 4. *Platelet total fatty acids (%) at the end of 3 weeks liquid formula diets (LFD) providing a linoleic acid supply of 0% (LFD IV) or 20% (LFD VI) of energy intake in six healthy females*

	14:0	14:1	16:0	16:1	18:0	18:1	18:2[a]	20:0
LFD IV								
Mean	0.7	2.0	11.0	0.8	15.2	18.4	4.5	0.7
SD	0.3	0.2	0.6	0.3	0.8	1.5	0.6	0.2
LFD VI								
Mean	0.6	2.1	10.8	0.8	16.6	15.7	8.3	0.7
SD	0.3	0.3	0.9	0.2	0.8	1.2	1.1	0.3

	20:1	20:3[a]	20:4[a]	22:1	22:6	24:0	24:1
LFD IV							
Mean	0.6	2.5	36.6	2.0	0.6	1.0	0.8
SD	0.1	0.9	2.1	0.3	0.1	0.3	0.3
LFD VI							
Mean	0.7	1.4	35.4	1.7	0.8	0.9	0.8
SD	0.3	0.7	2.1	0.3	0.2	0.1	0.2

[a]$N-6$ series.

after changing to a high linoleic acid intake is limited by the elapse of time until prostaglandin precursors are formed from linoleic acid. The increase of TNPDA-M is more pronounced if a high linoleic acid supply is given after a linoleic acid deficient diet; during the last days of the period with high linoleic acid intake, the amount of TNPDA-M in the urine seems to decrease and is at the end of this 2-week period in all subjects within the same range.

With low intake of polyunsaturated fatty acids a high activity of desaturating enzymes in animal liver has been reported (36). Desaturases are supposed to be the rate-limiting enzymes in the formation of arachidonic acid from linoleic acid (36). So far the influence of diet on the activity of desaturating enzymes has not been investigated in man, and no data are available for the rate of arachidonic acid synthesis under experimental conditions given here. Whether or not the increasing amount of linoleic acid in membrane lipids during high linoleic acid intake causes an inhibition of the desaturating enzymes, as it has been shown *in vitro* (41), remains to be established. The present authors cannot explain why prostaglandin metabolite excretion was diminished 24 hr after reduction of linoleic acid intake. As the arachidonic acid concentration in membrane phospholipids after such a short time probably has not changed, precursor substance concentration cannot be taken into account.

INFLUENCE OF LINOLEIC ACID INTAKE ON PLATELET FATTY ACID COMPOSITION AND PLATELET AGGREGATION

In vitro platelet linoleic acid content is changed according to its plasma level (9). Under *in vivo* conditions the plasma level of linoleic acid is influenced by linoleic acid intake (51). *In vitro* experiments and animal experiments have shown that an increase of linoleic acid reduces platelet aggregation tendency and thromboxane formation (3). Availability of arachidonic acid is thought to be a rate-limiting factor for thromboxane and prostaglandin formation (14). Therefore, platelet fatty acids and platelet aggregation tendency under the influence of the above described formula diets were investigated (see Table 2).

In this experiment, formula diets IV and VI were given to six healthy females for periods of 3 weeks in a crossover design, each three persons starting with one of the two formula diets. Analysis of platelet fatty acids and platelet aggregation studies were done under conventional diet before the experiment and at the end of weeks 1 and 3 of each formula diet period.

For platelet lipid analysis 20 ml blood was collected in plastic test tubes with 1 mg ethylenediaminetetraacetic acid per milliliter. Platelets were isolated by differential centrifugation and fatty acid methylesters were prepared as described elsewhere (3). Gas-chromatographic determination of fatty acids was done on two columns of different polarity (3). The percentage of fatty acids found in total platelet lipids at the end of the formula diet periods is given in Table 4. All experimental subjects showed an increase of linoleic acid in platelet lipids under high linoleic acid intake, on the average from 4.5 to 8.3%. In contrast to this increase of linoleic acid, an average decrease from 2.5 to 1.4% for dihomo-γ-linolenic acid was found (20:3, n-6). Mean arachidonic acid content amounted to 36.6% at the end of the 3-week formula diet without linoleic acid supply; the corresponding value after 3 weeks with high linoleic acid supply was 35.4% in platelet lipids. Oleic acid was slightly decreased; the saturated fatty acids were virtually unchanged under both formula diets (Fig. 17).

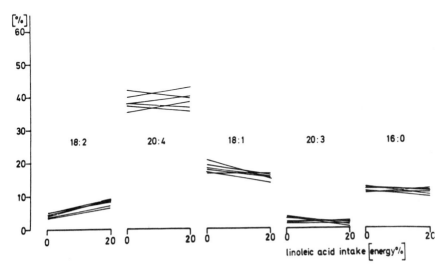

FIG. 17. Platelet total fatty acids (%) at the end of 3-week periods of formula diets, providing a linoleic acid supply of 0% (formula diet IV) or 20% (VI) of energy intake.

With a Born-type aggregometer *in vitro* platelet aggregation was studied, induced by a constant amount of adenosine diphosphate (ADP) or collagen sufficient to cause a monophasic, irreversible aggregation. Increase in light transmission was compared to the control values under conventional diet. With a linoleic acid supply of 20 energy %, a decrease of platelet aggregation tendency was found in all subjects. Those persons coming from the linoleic acid deficient diet revealed the effect already 1 week after their allotment to the high linoleic acid intake (Fig. 18). Experimental subjects who started with formula diet VI had a preceding linoleic acid intake of about 8% energy with conventional diet. These persons showed the decrease of *in vitro* platelet aggregation tendency only after 3 weeks (Fig. 19). ADP-induced platelet aggregation did not change with the linoleic acid deficient formula diet, compared to the values under free diet. But collagen-induced platelet aggregation (Figs. 18 and 19) increased in four of the six experimental subjects.

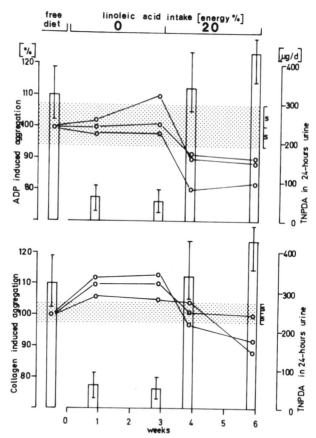

FIG. 18. Platelet aggregation (O——O) (% of the value on free diet) and TNPDA *(white columns)* in 24-hr urine (mean and range) in three subjects starting with the linoleic deficient formula diet. Shadowed area indicates the SD of the platelet aggregation on free diet. (From Adam et al., ref. 1a, with permission.)

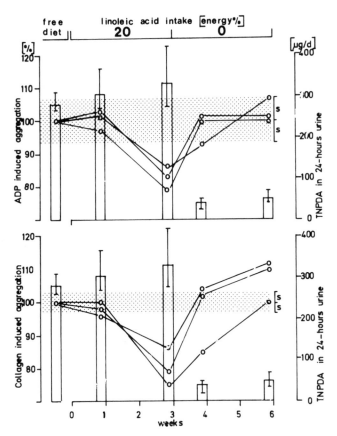

FIG. 19. Platelet aggregation and amount of TNPDA determined in 24-hr urine in three healthy females started on a formula diet with 20% energy linoleic acid intake (symbols correspond to Fig. 18). (From Adam et al., ref. 1a, with permission.)

These findings are in good agreement with the *in vitro* experiments of Chambaz et al. (9), showing that platelets have the ability to prevent arachidonic acid accumulation. In animal experiments high levels of linoleic acid reduced thromboxane formation (25) presumably by competing with arachidonic acid for thromboxane-synthesizing enzymes. This may cause a decrease of platelet aggregation, which was demonstrated above following high linoleic acid intake.

SUMMARY AND CONCLUSIONS

The effect of dietary fat on lecithin concentrations in plasma and lipoprotein fractions was evaluated with formula diets providing a fat supply of 25, 33, and 36% of energy. The variation of the p/s ratio was found to be less important than the amount of fat in the diet. Changes of lecithin and cholesterol in the plasma were similar, substantiated by a constant ratio of these lipids under all experimental conditions; however, the concentrations of sphingomyelin were neither affected by the amount nor by the composition of the dietary fat.

Lecithin is assumed to be the main pool for prostaglandin precursors. The effect of linoleic acid intake on fatty acid composition in HDL and LDL lecithin was investigated. High linoleic acid intake caused a decrease of arachidonic acid in HDL, but its concentration in LDL did not change. Assuming that HDLs are concerned with lipid transport from peripheral cells, this would indicate a decreased arachidonic acid formation in tissues. This finding is in good agreement with the reported inhibition of linoleic acid on the activity of desaturating enzymes in cell culture and animal experiments (24,41). Availability of the precursor substances appears to be a limiting factor for prostaglandin formation, which was evaluated by the determination of TNPDA, the main joint derivative of urinary prostaglandin metabolites (TNPDA-M). Following high linoleic acid intake an increase of TNPDA-M was found after 4 days. This may be a reflection of the time until linoleic acid has been transformed to arachidonic acid and is available in phospholipids for prostaglandin formation. A linoleic acid deficient diet causes a decrease of TNPDA-M within 24 hr. As changes of arachidonic concentration after such a short time cannot be taken into account, another influence of dietary linoleic acid on prostaglandin formation may be expected.

In vitro and *in vivo* experiments in animals provided evidence that linoleic acid concentrations may influence arachidonic acid formation either by competing for the metabolizing enzymes or by changing their activity (24,36). Moreover, inhibition of prostaglandin synthesis by a number of fatty acids, including linoleic acid, was reported *in vitro* (41), but in animal experiments a stimulation of prostaglandin biosynthesis by linoleic acid has been shown (38). The findings presented here in humans employing formula diets containing different amounts of linoleic acid are indicative of comparable effects in man.

REFERENCES

1a. Adam, O., Dill-Wiesner, M., Wolfram, G., and Zöllner, N. (1979): *Res. Exp. Med.*, 177:227–235.

1. Adam, O., Wolfram, G., and Zöllner, N. (1979): Quantitative evaluation of phospholipid fractions in serum by tubular thin-layer chromatography. In: *Recent Developments in Chromatography and Electrophoresis*, edited by A. Frigerio and L. Renoz, pp. 267–272. Elsevier, Amsterdam.

2. Adam, O., Wolfram, G., and Zöllner, N. (1979): Phosphatidfraktionen im Plasma des Menschen unter dem Einfluss von Formeldiäten mit modifizierten Fettanteilen. *Infusionsther. Klin. Ernaehr. Forsch. Prax.*, 6:176–180.

3. Adam, O., Wolfram, G., and Zöllner, N. (1980): Platelet fatty acids and prostaglandin turnover during defined linoleic acid intake with formula diets. *Artery*, 8:85–89.

4. Aizawa, Y., Yamada, K., and Hata, M. (1978): Double isotope derivative dilution method for the determination of prostaglandin F and E type metabolites in urine. *Prostaglandins*, 14:1165–1174.

5. Bierenbaum, M. L., Fleischmann, A. J., Raichelson, R. J., Hayton, Th., and Watson, P. B. (1973): Ten-year experience of modified-fat diets on younger men with coronary heart disease. *Lancet*, i:1404.

6. Bondjers, G., Olsson,G., Nyman, L. L., and Björkerud, S. (1977): High density lipoprotein (HDL) dependent elimination of cholesterol from normal arterial tissue in man. In: *Atherosclerosis*, Vol. 4, edited by G. Schettler, Y. Gotto, G. Kose, and G. Mata, pp. 70–71. Springer-Verlag, Berlin.

7. Bloj, B., Morero, R. D., Farias, R. N., and Trucco, R. F. (1973): Membrane lipid fatty acids and regulation of membranebound enzymes. *Biochim. Biophys. Acta*, 311:67–79.
8. Chajek, T., and Fielding, C. J. (1978): Isolation and characterization of a human serum cholesteryl ester transfer protein. *Proc. Natl. Acad. Sci. USA*, 75:3445.
9. Chambaz, J., Robert, A., Wolf, C., Béréziat, G., and Polonovski, J. (1979): Different acylation and accumulation in free form of arachidonic acid or its sodium salt in human platelets. *Thromb. Res.*, 15:743–754.
10. Danon, A., Heimberg, M., and Oates, J. A. (1975): Enrichment of rat tissue lipids with fatty acids that are prostaglandin precursors. *Biochim. Biophys. Acta*, 388:318–330.
11. Delcher, H. K., Fried, M., and Shipp, J. C. (1965): Metabolism of lipoprotein lipid in the isolated perfused rat heart. *Biochim. Biophys. Acta*, 106:10–18.
12. Dittmer, J. C., and Hanahan, D. J. (1959): Biochemistry of long chain fatty acids. II. Metabolic studies. *J. Biol. Chem.*, 234:1983–1989.
13. Van Dorp, D. A., Beerthuis, R. K., Nugteren, D. H., and Vonkeman, H. (1964): Enzymatic conversion of all-cis-polyunsaturated fatty acids into prostaglandins. *Nature (Lond.)*, 203:839–841.
14. Dusting, G. J., Moncada, S., and Vane, J. R. (1968): Vascular actions of arachidonic acid and its metabolites in perfused mesenteric and femoral beds of the dog. *Eur. J. Pharmacol.*, 49:65–72.
15. Ellis, C. K., Smigel, M. D., Oates, J. A., Oelz, O., Sweetman, B. J. (1979): Metabolism of prostaglandin D_2 in the monkey. *J. Biol. Chem.*, 154:4152–4161.
16. Friedmann, Z., Seyberth, H., Lamberth, E. L., and Oates, J. (1978): Decreased prostaglandin-E turnover in infants with essential fatty acid deficiency. *Pediatr. Res.*, 12:711–714.
17. Glomset, J. A., and Nerum, K. R. (1973): The metabolic role of LCAT: Perspectives from pathology. *Adv. Lipid. Res.*, 11:1–65.
18. Gjone, E., Nordoy, A., Blomhoff, J. P., and Wiencke, I. (1972): The effects of unsaturated and saturated dietary fats on plasma cholesterol, phospholipids and lecithin:cholesterol acyltransferase activity. *Acta Med. Scand.*, 191:481–484.
19. Gold, E. W., Fox, O. D., and Edgar, P. R. (1978): The effect of longterm corticoid administration on lipid and prostaglandin levels. *J. Steroid Biochem.*, 9:313–316.
20. Green, P. H. R., Glickman, R. M., and Saudek, Ch. D. (1979): Human intestinal lipoproteins. *J. Clin. Invest.*, 64:233.
21. Grundy, S. M. (1975): Effects of polyunsaturated fatty acids on lipid metabolism in patients with hypertriglyceridaemia. *J. Clin. Invest.*, 55:269–282.
22. Hamberg, M. (1973): Quantitative studies on prostaglandin synthesis in man. *Anal. Biochem.*, 55:368–378.
23. Hamilton, R. L., and Kayden, H. J. (1974): The liver and the formation of normal and abnormal plasma lipoproteins. In: *The Liver: Normal and Abnormal Functions*, edited by F. F. Becker, pp. 531–572. Marcel Dekker, New York.
24. Hassam, A. G., and Crawford, M. A. (1976): The differential incorporation of labelled linoleic, gamma-linolenic, dihomo-gama-linolenic and arachidonic acids into the developing rat brain. *J. Neurochem.*, 127:967–968.
25. Hornstra, G., and Haddeman, E. (1978): Diet-induced changes in arterial thrombosis not primarily mediated by arachidonate peroxidation. *Bibl. Haematol.*, 45:9–13.
26. Illingworth, D. R., and Portman, O. W. (1972): Independence of phospholipid and protein exchange between plasma lipoproteins in vivo and in vitro. *Biochem. Biophys. Acta*, 280:281–289.
27. Konturek, S. J., Mikoś, E., Pawlik, W., and Waluś, K. (1979): Direct inhibition of gastric secretion and mucosal blood flow by arachidonic acid. *J. Physiol.*, 286:15–28.
28. Kook, A. I., and Rubinstein, D. (1970): The role of serum lipoproteins in the release of phospholipids by rat liver slices. *Biochim. Biophys. Acta*, 202:396–398.
29. Lands, W. E. M. (1965): Lipid metabolism. *Ann. Rev. Biochem.*, 34:313.
30. Mahley, R. W., Weisgraber, K. H., Bersot, T. P., and Innerarity, T. L. (1978): Effects of cholesterol feeding on human and animal high density lipoproteins. In: *High Density Lipoproteins and Atherosclerosis*, edited by A. M. Gotto, N. E., Miller, M. F. Oliver, p. 149. Elsevier, Amsterdam.
31. Mead, J. F., and Fillerup, D. L. (1957): The transport of fatty acids in the blood. *J. Biol. Chem.*, 227:1009–1014.

32. Nelson, G. F., and Freeman, N. K. (1960): The phospholipid and phospholipid fatty acid composition of human serum lipoprotein fractions. *J. Biol. Chem.*, 235:578–583.
33. Nestel, P. J., and Miller, N. E. (1978): Mobilization of adipose tissue cholesterol in high density lipoprotein during weight reduction in man. In: High Density Lipoproteins and Atherosclerosis, edited by A. M. Gotto, N. E. Miller, and M. F. Oliver, p. 51. Elsevier, Amsterdam.
34. Nichaman, M. Z., Olson, R. E., and Sweeley, C. C. (1967): Metabolism of linoleic acid 1-¹⁴C in normolipemic and hyperlipemic humans fed linoleate diets. *Am. J. Clin. Nutr.*, 20:1070–1083.
35. Nowak, J., and Wennmalm, A. (1979): Human forearm and kidney conversion of arachidonic acid to prostaglandins. *Acta Physiol. Scand.*, 106:307–312.
36. Nugteren, D. H. (1965): The enzymic conversion of gamma-linolenic acid into homo-gamma-linolenic acid. *Biochim. Biophys. Acta*, 68:28.
37. Nugteren, D. H. (1975): The determination of prostaglandin metabolites in human urine. *J. Biol. Chem.*, 250:2808–2812.
38. Nugteren, D. H., van Evert, W. C., Soeting, W. J., and Spuy, J. H. (1980): The effect of different amounts of linoleic acid in the diet on the excretion of urinary prostaglandin metabolites in the rat. In: *Advances in Prostaglandin and Thromboxane Research Series. Vols. 6 and 7: Proceedings of the Fourth International Prostaglandin Conference*, edited by P. Ramwell, Raven Press, New York.
39. Oelz, O., Seyberth, H. W., Knapp, H. R., Sweetman, B. J., and Oates, J. A. (1976): Effects of feeding ethyl-dihomo-gamma-linoleat on prostaglandin biosynthesis and platelet aggregation in the rabbit. *Biochim. Biophys. Acta*, 431:268–271.
40. Ormsby, J. W., Schnatz, J. D., and Williams, R. H. (1963): The incorporation of linoleic 1-C¹⁴ acid in human plasma and adipose tissue. *Metabolism*, 12:812–820.
41. Pace-Asciak, C., and Wolfe, L. S. (1968): Inhibition of prostaglandin synthesis by oleic, linoleic and linolenic acids. *Biochim. Biophys. Acta*, 152:784–791.
42. Patil, G. S., Sprecher, H., and Cornwell, D. G. (1979): Correlations between surface area and the rate of enzymatic desaturation with methyl branched 8, 11, 14-eicosatrieon acid. *Lipids*, 14:826–828.
43. Redinger, R. N., Hermann, A. H., and Small, D. M. (1973): Effects of diet and fasting on biliary lipid secretion and relative composition and bile salt metabolism in the rhesus monkey. *Gastroenterology*, 64:610–621.
44. Schwartz, C. C., Halloran, L. G., Vlahcevic, R., Gregory, D. H., and Swell, L. (1978): Preferential utilization of free cholesterol from high-density lipoproteins for biliary cholesterol secretion in man. *Science*, 200:62.
45. Seyberth, H. W., Oelz, O., Kennedy, T., Sweetman, B. J., Danon, A., Fröhlich, J. C., Heimberg, M., and Oates, J. A. (1975): Increased Arachidonate in Lipids after Administration to Man: Effects on Prostaglandin Biosynthesis. *Clin. Pharmacol. Ther.*, 18:521–529.
46. Shaw, J. E., Gibson, W., Jessup, S., and Ramwell, P. W. (1971): The effect of PGE₁ on cyclic AMP and ion movements in turkey erythrocytes. *Ann. NY Acad. Sci.*, 180:241–245.
47. Stoffel, W., Därr, W., and Assmann, G. (1978): Pleomorphe Funktionen von hochungesättigten Phospholipiden im biologischen Membranen und Serumlipiden. *Med. Welt*, 29:124–132.
48. Subbiah, M. T. R. (1979): On the characterization of prostaglandin E₂ 9-keto-reductase from aorta and regional differences in its activity. *Proc. Soc. Exp. Biol. Med.*, 161:158.
49. Vergroesen, A. J., de Boer, J., and Thomasson, H. J. (1970): Influence of three dietary fats given at three caloric levels on serum lipids in man. In: *Atherosclerosis, Proceedings of the Second International Symposium*, edited by R. J. Jones. Springer-Verlag, Heidelberg.
50. Wiss, O, and Weber, F. (1965): Ernährungsphysiologische Beziehungen zwischen dem Vitamin E und den ungesättigten Fettsäuren. In: *Suppl 4, Z. Ernährungswiss.: Ernährungsprobleme in der modernen Industriegesellschaft*. Steinkopff-Verlag, Darmstadt.
51. Wolfram, G., Adam, O., and Zöllner, N. (1980): Der Einfluß von Menge und Art des Nahrungsfettes auf die Lipide in den HDL des Serums beim Menschen. *Verh. Dtsch. Ges. Inn. Med.*, 86:902–904.
52. Wood, P. D. S., Shioda, R., and Kinsell, L. W. (1966): Dietary regulation of cholesterol metabolism. *Lancet*, ii:604.
53. Zöllner, N., Adam, O., and Wolfram, G. (1979): The influence of linoleic acid intake on the excretion of urinary prostaglandin metabolites. *Res. Exp. Med.*, 175:149–153.

Phospholipids and Atherosclerosis, edited by
P. Avogaro, M. Mancini, G. Ricci, and
R. Paoletti. Raven Press, New York © 1983.

Platelet Phospholipids in Relation to Platelet Functions in Man and Animals

S. Renaud, L. McGregor, and R. Morazain

*INSERM, Unit 63, 69500 Bron, France, and Department of Nutrition,
University of Montreal, Canada*

Phospholipids represent the main component of all membranes. Membranes and particularly plasma membranes are involved in the various activities of all cells. In this regard, platelets are no different than other cells. However, in addition to the usual cell activities, platelets have specific functions which are directly related to the membrane phospholipids. These functions are the following:

1. The ability of platelets to aggregate, i.e., to form plugs involved in both hemostasis and thrombosis.
2. Their clot promoting activity, i.e., their essential role in the formation of fibrin to consolidate the platelet plug.

In response to various stimuli, particularly to thrombin, the membrane phospholipids supply the free arachidonic acid needed for prostaglandin synthesis (2), one of the steps in the mechanism of platelet aggregation.

In the coagulation process, platelets supply the so-called platelet factor 3. It seems that this term should be reserved to the clot promoting activity of the platelet lipoprotein surface (14). Nevertheless, even if the platelet phospholipids play only an indirect structural role in coagulation (14), they are essential for the clotting process. In addition, in man and in animals, minor changes in the fatty acid composition of these platelet phospholipids are responsible for drastic changes in the platelet function (both coagulation and aggregation) (6,15,26).

PHOSPHOLIPIDS FROM THE PLATELET PLASMA MEMBRANE

The positions of the five main phospholipid fractions from the platelet plasma membrane are illustrated in Fig. 1. This recent work (3) suggests an asymmetric distribution of phospholipids in the plasma membrane and confirms the studies by previous investigators (4,27).

In Fig. 1 are mentioned only the fatty acids in the 2-position of the glycerophospholipids, available for metabolic activities. The total arachidonic acid is es-

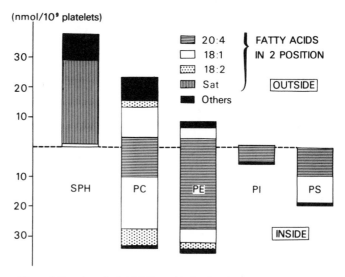

FIG. 1. Repartition of the phospholipid fatty acids in the 2-position, in the platelet plasma membrane. Sat, saturated; SPH, sphingomyelin; PC, phosphatidylcholine; PE, phosphatidyl-ethanolamine; PI, phosphatidylinositol; PS, phosphatidylserine. (Adapted from Chambaz et al., ref. 3.)

terified in this position and appears to be located almost entirely in the inner leaflet of the membrane. Since phospholipase A_2 appears also to be located on the inner layer of the platelet membrane (5), this might explain the efficient release of arachidonic acid on stimulation of platelets by an aggregating agent, such as thrombin, as an initial step in prostaglandin synthesis (2).

Concerning coagulation, phosphotidylserine, the most active phospholipid on clotting (7), appears to be entirely located in the inner part of the membrane (3,4,27). This asymmetric distribution might play a role in regulating the coagulation process (30).

PROCOAGULANT AND ANTICOAGULANT ACTIVITIES OF PHOSPHATIDYLSERINE

As already mentioned, the main platelet phospholipid with clot promoting activity seems to be the phosphatidylserine (PS) although the other fractions might have some additional effects (7). A surprising result in this regard is that PS has been shown to have anticoagulant activities (16,28). Apparently an intrinsic coagulant activity could be observed with phospholipid particles of certain size and electric charge; others of much smaller size, such as PS well solubilized with deoxycholate, have intrinsic anticoagulant activity (28).

In the studies briefly reported below, the present authors attempt to determine the following:

1. If the anticoagulant activities of PS, adequately solubilized with deoxycholate or via sonication, could be obtained for levels of PS normally present in blood or in platelets.

2. If the same activity might also be observed with PS extracted from platelets since most of the work on anticoagulant properties of PS has been performed with phospholipids extracted from beef brain.

Figure 2 shows the results obtained when beef brain phosphatidylserine (kindly supplied by Dr. Nishizawa) is added to rat platelet-poor plasma. The beef brain PS was prepared as reported elsewhere and exposed for several days to air since this treatment increased the anticoagulant activity (16). In both the recalcification and stypven time [performed as in previous studies (22)], an increased amount of PS added to plasma shortened the clotting time until it was well above a concentration normally found in platelet-rich plasma. At concentrations (125–250 µg/ml) ten times higher than normal, the clotting time was prolonged, but real anticoagulant activities were observed for concentrations that were from 40 to 100 times the physiologic range found in platelet-rich plasma.

In Fig. 3, the results obtained under similar conditions are reported, with PS plus Phosphatidylinositol (PI) carefully prepared, half of the material being oxidized for 6 weeks by air exposure. At any concentration tested (the highest was 40 times

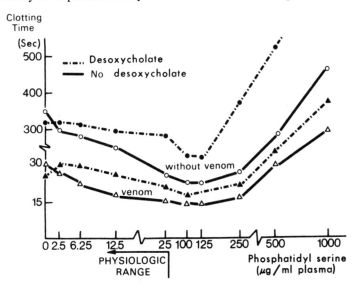

FIG. 2. Clotting activity of oxidized phosphatidylserine (PS), extracted from beef brain, added to a pool of platelet-poor plasma from normal rats, 10 min before starting the test. Prior to its addition to plasma, PS was solubilized in incomplete Tyrode solution, as in previous studies (6,23) either by including sodium desoxycholate (2 mg/ml) in the solution or by sonicating for 15 sec. The tests performed in duplicate, in a recording coagulometer, were started by adding to plasma CaCl₂ (0.02 M) not containing or containing Russell's viper venom (1/100,000) (stypven time) (10).

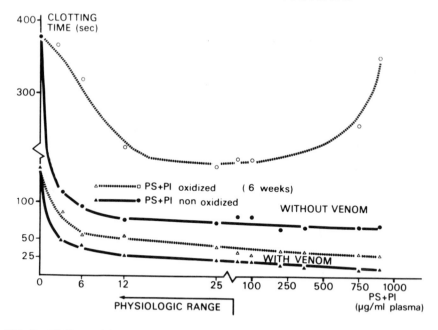

FIG. 3. Clotting activity of oxidized or nonoxidized PS + PI from rat platelets. These phospholipid fractions were prepared as reported elsewhere (3). Half of the material obtained was exposed to air in an opened test tube for 6 weeks. The tests were performed as in Fig. 2, except that the phospholipids were solubilized by sonication only.

the normal amount found in platelet-rich plasma) the nonoxidized PS + PI fractions presented procoagulant activity in both the recalcification and the stypven time. By contrast, the oxidized platelet PS + PI showed a similar biphasic activity on clotting (solely in recalcification) to that observed with the beef brain PS, also oxidized by air exposure. Consequently, at least in this system, nonoxidized platelet PS or PS + PI never exhibited any anticoagulant activity, whatever concentration was utilized. By contrast, the procoagulant activity that was always observed under these conditions confirmed previous work (7,13).

RELATIONSHIP BETWEEN THE CLOTTING TIME AND THE PROCOAGULANT ACTIVITY OF PLATELETS

In these studies, the recalcification plasma clotting time (PCT) of platelet-rich plasma (PRP) in siliconized or plastic material (19,20) was used as an evaluation of the blood clotting activity. Provided the blood centrifugation is performed in the minutes following blood removal, this test gives reproducible results for several hours with the plasma stored at 25°C. In contrast, if the same determination is performed on whole blood, it would have to be done minutes after blood removal, since the clotting time, even on citrated blood, shortens very rapidly with time. Consequently, the test has to be done almost immediately after blood removal, and this is usually not feasible, particularly for serial determinations.

On the other hand, as already mentioned, the PCT performed on PRP stored at 25°C is stable with time. Since, as shown in Fig. 4, it gives exactly the same results as the whole blood clotting time, it can be said that the PCT evaluates the whole blood clotting activity. In addition, this test can be performed in a recording aggrego-coagulometer (Rubel-Renaud, U.S. Patent 4.116.564).

A third test, the factor 3 clotting test (F_3-CT), devised more than 10 years ago (19), also reproduces completely the results obtained with the PCT. It evaluates the clotting activity of platelets washed and resuspended in a standard platelet-poor plasma (20). The close relationship between the two tests is illustrated in Fig. 5, on 51 normal subjects. In addition, in recent studies involving more than 900 farmers from France, England, and Belgium in which the PCT and the F_3-CT have been performed simultaneously, the correlation coefficient (r) between the two tests within each group ranges from 0.95 to 0.99 on an individual basis. In the F_3-CT, only the platelets are different from one test to another since the platelet-poor plasma comes from a pool, prepared once a year and kept frozen.

This extremely close relationship between the PCT and the F_3-CT has been reproduced recently in an epidemiologic study performed in Belgium (M. Verstraete, *personal communication*).

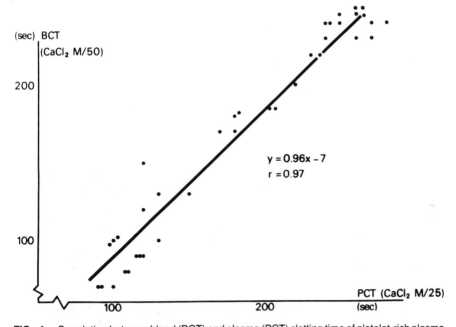

FIG. 4. Correlation between blood (BCT) and plasma (PCT) clotting time of platelet-rich plasma (PRP) from rats fed for 10 weeks either laboratory chow or a hyperlipemic diet as in previous studies (3,16). For both tests, blood was collected in siliconized syringes containing sodium citrate (3.8%) (one volume citrate to nine of blood). The tests were started by adding 0.1 ml of a $CaCl_2$ solution to the blood or plasma (0.1 ml) diluted with (0.1 ml) saline 0.95%, in a plastic cuvette. In the minutes following the blood removal, the BCT was performed and a second sample of blood was centrifuged to obtain the PRP which was stored at 25°C and utilized 1 or 2 hr later for the PCT determination.

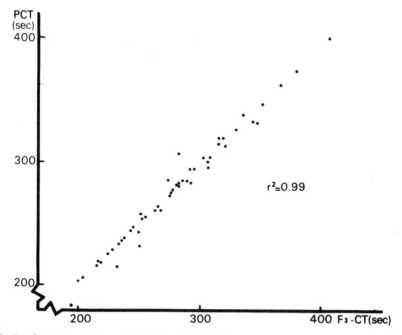

FIG. 5. Correlation between the PCT and the F_3-CT in 51 normal farmers from Var and Moselle in France (24). Both tests were performed in a recording aggrego-coagulometer.

These results suggest that the clotting activity of blood depends primarily on the clot promoting activity of platelets as already suggested (21,24). In other terms, the so-called platelet factor 3 should be the rate limiting factor of coagulation. It should be also the main factor involved in hypercoagulability.

Of interest is that factor 3 is the only clotting factor with a lipid moiety, mostly phosphatidylserine; as already mentioned, the composition of PS can be modified by dietary fats. In studies of animals fed different fats, the PCT also correlated perfectly with the clotting activity of PS extracted from the platelets (Fig. 6). The difference in the clotting activity did not appear to be due to changes in the concentration of this phospholipid fraction, but rather to changes in its fatty acid composition. This might be considered as the main mechanism through which dietary saturated fats induce a hypercoagulable state.

RELATIONSHIP BETWEEN THE CLOTTING ACTIVITY OF PLATELETS AND THEIR SUSCEPTIBILITY TO AGGREGATION

In human and animal studies, a significant correlation has been consistently found between the PCT (or the F_3-CT) and the susceptibility of platelets to aggregate, mostly via thrombin. This was particularly striking in a recent experiment in rats fed different fat mixtures (15). This can be more easily observed on an individual basis in humans. Table 1 summarizes the correlations recently obtained in farmers

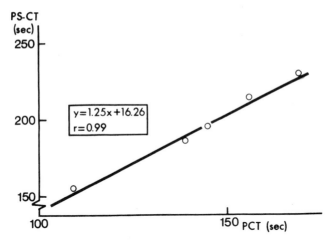

FIG. 6. Correlation between the PCT and the clotting activity of platelet PS (+ PI) from the same animals, fed different fat mixtures (Courtesy of Thrombosis Research) (6).

TABLE 1. *Correlations* (r) *between the clotting activity of platelets (F$_3$-CT), the clotting time of PRP (PCT) and the aggregation to thrombin and ADP in three different studies in man*[a]

	PCT	THR	ADP	N
F$_3$-CT	0.99[d]	0.53[d]	0.45[c]	52
	0.99[d]	0.65[d]	0.31[c]	86
	0.99[d]	0.62[d]	0.27[b]	63

[a]F$_3$-CT, factor 3 clotting test; PRP, platelet-rich plasma; PCT, plasma clotting time; N = number of subjects; THR = thrombin; ADP = adenosine diphosphate-induced aggregation.
[b]$p < 0.05$; [c]$p < 0.01$; [d]$p < 0.001$.
Adapted from Renaud et al. (23-25).

from France and Great Britain (24–26). In the three different studies reported in Table 1, the F$_3$-CT is significantly ($p < 0.001$) correlated not only with the PCT but also with the aggregation induced by thrombin. With adenosine diphosphate (ADP)-induced aggregation, the correlation coefficients, although still statistically significant, were much lower than with thrombin.

Consequently, there is a close relationship between the clot promoting activity of platelets and their response to thrombin. Since thrombin is an enzyme formed in the clotting process, this might suggest that once the platelets become more susceptible to small amounts of thrombin generated during the process, factor 3 would be more easily available and a more rapid formation of fibrin would ensue. However, this would not explain why phospholipids, extracted from platelets which are more active on coagulation, shorten the clotting time, in a similar way to the platelets, when solubilized by sonication in a standard platelet-poor plasma. This phenomenon has been observed in animals fed different fats (6,23) as well as in coronary patients (22). Thus, another possibility might be that the same modifications within the phospholipid molecules (essentially changes in the fatty acid composition), which accelerate the enzymatic process of coagulation, also accelerate an enzymatic process involved in aggregation, such as the liberation of free arachidonic acid or prostaglandin biosynthesis. A third possibility suggested by recent studies (12) would be that the main fatty acid, i.e., 20:3ω9 (nomenclature designating fatty acids by the position of the first double bond from the terminal methyl group) apparently involved in the increased clotting activity of platelet phospholipids (present in sizeable amounts in platelets, solely when the diet is highly saturated) would also form proaggregating substances under thrombin stimulation.

FATTY ACID COMPOSITION OF THE PLATELET PHOSPHOLIPIDS AND PLATELET FUNCTIONS

The marked influence of dietary fats on platelet functions in man and animals, both on coagulation and aggregation, has been observed by several investigators (9,10,15,17,18,20,25,26). Feeding different levels of saturated fat does not usually induce significant changes in the level of saturated fatty acids from the plasma (29) or the platelet (15,17,26) phospholipids which might explain changes in the platelet functions.

The result is a slight increase in the monoemes and a sizeable increase in 20:3ω9 (and 22:3ω9), a fatty acid derived from $C_{18:0}$ by desaturation and elongation, specifically increased in essential fatty acid deficiency (8). The close relationship between the level of 20:3ω9, the intake of long-chain saturated fatty acids, and the susceptibility of platelets to aggregate is illustrated in Fig. 7. A relationship has been previously observed between the level of this fatty acid and the clotting activity of platelet PS + PI (6). Close correlations between the level of 20:3ω9 in the platelet phospholipids, the clotting activity of platelets, and their susceptibility to thrombin-induced aggregation have also been recently found in extensive studies in British (26) and French farmers (*unpublished data*). In addition, in recent studies (12) we have observed platelets with their phospholipids enriched in 20:3ω9 by *in vitro* incubation with this fatty acid bound to albumin exhibited a marked increase in their response to thrombin-induced aggregation. This potentiating effect of 20:3ω9 was apparently due to the production of a monohydroxy derivative through the lipoxygenase pathway.

Of special interest concerning the possible adverse effects on platelet functions of 20:3ω9 in platelet phospholipids is that in atherosclerotic patients an increase in the monoemes and in 20:3ω9 has been reported in plasma cholesteryl esters (11). In the same patients, there was, most probably, a similar increase in the fatty acids from platelet phospholipids since the fatty acid composition of plasma cholesteryl esters and of platelet phospholipids seems to be closely correlated (*unpublished observations*).

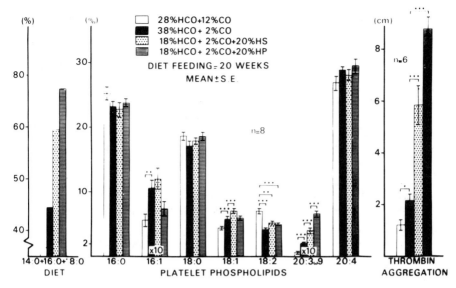

FIG. 7. Relationship, in rat, between the level of the three main saturated fatty acids (14:0 + 16:0 + 18:0) (from the human diet) and the resulting changes in the fatty acid composition of the platelet phospholipids and thrombin-induced aggregation. HCO, hydrogenated coconut oil; CO, corn oil; HS, hydrogenated sunflower oil; HP, hydrogenated palm oil; $^*p < .05$; $^{**}p < .01$; $^{***}p < .001$.) (Adapted from McGregor et al., ref. 14, with permission.)

Consequently, changes in the fatty acid composition of the platelet phospholipids might be one of the main mechanisms through which saturated fats predispose to coronary heart disease (CHD) for the following reasons.

1. These changes result in a marked increase in platelet functions involved in both coagulation and aggregation.

2. In recent studies performed in different countries, platelet aggregation (1,24–26) and platelet clotting activity (24–26) (a) appeared to be related to the known incidence of CHD in the region or the country investigated, and (b) were markedly influenced by the environmental factors (dietary intake of fat, calcium, and alcohol, as well as cigarette smoking) associated with CHD (25).

ACKNOWLEDGMENTS

The authors are greatly indebted to the CETIOM Organization and to Astra-Calvé for financial support, and to Dr. E. E. Nishizawa, from the Department of Pathology, McMaster University, Hamilton, Canada, for supplying the beef brain phosphatidylserine utilized in the studies reported here.

REFERENCES

1. Agradi, E., Carvalho, A., Dougherty, R., Ferro-Luzzi, A., Galli, C., Galli, G., Gianfranceschi, G., Iacono, J., Paoletti, R., and Sautebin, L. (1978): Epidemiological studies on dietary lipids, human plasma lipids and platelet lipids and function. In: *International Conference on Athero-*

sclerosis, edited by L. A. Carlson, R. Paoletti, C. R. Sirtori, and G. Weber, pp. 441–448. Raven Press, New York.

2. Bills, T. K., Smith, J. B., and Silver, M. J. (1977): Selective release of arachidonic acid from the phospholipids of human platelets in response to thrombin. *J. Clin. Invest.*, 60:1–6.
3. Chambaz, J., Wolf, C., Pepin, D., and Bereziat, G. (1980): Phospholipid and fatty acid exchanges between human platelets and plasma. *Biol. Cell.*, 37:223–230.
4. Chap, H. J., Zwaal, R. F. A., and Van Deenen, L. L. M. (1977): Action of highly purified phospholipases on blood platelets. Evidence for an asymmetric distribution of phospholipids in the surface membrane. *Biochim. Biophys. Acta*, 467:146–164.
5. Derksen, A., and Cohen, P. (1975): Patterns of fatty acid release from endogenous substrate by human platelet homogenates and membranes. *J. Biol. Chem.*, 250:9342–9347.
6. Gautheron, P., and Renaud, S. (1972): Hyperlipemia induced hypercoagulable state in rat. Role of an increased activity of platelet phosphatidyl-serine in response to certain dietary fatty acids. *Thromb. Res.*, 1:353–370.
7. Gautheron, P., Dumont, E., and Renaud, S. (1974): Clotting activity of platelet phospholipids in rat and man. *Thromb. Diath. Haemorrh.*, 32:382–390.
8. Holman, R. T. (1960): The ratio of trienoic-tetraenoic acids in tissue lipids as a measure of essential fatty acid requirement. *J. Nutr.*, 70:405–410.
9. Hornstra, G. (1973): Experimental studies. Dietary fats and arterial thrombosis. In: *Dietary Fats and Thrombosis*, edited by S. Renaud and A. Nordoy, pp. 21–52. Karger, Basel, Switzerland.
10. Iacono, J. M., Binder, R. A., Marshall, M. W., Schoerne, N. W., Jencks, J. A., and Mackin, J. A. (1975): Decreased susceptibility to thrombin and collagen platelet aggregation in man fed a low fat diet. *Haemostasis*, 3:306–318.
11. Kingsbury, K. J., Brett, C., Stovold, R., Chapman, A., Anderson, J., and Morgan, D. M. (1974): Abnormal fatty acid composition and human atherosclerosis. *Postgrad. Med. J.*, 50:425–440.
12. Lagarde, M., Burtin, M., Sprecher, H., Dechavanne, M., and Renaud, S. (1983): Potentiating effect of 5,8,11-eicosatrienoic acid on human platelet aggregation. *Lipids* (in press).
13. Marcus, A. J., Ullman, H. L., Safier, L. B., and Ballard, H. S. (1962): Platelet phospholipids. Their fatty acid and aldehyde composition and activity in different clotting systems. *J. Clin. Invest.*, 41:2198–2212.
14. Marcus, A. J. (1978): The role of lipids in platelet function: with particular reference to the arachidonic acid pathway. *J. Lipid Res.*, 19:793–826.
15. McGregor, L., Morazain, R., and Renaud, S. (1980): A comparison of the effects of dietary short and long chain saturated fatty acids on platelet functions, platelet phospholipids, and blood coagulation in rats. *Lab. Invest.*, 43:438–442.
16. Nishizawa, E. E., Hovig, T., Lotz, F., Rowsell, H. C., and Mustard, J. F. (1969): Effect of a natural phosphatidyl serine fraction on blood coagulation, platelet aggregation and haemostasis. *Br. J. Haemat.*, 16:487–499.
17. Nordoy, A., and Rodset, J. M. (1971): The influence of dietary fats on platelets in man. *Acta Med. Scand.*, 190:27–34.
18. O'Brien, J. R., Etherington, M. D., and Jamieson, S. (1976): Acute platelet changes after large meals of saturated and unsaturated fats. *Lancet*, i:878–880.
19. Renaud, S. (1969): The recalcification plasma clotting time. A valuable general clotting test in man and rats. *Can. J. Physiol. Pharmacol.*, 47:689–693.
20. Renaud, S., and Lecompte, F. (1970): Hypercoagulability induced by hyperlipemia in rat, rabbit and man. Role of platelet factor 3. *Circ. Res.*, 27:1003–1011.
21. Renaud, S. (1973): Role of platelet factor 3 activity in hypercoagulable state. *Thromb. Diath. Haemorrh.*, 30(Suppl. 56):13–20.
22. Renaud, S., Gautheron, P., Arbogast, R., and Dumont, E. (1974): Platelet factor 3 activity and platelet aggregation in patients submitted to coronarography. *Scand. J. Haematol.*, 12:85–92.
23. Renaud, S., and Gautheron, P. (1975): Influence of dietary fats on atherosclerosis, coagulation and platelet phospholipids in rabbits. *Atherosclerosis*, 21:115–124.
24. Renaud, S., Dumont, E., Godsey, F., Suplisson, A., and Thevenon, C. (1978): Platelet functions in relation to dietary fats in farmers from two regions of France. *Thromb. Haemostasis*, 40:518–531.
25. Renaud, S., Dumont, E., Godsey, F., Morazain, R., Thevenon, C., and Ortchanian, E. (1980): Dietary fats and platelet function in French and Scottish farmers. *Nutr. Metab.*, 25(Suppl. 1):90–104.

26. Renaud, S., Morazain, R., Godsey, F., Dumont, E., Symington, I. S., Gillanders, E. M., and O'Brien, J. R. (1981): Platelet functions in relation to diet and serum lipids in British farmers. *Br. Heart J. (in press).*
27. Schick, P. K., Kurica, K. B., and Chacko, G. K. (1976): Location of phosphatidylethanolamine and phosphatidylserine in the human platelet plasma membrane. *J. Clin. Invest.*, 57:1221–1226.
28. Silver, M. J., Turner, D. L., Rodalewicz, I., Giordano, N., Holburn, R., Herb, S. F., and Luddy, F. E. (1963): Evaluation of activity of phospholipids in blood coagulation in vitro. *Thromb. Diath. Haemorrh.*, 10:164–189.
29. Wilson, W. S., Hulley, S. B., Burrows, M. I., and Nichaman, M. Z. (1971): Serial lipid and lipoprotein responses to the American Heart Association fat-controlled diet. *Am. J. Med.*, 51:491–503.
30. Zwaal, R. F. A. (1978): Membrane and lipid involvement in blood coagulation. *Biochim. Biophys. Acta*, 515:163–176.

Subject Index

Subject Index

A

Absorption, intestinal
of fat, lecithin role in, 33–55; *see also* Digestion of fat
of phospholipids, 29–30
of polyene phosphatidylcholine, 66–71, 176–179

Acetylcholine in brain
choline affecting, 18
exogenous phospholipids affecting, 29
lecithin affecting, 205

Acid soaps, and intestinal emulsification, 43–44

S-Adenosylmethionine, in methylation pathway for phosphatidylcholine synthesis, 7, 8

Aging, and lecithin affecting cerebral function, 204–207

Alkenylacyl-GPC, 2
structure of, 3

Alkylacyl-GPC, 2
structure of, 3

Alzheimer's disease, neuronal changes in, 204

Amphipathic helical regions of apolipoproteins, 102

Amphipathic nature of phospholipids, 144

Amphiphilic nature of phospholipids, 91

Anemia, hemolytic, phosphatidylcholine infusions in, 88

Apolipoproteins, 99, 100
affinity of A-I and A-II for HDL lipids, 168–172
amphipathic helical regions of, 102
apo A/lecithin complex, 103–104
apo C-III/lecithin complex, 104
binding of phospholipids to, 211
interaction with lysolecithin, 105
interaction with phospholipid vesicles, 93–94
in liver perfusate, 137–138
size of, and rate of lipid-protein association, 107
structure and properties of, 102

Arachidonic acid
in platelet phospholipids, 219–220
and prostaglandin formation, 19, 247
release from platelets, 262

Arterial disease, erythrocyte deformability in, 84–89

Arterial plaque, phospholipids in, 212

Arterial wall metabolism, lipoproteins affecting, 201

Assays of phospholipids in HDL, 191–195

Atherosclerosis
antiatherosclerotic effect of phospholipids, 28
in animals, 197–200
in humans, 203–204
mechanism of, 201–203
and fatty acids in plasma cholesteryl esters, 268

B

Base-exchange reactions, and interconversion of phospholipid molecules, 7–8

Bile salts, interaction with pancreatic lipase, 46, 47

Brain function, phospholipids affecting, 18, 29, 204–207

C

Calcium, micellar complex with phospholipid, 26

Cerebral function, phospholipids affecting, 18, 29, 204–207

Cholesterol
cellular excretion affected by lecithin, 146
crosslinking after photolysis, 123
and dimyristoyl lecithin in vesicles, HDL incubated with, 164–167
in erythrocyte membranes, 81
affecting deformability of cells, 83